Women and Health: ~~Biological and Social~~ Perspectives

Don't Kill Your Baby

Public Health and the Decline of Breastfeeding in the Nineteenth and Twentieth Centuries

Jacqueline H. Wolf

The Ohio State University Press
Columbus

Library of Congress Cataloging-in-Publication Data

Wolf, Jacqueline H.
    Don't kill your baby : public health and the decline of breastfeeding
in the nineteenth and twentieth centuries / Jacqueline H. Wolf.
        p.   cm. — (Women and health)
Includes bibliographical references and index
    ISBN 0-8142-0877-0 — ISBN 0-8142-5077-7 (alk. paper)
    1. Breastfeeding—Illinois—Chicago—History.   2.
Infants—Illinois—Chicago—Nutrition—History.   3.
Motherhood—Illinois—Chicago—History.   4. Public
health—Illinois—Chicago—History.   I. Title.
    RJ216 .W719 2001
    649'.33'0977311—dc21   2001001846

Text design by Bookcomp, Inc.
Cover design by Dan O'Dair.
Type set in 11 point Apollo by Bookcomp, Inc.
Printed by Thomson-Shore.

The paper used in this publication meets the minimum requirements of the American
National Standard for Information Sciences—Permanence of Paper for Printed Library
Materials. ANSI Z39.48-1992.

9   8   7   6   5   4   3   2   1

To Sam
for the support

and

To Cora
for the inspiration

Contents

Acknowledgments

Generous and knowledgeable people helped me to hone many skills and to become a better historian as I worked on this book.

The Department of History at the University of Illinois at Chicago was home for nine years when I was a graduate student. I owe very special thanks to Perry Duis, an inspirational and wonderfully generous dissertation adviser. I am also grateful to Burton Bledstein, Gerald Danzer, George Huppert, Richard John, Michael Perman, Leo Schelbert, Daniel Scott Smith, and Mary Kay Vaughan for many years of advice and encouragement.

Norman Gevitz, Rima Apple, and Lawrence Gartner will always be my personal models of what collegiality is all about. Norm has been both my harshest critic and biggest booster since I first sent him my dissertation proposal for comment in 1994. While others had already approved the proposal, he insisted I rewrite and rethink. I can never thank him enough for his rigorous demands then and his ongoing guidance (and rigorous demands) now. "Rdapple" first sent me e-mail in 1995 after I presented a paper before the Society of Medical History of Chicago. As a budding historian of infant feeding I had read all of Rima Apple's work avidly, but had never met her. Ever since our first contact via that e-mail—she wanted to see a copy of the paper I had presented the night before—Rima has helped me in more ways than I can count. I owe her a special debt. Larry Gartner, longtime chair and now professor emeritus of the pediatrics department at the University of Chicago, has taken an enthusiastic interest in my work ever since we met through the Society of Medical History of Chicago. He read every page of an early version of this work, thoughtfully criticizing it and giving it an invaluable "medical scan."

Some very competent archivists made my visits to assorted Chicago-area archives particularly productive. I especially want to thank Stuart Campbell of the Rush-Presbyterian-St. Luke's Medical Center Archives, Archie Motley of the Chicago Historical Society, Jane Kenamore, formerly of the American Medical Association Archives, and Sue Sacharski of the Northwestern Memorial Hospital Archives.

My brother Kevin Wolf, The Actuary, spent endless hours over countless months helping me unravel the mysteries of Excel so I could complete the tables and graphs at the end of this book. I thank him for his time and the patience he showed his statistically challenged sister.

My colleagues in the Department of Social Medicine at the Ohio University College of Osteopathic Medicine provide daily support, guidance, constructive criticism, and laughs in just the right doses. Bruce Dubin, Judith Edinger, Ann Fingar, Norman Gevitz, Gillian Harper Ice, and Cheri McFee deserve special mention.

As I neared completion of this book, I became increasingly nervous about its clarity, a malady I presume afflicts many authors. To ease my mind, I prevailed on several friends and colleagues to read the entire manuscript and comment. Ann Fingar, Jim Fingar, Debbie Jones, Susan D. Jones, Susan Matthews, and Vicki Turow all took time from their busy lives to read the manuscript carefully and offer me lots of encouragement and helpful criticism. I can never thank them enough for that and for the years of invaluable friendship that made me confident that I could count on their last-minute help for the asking.

My brother Rob Wolf will always have my admiration and gratitude. With his customary humor and skill, he answered many a hurried call for advice on everything from the book title to how to craft writing to appeal to assorted audiences. Thanks also to Janet Golden, who was always there to reassure a nervous author. I felt better just knowing that e-mail from her was never more than minutes away.

I am grateful to the editors of Oxford University Press, *Journal of Social History,* and The Haworth Press for permission to reprint material previously published as "'Don't Kill Your Baby': Feeding Infants in Chicago, 1903–1924," *Journal of the History of Medicine and Allied Sciences* 53 (July 1998): 219–53; "'Mercenary Hirelings' or 'A Great Blessing'?: Doctors' and Mothers' Conflicted Perceptions of Wet Nurses and the Ramifications for Infant Feeding in Chicago, 1871–1961," *Journal of Social History* 33 (Fall 1999): 97–120; and "The Social and Medical Construction of Lactation Pathology," *Women and Health* 30 (Fall 2000): 93–109.

Since my first days of graduate school, my husband, Sam Wilen, has shared my enthusiasm for my classes and research. As I embarked on dissertation writing and eventually book writing, he read and commented on draft after draft of each chapter. As a perpetual student himself, he understood the demands of scholarship and never failed to reassure me when I fretted over this and that. If I had not had the pleasure of breastfeeding our daughter,

Cora, I never would have thought of studying the history of infant feeding in the first place. Her birth and the privilege and delight of sharing the life of a child (as well as the anxiety of caring for a child) have inspired what will probably be my lifelong scholarly interests—the history of women's and children's health and medicine. Thanks to Sam and Cora for everything, always.

Chronology of Events
in Infant Feeding History

1856
Gail Borden opens the first canned milk factory in the United States.

1866
London chemist Gustav Mellin invents Mellin's Food.

1868
Henri Nestlé sells his powdered infant food in Switzerland, Germany, France, and England.

1873
Nestlé's Food first sold in the United States.

1877
Chicago requires milk dealers to obtain licenses.

1878
Nestlé's manufactures condensed milk.

1885
The Bowman brothers open the Bowman Dairy in Chicago.
Arthur Meigs publishes *Milk Analysis and Infant Feeding,* introducing the Meigs Mixture as an infant food.
John Meyenberg opens the Helvetia Milk Condensing Company in Highland, Illinois.

1888
Harvard pediatrician Thomas Rotch introduces percentage feeding.

1889
New England physicians complain that more than half of all mothers are unable to "properly nurse their offspring."
Inaugural meeting of the American Pediatric Society.
Dr. Henry Koplik opens the first milk station in the United States in New York.

1891
George Walker and G. E. Gordon open the first Walker-Gordon milk laboratory.

1892

Chicago Health Commissioner attributes Chicago's high infant mortality to the city's unsanitary cows' milk and Chicago's milk reform movements begin.

New Jersey doctor Henry Coit invents certified milk.

1893

Chicago passes its first pure milk ordinance and establishes the Bureau of Milk Inspection.

Merchant and philanthropist Nathan Straus opens his first pasteurized milk station in New York.

1895

The Illinois State Board of Health agrees to supply state inspectors to enforce Chicago's milk regulations outside Chicago's jurisdiction.

Walker-Gordon opens a milk laboratory in Chicago.

1897

The Chicago Department of Health correlates cause of death with age at death for the first time in their compilation of vital statistics.

18 percent of Chicago's babies die before their first birthday.

53.7 percent of the dead die from diarrhea.

Chicago Pediatric Society formed.

1902

Milk laboratories and percentage feeding begin to decline in popularity after an article in the *Boston Medical and Surgical Journal* proves infant formulas are commonly inaccurate.

1903

The Children's Hospital Society of Chicago establishes the Chicago Milk Commission.

1904

Inspectors find that one-fourth of Chicago's dairies still feed distillery waste to their dairy cattle.

Chicago requires dairies to seal milk containers.

Isaac Abt contends in a *Chicago Tribune* column that two-thirds of mothers are unable to breastfeed.

1905

The Chicago Visiting Nurse Association, the Northwestern Settlement House, and the Chicago Relief and Aid Society establish "baby tents" in neighborhoods to care for babies with digestive ailments.

The Bowman Dairy begins to pasteurize all its milk voluntarily.

1906

First federal Pure Food and Drugs Act passed by Congress.

1907

12.7 percent of Chicago's babies die before their first birthday. 39.2 percent of the dead die from diarrhea.

Chicago Department of Health sends seventy-five medical inspectors door-to-door to talk to mothers about infant care.

1909

Chicago Department of Health conducts its first field survey of mothers with newborns.

The Chicago Medical Society sets up the Chicago Medical Society Milk Commission to certify milk for the city.

Chicago's Children's Memorial Hospital hires its first wet nurse.

1910

Chicago Department of Health hangs its first posters in Chicago neighborhoods urging mothers to breastfeed.

Five hundred public health nurses visit the homes of 23,984 newborns in Chicago.

The Chicago Infant Welfare Committee forms, consisting of the Department of Health, United Charities, and the Visiting Nurse Association.

The Wet Nurse Directory opens in Boston.

1911

The Chicago Milk Commission shuts down its milk stations after Board members agree with criticism that their stations discourage breastfeeding.

The Chicago Milk Commission replaces itself with the Chicago Infant Welfare Society.

The Chicago Infant Welfare Society sponsors Chicago's first Little Mothers' Club classes.

1912

11.8 percent of Chicago's babies die before their first birthday. 39.4 percent of the dead die from diarrhea.

Chicago Department of Health field nurses report that only 39 percent of Chicago's newborns are exclusively breastfed.

Chicago requires dairies to bottle milk in individual containers.

1913

The Chicago Department of Health opens four infant welfare stations to augment the thirteen run by the Infant Welfare Society.

Sarah Morris Children's Hospital opens in Chicago with a wing devoted to housing wet nurses and their babies.

1914

The Chicago Infant Welfare Society orchestrates its first Baby Week campaign.

1916

12.2 percent of Chicago's babies die before their first birthday. 42 percent of the dead die from diarrhea.

The Chicago Infant Welfare Society now operating twenty-two infant welfare stations.
Chicago requires dairies to pasteurize all milk sold in the city.

1917
Baby tents closed.

1918
U.S. Children's Bureau declares 1918 "Children's Year."

1920
9.9 percent of Chicago's babies die before their first birthday. 33.1 percent of the
    dead die from diarrhea.
Chicago requires shippers to keep all milk cold during shipping.

1921
Congress enacts the Sheppard-Towner Maternity and Infancy Protection Act.
The Chicago Board of Education makes Little Mothers' Club classes part of the
    regular curriculum for 7th and 8th grade girls.

1923
The Chicago Department of Health begins sending breastfeeding pamphlets to
    every new mother.
The Chicago Department of Health now operating twenty-five infant welfare
    stations (up from four in 1922). The IWS infant welfare stations and the
    Chicago Department of Health infant welfare stations together care for
    almost 57 percent of Chicago's babies.

1924
Chicago Health Commissioner Herman Bundesen expands the health department's
    pamphlet "Our Babies" and sends it to every Chicago mother shortly after she
    gives birth.
Every infant in Chicago gets regular home visits from a health department field nurse.

1926
55.1 percent of Chicago mothers give birth in hospitals.
Chicago requires dairy farms to test all their dairy cattle for bovine tuberculosis.

1929
At least twenty American cities house human milk stations.
Congress repeals the Sheppard-Towner Act.

1930
5.3 percent of Chicago's babies die before their first birthday. 11.1 percent of the
    dead die from diarrhea.
68 percent of Chicago's mothers give birth in hospitals.

1931
The Code of the Chicago Board of Health requires that every hospitalized prema-
    ture baby be fed human milk.

1938

Chicago Department of Health opens its Mothers' Breast Milk Station.

1939

3.1 percent of Chicago's babies die before their first birthday. 1.4 percent of the dead die from diarrhea.

1940

Fifty-five men work in medical relations for Pet Milk to pitch Pet Milk as an infant food to physicians.

1950

88 percent of Chicago's mothers give birth in hospitals.

1955

29.2 percent of one-week-old infants in the United States are either breastfed or mixed fed; 4.1 percent consume cow's milk; 23.2 percent consume some type of formula; and 45.9 percent consume evaporated milk.

1956

La Leche League holds its first meeting in a Chicago suburb.

1961

The Chicago Department of Health closes its Mothers' Breast Milk Station.

1962

Pet Milk employs a nationwide staff of "medical detail men" to sell Pet Milk as an infant food to physicians.

1963

The second revised edition of La Leche League's *The Womanly Art of Breastfeeding* is released and eventually sells 1,172,200 copies.

1972

22 percent of newborns leave the hospital breastfeeding.

1982

62 percent of newborns leave the hospital breastfeeding.

1989

52 percent of newborns leave the hospital breastfeeding.

1997

The American Academy of Pediatrics issues new breastfeeding guidelines.

2000

The Department of Health and Human Services issues its "Blueprint for Action on Breastfeeding."

Introduction

For every one hundred babies born in the United States in the late nineteenth century, close to thirteen of them died before their first birthday.[1] Since many of the dead died of diarrhea, physicians laid much of the blame on an entirely preventable cause: the growing use of cows' milk as an infant food. "Nature gave infants as their birthright mother's milk . . . without a chance for contamination, without 100 miles intervening for the milk man to bring it," railed one doctor at a meeting on infant mortality.[2]

By the 1910s, when the Chicago Department of Health estimated that fifteen bottle-fed babies were dying for every one breastfed baby, alarmed public health workers traversed neighborhoods hanging posters imploring mothers to breastfeed.[3] One of the posters, designed in 1910 and headlined "Don't Kill Your Baby," proclaimed "Mother's Milk is Best of All." A 1911 placard advised "To Lessen Baby Deaths Let Us Have More Mother-Fed Babies. You can't improve on God's plan. For Your Baby's Sake—Nurse It!"[4] While these pleas, especially "Don't Kill Your Baby," sound to early twenty-first-century ears like the hyperbole of what has been derisively referred to as a "breastfeeding fanatic," at the time the phrase was a sober and supportable warning to women. Physicians viewed bottle-feeding, justifiably according to mortality statistics, as tantamount to infanticide.

The link between infant feeding method and infant health was unmistakable at the end of the nineteenth century. The extraordinary number of infants who succumbed to diarrhea usually died during the summer, when food spoiled quickly. Unrefrigerated for the two to three days it took to travel from rural dairy farmer to urban consumer, cows' milk was the invariable cause of these deaths. Shipped and stored in large, uncovered vats, milk not only soured but was susceptible to adulteration by farmers, shippers, dealers, and peddlers. In this era before refrigeration, pasteurization, pure food laws, and the sealing of milk in individual bottles, whether a mother breastfed her baby was often the single most important factor determining an infant's survival.

This scenario raises obvious questions. Why, in an age when cows'-milk feeding posed such an obvious threat to babies, were mothers in ever-increasing numbers either supplementing their breast milk with cows' milk, weaning babies within a few weeks or months of birth, or, to a lesser extent, never breastfeeding at all? Mothers wanted healthy babies at least as fervently as physicians did. No mother set out to harm her baby by withholding breast milk. Clearly, forces more powerful than public health admonitions influenced mothers. What were they? How did mothers' choices shape physicians' activities and how did physicians' activities inspire mothers' choices? How did women's very public complaints of inadequate breast milk, their primary explanation for choosing bottles, affect physicians' attitudes toward human milk? In what ways did the myriad efforts to improve mothers' milk substitutes—making the milk of wet nurses more accessible, cleaning up the cows' milk supply, modifying cows' milk to approximate mothers' milk, and manufacturing commercial infant foods—hasten the move to bottle-feeding? How did a health practice detrimental to health, like bottle-feeding, come to be viewed as the normal and necessary way of doing things?

In her groundbreaking book *Mothers and Medicine: A Social History of Infant Feeding, 1890-1950,* Rima Apple explores some of these questions. Yet her central query—in essence, Why were women bottle-feeding?—led her down different avenues than I explore in this book. Apple focuses primarily on the activities and philosophies of physicians and commercial infant food companies as the determinants of women's infant-feeding practices. She argues that, in particular, the ideology of "scientific motherhood" stressed the importance of medical expertise in child rearing and that infant formulas, created and blessed by science, provided a persuasive rationale for medical intervention between mothers and their babies.[5]

I approached the history of infant feeding with a different central question. Intrigued by the high infant mortality rate from diarrhea in Chicago in the 1890s, I wondered, Why weren't women breastfeeding? That question produced a very different answer than Apple found. I contend that, rather than being instrumental in altering women's infant-feeding habits, physicians' experimentation with breast milk substitutes and even the products of commercial infant food companies were actually a reaction to changes in infant-feeding practice already instituted by women. The ensuing interactions between mothers and a host of players, including physicians, public health workers, wet nurses, dairies, and infant food companies, hastened the move to bottles. In perusing the statistics compiled by Chicago public health officials, who wanted to know beginning in 1907 precisely what mothers fed their newborns, I also found that mothers' preference for bottles over breasts was not cemented in the 1930s and 1940s, as Apple and others contend, but by the 1910s.

I argue that women—all women, for the increasingly common preference for cows' milk crossed class and ethnic lines—and not physicians instigated the move from breast to bottle. Economic pressure and class conflict, as well as changing views of time, efficiency, self-control, health, medicine, sex, marriage, and nature—in short, the social change concomitant with urbanization—prompted women to doubt the efficacy, propriety, and necessity of breastfeeding. By the 1890s women no longer breastfed their babies according to the historical norm, through infants' second summer in the seventeenth century and for at least a year but often longer in the eighteenth century.[6] Instead, although mothers for the most part still breastfed for a time immediately after giving birth, they often weaned their babies at or well before their babies' third month or supplemented their breast milk with cows' milk and worse. Dismayed physicians translated these new habits into one alarming fact. Mothers exposed babies under the age of one—and usually under the age of three months—to the spoiled, adulterated, bacteria-ridden cows' milk common to urban areas.

Before the plethora of sick bottle-fed babies, infant feeding was of little interest to doctors. Only the few physicians who cared for orphaned infants in foundling homes gave the matter any thought, and their work to improve human milk substitutes was strictly in the interest of motherless infants.[7] It was mothers' move from breast to bottle-feeding, and municipalities' statistical compilations listing the numbers of concomitant sick and dead babies, that sparked physicians' interest in developing human milk substitutes for all babies, not just the unfortunates without a mother.

The medical community was not particularly enthusiastic about this task. Doctors had long witnessed the dire impact of cows'-milk feeding on babies and few wanted any part of it. Isaac Abt, who practiced medicine for fifty years beginning in the late 1890s and is now known as "the father of pediatrics in Chicago," complained of examining babies "who were so emaciated that they looked like ancient, wrinkled dwarfs. Their condition was due to malnutrition . . . not because the babies lacked food, but because they were not getting the right food. Some of them rallied when they were put on breast milk, but the majority died."[8]

Physicians often witnessed such tragedies and denounced bottle-feeding accordingly. Their most common and pointed denunciation of bottle-feeding was to coin the term "artificial food," a neutral expression today but originally intended as a damning phrase. Mothers who breastfed, physicians contended, provided babies with their "natural sustenance." Mothers who fed their babies something other than human milk did the irresponsible opposite: they forced an "unnatural makeshift," an "artificial food" upon their pitiable infants. Perhaps because the term disparaged bottle-feeding so harshly, mothers who did not breastfeed chose to use less charged terms, referring to artificial feeding as "hand feeding" or simply "feeding." When a mother said she "fed" her baby, she meant that she fed her baby something other than her own milk.

Despite their penchant for breast milk, physicians could not ignore the consequences of artificial feeding in an era when high infant mortality was fast becoming a clearly defined social problem. Thus, they responded to the crisis in two seemingly contradictory ways. Strong and steady advocates of human milk, they orchestrated municipal breastfeeding campaigns imploring women to breastfeed. But at the same time, because they faced the immediate task of caring for the sick babies dubbed "feeding cases" by visiting nurses,[9] they also worked alongside reformers, government officials, dairy farmers, and dairy owners to clean up the urban milk supply and to improve artificial food. These latter efforts altered public perception of cows' milk from a potentially deadly substance for infants to a consistently safe and beneficial one, and paradoxically predisposed even more women to feed their babies cows' milk.

As physicians toiled to improve human milk substitutes in response to women's changing infant-feeding practices, they also attempted to solve a medical mystery. Most of the women who introduced cows' milk to their babies early in life contended that they did so because their own milk was so quantitatively or qualitatively inadequate that it could not possibly sustain their babies. What, doctors wondered, was the cause of this apparent epidemic of lactation failure? Physicians' assorted explanations for the phenomenon—the most popular was that urbanization so unnerved and weakened women that many of their body parts were doomed to fail—appeared not only in medical journals but in women's and infant-care magazines. This public discussion convinced even more women that breastfeeding was an activity likely to end in failure, and as such could be as potentially dangerous to an infant's health as cows' milk, the same cows' milk that, thanks to the clean-milk campaigns, was beginning to look a lot safer anyway.

Eventually, lactation-failure theories profoundly influenced pediatricians. Colleagues derided these new specialists of the 1890s as unnecessary, inconsequential "baby doctors." Although that first generation of pediatricians never stopped urging mothers to breastfeed, by 1900 their desire to prove their utility to colleagues made them equally vested in believing that human milk could be less than optimal. If women could no longer sustain their babies with their bodies alone, physicians, and pediatricians in particular, had no choice but to place themselves between mothers and babies. Here was a clearly vital purpose for pediatricians. The medical management of motherhood, described so well by Apple, ensued.

This study of changing infant-feeding practices sheds light on how women, particularly mothers, influence medical practice, and how normal and necessary medical practice comes to be defined and accepted. The relationship between mothers and physicians has been, and continues to be, a complex one. Women initiated the move from breast to bottle as they embraced complex social, cultural, economic, and intellectual change concomitant with urbanization, change that on the surface had little to do with infant feeding yet affected it profoundly. Babies sickened by adulterated cows' milk and mothers' complaints that they had inadequate breast milk persuaded doctors to dilute their advocacy for breastfeeding and devote at least some of their energy and expertise to cleaning up the urban milk supply and formulating, if not safe, at least safer artificial food. The ensuing dialogue between mothers and physicians generated the development of and strong faith in the dairy and formula industries and changed the most fundamental way that mothers interact with and care for their infants.

♦

Much of this book focuses on events in Chicago, although cows' milk and the problems and solutions triggered by its use as an infant food were by no means unique to that city. Until municipalities passed and enforced laws governing the production of milk, cities throughout the United States saw babies die in high numbers from diarrhea. Yet Chicago is an ideal locale to study the change in infant-feeding practices occurring in late nineteenth- and early twentieth-century urban America, for three reasons. First, Chicago's late nineteenth-century problems—poverty, a poor housing stock, lack of planning as a municipality, and, consequently, a host of public health woes, including a high infant death rate—were representative of those in other big cities. Second, Chicago housed a group of energetic reformers who attempted to lower the infant death rate from diarrhea by employing solutions already tested in some other cities. But perhaps most important, Chicago also housed a uniquely high-profile community of pediatricians who were at the national forefront of the infant feeding debate. Consequently, Chicago's infant welfare reformers were both followers and leaders in the infant-food arena, and their efforts to lower the number of infant deaths from diarrhea reflected both time-honored methods and innovative ones eventually copied by public health advocates in other cities. The history of changing infant-feeding practices in Chicago is thus representative of the history of infant feeding in much of the urban United States.[10]

I have organized this book topically. Each chapter covers roughly the same time period—from the last quarter of the nineteenth century through the 1930s—and examines how the actions and reactions of a different set of players in the infant-food drama impacted mothers' choices. The first chapter examines the sociocultural forces that prompted women to modify centuries-old infant-feeding practices. The second chapter examines the most serious consequence of women's decisions: high infant mortality from diarrhea caused by spoiled and adulterated cows' milk, and the subsequent efforts of Chicago reformers to provide pure milk to consumers and the impact of those efforts on mothers. The third chapter describes private physicians' debates and theories prompted by the "feeding question"—a question posed to physicians by mothers' new infant-feeding practices, women's professed inability to successfully breastfeed, and infants' subsequent illnesses and deaths. The fourth chapter looks at infant feeding from the perspective of public health workers. How did the Chicago Department of Health and the city's widely used medical charities respond to the "feeding question"? What did they teach a vast audience of mothers about infant feeding? How did mothers react to the educational efforts? The last two chapters describe the medical community's proposed alternatives to breastfeeding—wet nursing and artificial feeding—and how those options hastened the move to bottles. A chapter-length epilogue examines the profound change in physicians' thinking beginning in the 1930s as they began to overtly sanction artificial food. Mothers and physicians did not rediscover breastfeeding, and the extraordinary health exhibited by breastfed babies, until the mid-1970s.

Yet, as I make clear in the epilogue, even this "new" late twentieth-century discovery of the importance of human milk to human health is plagued by an ongoing discomfort with breastfeeding and a mistrust of human milk, a discomfort and mistrust that I trace back to the 1880s and 1890s. Today, customers complain to store managers that mothers who "openly nurse" ruin their shopping experience.[11] States have to pass laws giving mothers the right to breastfeed in public.[12] In doing so, many states have had to clarify the terms used in antiobscenity statutes to exclude breastfeeding from being construed as an "unnatural and lascivious act," or an "exposure of sexual organs," or a "lewd, lascivious or indecent assault or act upon or in the presence of a child."[13] In February 1999 the Ohio legislature considered a statute giving a mother the right to breastfeed in any public space "except the private home or residence of another if the mother's breast-feeding is likely to be viewed by and affront the owner or any occupant of the private home or residence." The ambivalence suggested by this proposed statute is typical of the breastfeeding-is-good/breastfeeding-can-be-bad dichotomy introduced by women and corroborated by physicians beginning in the late nineteenth century.

In addition to the discomfort generated by lactating women and breastfeeding babies today, there remains widespread doubt that exclusively breastfeeding a baby will even "work." Since the late nineteenth century, an extraordinary number of mothers who start to breastfeed have complained either that they do not have "enough" milk or that their milk is "not good enough" to continue to breastfeed. Recently, horrific front-page news stories about exclusively breastfed infants dying of starvation or suffering permanent damage from dehydration corroborate this fear.[14] These news reports inspired the television dramas *Chicago Hope* and *Law and Order* to feature story lines depicting babies killed by insufficient breast milk. That a conscientious mother should anticipate and prepare for lactation failure has become virtually axiomatic.

The notion that something can easily go wrong with breastfeeding has dissuaded many mothers from nursing their infants in the last 120 years. Since the end of urban breastfeeding campaigns in the 1920s, neither the medical community nor mothers have widely acknowledged the profound repercussions of the move to bottles. Artificial feeding reshaped the needs of the human infant, redefined the health of the "normal" human infant, and changed the most basic way that mothers and their babies interact. This book is an attempt to explain how breastfeeding, which women and physicians once accepted as the essence of motherhood and essential to infants' health and well-being, came to be viewed with distaste and mistrust.

1

"It Takes Quite a Little Courage to Stand Out": Mothers Move from Breast to Bottle

In 1873 Chicagoan Nettie Fowler McCormick noted in her diary that after she had a "wonderful escape from a serious disaster," her baby Harold grew ill—"I think from the disordered state of my milk consequent upon the shock."[1] McCormick's private, fleeting worry that her breast milk could spoil internally and harm her son was probably not uncommon. That particular concern, however, would remain neither momentary nor private. By the end of the century, discussion of human milk's propensity to be quantitatively or qualitatively inadequate was rife among mothers and physicians, and a staple of women's and infant-care magazines and medical journals.

Changing infant-feeding habits generated all the talk. By the 1890s women no longer breastfed through their babies' second summer, the norm in the seventeenth century, or even for a year, the recommended minimum in the eighteenth century.[2] Instead, mothers customarily weaned their infants at or before three months of age. Many never breastfed exclusively even for a short time and chose instead to give their babies other food, usually cows' milk, in addition to breast milk beginning soon after birth. The most common explanation that mothers gave for this change of habit was a simple one: they did not have adequate milk, either quantitatively or qualitatively, to breastfeed. Women reported that their breasts were failing their babies, and in short order physicians agreed that the human mammary gland and human milk were fast becoming unreliable.

The perception among mothers that they had neither enough milk nor good enough milk was so ubiquitous by the 1880s that New England physicians reported in 1889 that more than half of all mothers were unable to "properly nurse their offspring." One Massachusetts doctor lamented, "The women of no race or nation in the history of the world in such large numbers, as far as we can learn, have ever reached such an anomalous relation in respect to offspring." By 1912 the habits of early weaning and mixed feeding were entrenched cultural phenomena. Disconcerted physicians complained bitterly that breastfeeding rates had been declining steadily since the mid-nineteenth century "and now it is largely a question as to whether the mother will nurse her baby at all."[3]

A number of unrelated factors in the late nineteenth and early twentieth centuries altered mothers' perceptions of breast milk and breastfeeding and contributed to this dramatic change in practice. Some factors were economic. An abundance of immigrants willing to work as servants enabled upper-class women to resume their social lives almost immediately after giving birth, precluding breastfeeding. Women living in congested urban neighborhoods often worked outside the home, leaving their babies with older children and bottles.

Other factors were social. Immigrant women, divorced from traditional knowledge, fell under the influence of Americanized daughters and the lure of American food products. As women ceased attending and observing each other's births, biological functions like parturition and lactation became shrouded in mystery and anticipated with fear and mistrust. As women and men sought romantic marriages, breasts became sexualized and that sexualization diminished breasts' physiological importance. Women's enthusiastic, wholesale adoption of feeding schedules likewise prompted bottle use. Mothers embraced infant-feeding schedules as a means of easing the complexities of urban domestic life and teaching their infants self-control. Unbeknownst to women at the time, however, adequate milk supplies depend on an infant's frequent sucking, as all mammalian milk supplies are governed by the axiom "supply equals demand." Thus feeding schedules, usually characterized by long intervals between feedings, quickly diminish mothers' milk supplies. These schedules were the likely source of mothers' complaints of inadequate milk.

Still other factors were neither economic nor social, but quasi-medical. By the end of the nineteenth century, municipal health departments were teaching the germ theory of disease to the masses via a barrage of posters, pamphlets, and newspaper articles. The alarming message—that invisible, life-threatening creatures menaced everyone—was aimed largely at women as the preparers of food and the caretakers of infants. In this post–germ theory atmosphere, women began to view their breast milk warily. Given their new understanding of bacteriology, their new responsibility to keep germs at bay, and the accompanying dictum that only mothers who failed to properly prepare food and sanitize their homes had unhealthy babies, many women began to fret that their milk was not up to the task of keeping a baby alive.

As mothers modified what had been the custom of prolonged breastfeeding, they exposed their babies at younger and younger ages to assorted artificial foods, most of which had cows' milk as their primary, if not sole, ingredient. By the 1890s it was common for mothers to consult physicians about infants sickened by the spoiled, adulterated cows' milk common to the nineteenth-century city. Physicians did not introduce women to the "feeding question"—a passionate, decades-long debate on how best to sustain the many infants suffering from the dearth of human milk. Rather, mothers themselves posed the query to physicians and physicians scurried for an answer.

Doctors faced this medical conundrum reluctantly, for no reliable remedy other than human milk existed for the baby sickened by artificial food. As John Cook, the founder and first president of the Chicago Pediatric Society, wrote wearily in 1904, "No physician's resources are ever more sorely taxed than on the summer day when his advice is asked concerning the [bottle-fed] baby that cannot retain its food, or if it does retain it, it is not digested."[4] Cook's assessment was borne of experience, for when mothers did feed their babies artificially the practice proved almost uniformly disastrous.

One mother reported a typical tale to a women's magazine in 1907. Her son, seven and a half pounds at birth, initially thrived on her breast milk, weighing a hefty twenty pounds when he was five months old. Then her "milk began to give out." Despite her best efforts, she "had to wean him." Desperate, she replaced her breast milk with one artificial food after another—mothers often experimented frantically in such situations—"but he dragged along all summer." At ten months of age he seemed to vomit for five straight weeks. She explained, "The doctors' treatment was not able to stop it and he kept growing worse." When he was two years old the boy weighed only thirteen and a half pounds.[5]

The outline of this story was so common—this particular tale is unusual only because the child had not yet died—that the medical community unanimously condemned artificial food use. Yet mothers' reports of inadequate human milk alarmed physicians, and consequently, physicians' appeals to breastfeed were often accompanied by cautionary tales of the potential inadequacy of human milk. Mothers were left with a decidedly mixed message. This type of mother-physician interaction hastened a practice that mothers dreaded and physicians deplored: artificial feeding.

♦

Mothers who ceased breastfeeding in the traditional sense participated in one of three practices. Some, though probably not many, never breastfed their babies at all. Others, although they initially breastfed, weaned their babies early, most commonly, according to physicians' complaints and women's admissions, at or before three months of age. Still others relied on mixed feeding. Some mothers who supplemented their breast milk with artificial food did so because they feared their milk supply was waning, a practice that some physicians occasionally encouraged given mothers' increasing complaints of inadequate milk. The eminent pediatrician Henry Dwight Chapin, for example, worried that even the best breast milk diminished in both quantity and quality by a baby's eighth or ninth month. Therefore he suggested, as a bulwark against the inevitable, that mothers give their babies one or two bottles daily soon after birth. He explained, "The baby will then be educated in its use, the mother will have more time to herself, and in case of her being ill, sudden weaning will not be necessary. If this method is employed, the change from breastfeeding to bottle feeding will not cause inconvenience."[6]

Most often, however, mixed feeding was a mother's unconscious act. Historian Molly Ladd-Taylor reports that although most immigrants nursed their babies, they concurrently fed their infants table food; as one mother put it, "just the same as I eat myself."[7] The habit was so common in Chicago that F. W. Reilly, the assistant commissioner of health, warned mothers in 1895 that "it is a sin to give any infant one morsel of solid food of any kind, or anything but breast milk" before a baby cuts his first teeth. He admonished women that their habit of holding their babies on their laps at the dinner table and nonchalantly "giving them a little of this, that and the other . . . which the little stomach is not fitted for" harmed babies "just as surely, though not as quickly, as if they had been fed poison out of a drug store."[8] Mothers constantly swapped infant-care advice, however, and the talk fueled mixed feeding. As one young mother explained to *American Motherhood* magazine in 1907, "People tell me that if I feed him a little of everything I eat, he won't be so apt to have colic."[9] The president of the Chicago Infant Welfare Society Auxiliary complained in 1915 that mothers habitually compared their babies' weight, likening fat babies to healthy babies, "and with this end in view they feed them coffee, sausage, doughnuts, pancakes, etc."[10]

Even mothers aware of the potential dangers of human milk substitutes rarely, if ever, equated giving table food to a nursing infant with artificial feeding. Consequently, they were notoriously unreliable reporters when physicians asked them whether they exclusively breastfed their babies. Isaac Abt recalled quizzing the mother of one terribly sick infant about what she had given her son to eat. "Nothing. Nothing but the breast," she assured Abt. Suspicious, Abt called his assistant, Issy, over for help. Issy gently prodded the mother. "When you eat your dinner, you hold the baby on your lap, I suppose?" Mother agreed. Issy persisted. "And when you have soup, don't you give him a taste?" The mother admitted to "just a sip." What about potatoes, Issy asked, "of course you let him have them?" Mother nodded. "He licks my spoon, maybe." Encouraged, Abt's aide added, "And nice, rich gravy—don't you let him have a little gravy on bread?" Mother replied, "A little bit. He always cries for it."[11]

Women's diaries and children's medical records corroborate physicians' complaints that even women who breastfed exclusively usually weaned their babies at or well before three months of age. As one new mother said matter-of-factly of her three month old in 1884, "I feed her a little now." Likewise, Josephine Laflin "decided to feed" her ten week old in 1903. When Katherine Shedd Bradley had her second baby in 1920 he weighed only three pounds ten ounces. The doctor told her that this baby—her first child, born in 1913, apparently was not breastfed—"must have Mother's milk." Bradley reported having "lots of milk" and her son's weight increased steadily. "David gained 2½ ozs. Wonderful" was a typical entry in her diary in the weeks following her son's birth. When David was thirteen days old, doctors discharged Bradley, but not David, from the hospital. To ensure that her baby continued to consume only breast milk, Bradley dutifully expressed her milk several times daily and her husband delivered it to the hospital. She continued to record her baby's weight meticulously: David weighed four pounds seven ounces at three weeks. Finally, in July, shortly after he was three months old, he weighed "9 lbs. at last" and his happy and grateful mother did what most women had been doing for several decades when their baby reached three months of age. She "put him partly on [a] bottle."[12]

Mothers rarely sought medical opinion before weaning their babies, and exasperated physicians protested that mothers' decisions to wean were invariably "injudicious."[13] Chicago physician Charles Warrington Earle complained in 1892, "Hardly a week passes that I am not called in families where I find the baby weaned and upon an insufficient artificial food, frequently unsterilized. The long list of maladies which frequently result therefrom, have in many cases already commenced." Earle admitted that "in some instances" weaning was at a doctor's behest, but insisted that it was far more common to find that "the mother had what to her was a reasonable excuse for weaning the baby."[14] Chicago pediatrician Frank Spooner Churchill likewise complained that mothers weaned their babies without a physician's approval and rarely summoned doctors "soon enough to prevent the ravages caused by improper feeding . . . [mothers] do not seek medical advice until some pressing condition . . . drives them to the clinic."[15]

Women themselves confirmed that they customarily weaned without consulting doctors. In letters to magazines detailing their misadventures with artificial food, mothers rarely mentioned any contact with a physician. One mother, "obliged to wean" her four-and-a-half-month-old son who was in "splendid condition," replaced her breast milk, in growing desperation, with one artificial food concoction after another. Nothing nourished him. Her baby grew "thin and sickly and fretful." Finally, she reported happily, she discovered Mellin's food mixed with Anglo-Swiss condensed milk. The mixture "worked to a charm" and made her son, once again, a "happy, well-satisfied baby, gaining steadily in flesh, and so he has continued ever since." Another mother wrote that her "supply of breast milk failed" when her daughter was three months old and attempts to feed her cows' milk were "unsuccessful." This mother thumbed through magazines until she discovered Lacto-Preparata, on which her baby thrived "as she did when she had her natural food."[16]

Entries in women's diaries likewise suggest that women rarely consulted a physician before weaning. Anita McCormick Blaine, for example, interviewed three doctors shortly before her son's 1890 birth. Each physician urged her to breastfeed. Blaine consequently breastfed her son, who behaved "as if he was enjoying a delicious six course dinner." By her son's fourth month, however, Blaine had him on a mixed diet, and, judging by her faithful recording of her numerous conversations with physicians previously, she apparently did not consult a doctor in the matter. The baby continued to receive some breast milk through his tenth month.[17] Josephine Laflin also describes numerous discussions with physicians before, during, and after the birth of her third son—whom she described as "a ready nurser"—in 1903. But when she chose to stop breastfeeding her baby at two and a half months she merely wrote, "Decided to feed Lloyd and wean him as soon as convenient."[18]

By the 1920s attitudes had changed dramatically and parents regularly conferred with physicians—the wealthy with private physicians and the poor with the physicians who volunteered their services at infant welfare stations—about all aspects of their children's health, including weaning. By then, ironically, many physicians had reversed their position on early weaning. When Katharine Kerr Moore began to wean her ten-month-old son Marvin in 1922, he immediately became ill and she blamed her doctor for the calamity, just as physicians had blamed women for similar crises a generation earlier. A frightened Moore wrote to her mother, "These modern doctors seem in a big hurry to get the babies weaned and to eating. . . . Got a book from the library on the subject written about 10 years ago, which says that a baby should not have even cracker or toast until 14 or 15 months old."[19]

When mothers did begin to turn to physicians for help with their infants, the interaction was often fraught with antagonism, which might account for the lingering reluctance to consult doctors about events like weaning. While mothers like Moore expressed frustration with the know-how of "these modern doctors," doctors traditionally doubted mothers' competence. Chicago physician Thomas Allen warned his colleagues in 1908, "As to the mother's ability and wisdom in feeding an infant . . . the only safe attitude for the physician to take is that the mother knows nothing about it, and this holds true whether she be a primipara or a multipara." Charles Warrington Earle condemned bottle-feeding as mothers' deadly experiments. "The matter is left too largely to the people until a food of their selection has produced its deleterious effects," he protested in 1891, "and then we are called, only to find a child emaciated, impoverished and with a digestive apparatus so thoroughly out of repair that the child dies before we can bring about a normal condition of digestion."[20]

Servants Take Charge

Because the suffering described by Earle was so prevalent, mothers' changing infant-feeding habits were the subject of much social and medical commentary, none favorable. One writer complained in 1883, "Horses and cattle are carefully fed with the food that suits them best . . . greater care is bestowed upon them than the majority of parents give to their children. . . . the wonder comes to be, not that so many children die, but that so many survive their early mismanagement."[21]

Critics aimed these caustic remarks almost exclusively at wealthy mothers who hired servants to care for their babies. One infant-care expert admonished well-to-do women in 1881, "It is too much the modern custom to bring up children by hand, as it is called, even when there is nothing to prevent the mother from nursing." The writer accused the mothers of hand-fed babies of "indolence, selfishness and a determination not to give up visiting and pleasure-seeking at all hours." Another writer derided "the society woman . . .

whose many social functions call her constantly from her babe's cradle, leaving the little helpless mortal to the care of a hireling." A physician writing in a popular women's magazine in 1909 about the benefits of human milk admonished, "The mother who permits social 'duties,' laziness or any other such excuse or motive to interfere with her highest of privileges is a woman unfit to bring human beings into the world." In 1911 a physician writing for the Chicago Department of Health scolded, "The mother who can nurse her baby but will not do so, because it interferes with her social and other pleasures, is guilty of a neglect that is little short of criminal."[22]

Many wealthy mothers apparently did sustain full social calendars in the months immediately after giving birth. Katherine Shedd Bradley hired a nurse after the 1913 birth of her first baby and continued to shop and visit friends at much the same hectic pace as before her baby was born. In 1912, when her daughter was considerably less than a year old, Preston Owsley Morton accompanied her husband on a one-month cruise of assorted Caribbean islands. Their baby remained in Chicago.[23]

When a mother hired a nurse to help her care for her baby, it evidently was the norm for the nurse to take complete charge of the infant, thus precluding breastfeeding. One nurse caring for a five-month-old born to a Chicago family threatened to quit when other members of the household tried to help her calm the crying baby. Furious, she warned the baby's father that she would "not be interfered with." The baby was her domain and she would not permit anyone, presumably even the baby's mother, to intercede. Another father, hunting for a nurse to care for his fourth child, reported that nurses had cared for all his children, hence his wife "knew nothing about feeding them." Josephine Laflin complained in her diary that Miss Kunz, the Chicago nurse who cared for her newborn second son in 1898, "was most scientific and watchful in her care of baby and me, but her face was like marble, her demeanor like an iceberg and she was as devoid of sympathy as a machine. She kept baby in another room day and night, would scarcely allow me to look at him and never spoke of him." Despite this lament, however, five days after her son's birth Laflin hired an additional nurse to help the exhausted Miss Kunz with the baby. Predictably, although Laflin had "hoped with all my heart that I might be able to nurse baby and every thing seemed propitious at first," she was soon disappointed "and it was heart breaking." Miss Kunz proceeded to purchase modified cows' milk formula for the baby from the local Walker-Gordon milk laboratory. The formula, fortunately, "seemed to agree perfectly" with Laflin's son. It (and, presumably, Miss Kunz) also permitted Laflin to travel with her husband from Chicago to New York to greet her in-laws when they returned from an extended European vacation. Laflin wrote in her diary, "I gave them a genuine surprise for they never thought of my being able to leave Baby so soon."[24]

Crossing Class Lines

The abandonment of breastfeeding was not unique to the well-to-do, however. The increasingly common practices of supplementing or wholly replacing breast milk with artificial food crossed class lines: poor and working mothers as well as middle- and upper-class mothers all embraced the practice. Isaac Abt, who volunteered his services to several medical charities in Chicago, recalled in his autobiography, "Most of the peasant mothers and poor women of the city nursed their babies; yet there were many who were artificially fed and physicians everywhere were searching for a satisfactory food."[25] The Chicago Department of Health responded to the changing infant-feeding habits of immigrant mothers by disseminating literature and posting notices in myriad languages about the importance of breastfeeding.[26]

Artificial feeding was so common in the city's congested neighborhoods that in the summer of 1908 alarmed health department officials sent physicians and nurses door-to-door in these areas to discuss infant feeding with new mothers.[27] Nurses and doctors recorded the results of their interviews on printed forms and statisticians compiled the data. Even though all the interviews took place shortly after a woman gave birth, when she was most likely to be breastfeeding, the vast majority of women questioned were not exclusively breastfeeding their babies. In 1912, for example, Chicago Department of Health field nurses reported that, of the women they interviewed, 11,923 breastfed their newborns, 5,538 offered their newborns some type of "mixed feeding," 7,611 fed their newborns cooked (pasteurized or sterilized) cows' milk, and 5,829 fed their newborns raw (unpasteurized) cows' milk. These 30,901 babies represented 55 percent of the babies born in Chicago that year. Only 39 percent of them were exclusively breastfed. The remainder consumed, either partially or wholly, some type of artificial food. (See appendix C.)[28]

When poor and working-class women did not exclusively breastfeed their newborns, critics attributed their decision, not to the narcissism they saw in middle- and upper-class mothers, but to ignorance. A Chicago doctor charged in 1891 that the infants of poverty-stricken parents often had chronic diarrhea because their mothers fed them "partially spoiled fruit, pickles, peanuts, cheap candies and cakes . . . and the wonder is that any of

```
Ward..............Street.....................................No.....................
House.....................Ft..............Rr...............Flat...................
Ft................Mid..............Rr...............Floor..................1-2-3-B
NAME.........................................................................
Place Mother's Birth............................Occupation....................
Place Father's Birth............................Occupation....................
Children:  Alive...............Ages................Youngest Child Sex...........
           General Condition.......................................Dead.........
           Ages at Death................Second Child Sex.....................
           General Condition.......................Abortions..................
Feeding Youngest:  Breast...............Breast and.............Comm...........'s
                   Pat. Fd...........Cow's Milk only..................Cow's
                   and.............Cond. Milk.............Water...........
Feeding Next Youngest:
    If the Mother is Nursing what does she take to make milk?
Feeding:  Regular..........................Too often...............Night
          Feedings............................How many?..............
Milk:  Boiled...............Pasteurized.................Covered...............
       Kept on Ice....................In Water...............
Bathing:  Sponge.................Tub..................How often?................
Clothing:  Too much...........................Too little..................
Stool:  Color  ...............Consistency..................Blood...............
        Mucous..................No. in 24 Hours..........
Sickness in House:  Cases Diarrhea.................Tuberculosis...............
        Chronic Cough..............Contagious.............Skin...........
```

LIVING ROOMS	PERF.	ALLOW	SURROUNDINGS	PERF.	ALLOW
Cleanliness: Deduct when Unclean Floors 4, Walls 3, Ceilings 3, Ledges 3, Windows 2.	15		**Accumulations:** Within 50 feo*: Garbage — Rubbish	15	
Ventilation: Adjustable Windows 6, No Odor 4.	10		**Yard and Areas:** Space available.	15	
Lighting: Deduct 2 Points for every 3 per cent. less than 15 per cent. of Floor Space.	10		**Plumbing on Premises:** Deduct when Leaking 4: Clogged 4: Odor 2.	10	
Presence of Flies:	15			**40**	
Crowding: Rooms, No.................. Men ....Women. .... Children...................... Boarders......................	10		**Plus Living Rooms 60** **Final Score . . . 100**		
	60				

Figure 1 1908 Field Survey Form. Artificial feeding and high infant mortality were so common in Chicago's congested neighborhoods that in the summer of 1908 alarmed health department officials sent physicians and nurses door-to-door in these areas to discuss infant care, and particularly infant feeding, with new mothers. Nurses and doctors recorded the results of their interviews on this printed form. *Source: Report of the Department of Health of the City of Chicago for the Years 1907, 1908, 1909, 1910,* 175.

these children live, not that so many of them die."[29] Workers for the Chicago Milk Commission (CMC)—a medical charity organized in 1903 to disseminate clean cows' milk in poor neighborhoods to families with babies—claimed that they observed babies as young as four days old consuming beer, whiskey, sausage, pork, and watermelon or "as several mothers . . . expressed it 'any old thing.'" CMC volunteers consequently reported teaching neighborhood mothers a number of lessons, such as "the 'nasty yellow stuff' on top of the milk is fit for use [a reference to cream, which rises to the top in whole milk that is not homogenized] and a nipple full of live maggots should not be given to the baby." Mary Plummer, secretary of the Milk Commission, chided, "Never to have seen cream before is a volume in itself."[30] *Babyhood* magazine echoed the complaints of Chicago's medical and philanthropic communities when it reported that poor babies in New York were "fed with tea or some other dark decoction from nursing-bottles and nipples which had not been cleansed this year." The magazine described infants, not more than two or three months old, who gummed bread and cake "held with a tight grip by puny fingers from which it would seem as if the bones must soon protrude." *Babyhood*'s editor urged "rescuing the little ones permanently from the care of their mothers."[31]

In contrast to their unrelenting criticism of middle- and upper-class women, social critics did voice occasional sympathy for the poor and working-class women who did not breastfeed. The Chicago Department of Health defended these women, arguing that overwork so exacerbated the "normal" difficulties of breastfeeding that it was little wonder that some of these women turned to bottles.[32] One physician explained that "poorer mothers do not refrain from or cease nursing because of social duties, nor is unwillingness the dominant cause of their failure." Rather, he contended, they did not breastfeed for reasons largely beyond their control—poor diet, overwork, worry borne of their difficult lives, ignorance, the "promises of proprietary food advertisements," and "being turned out from a maternity hospital almost too weak to walk steadily and returning to a home lacking in hygiene."[33]

A. Belcham Keyes, a physician and secretary of the Children's Hospital Society of Chicago, recognized that a poverty-stricken mother's exhaustion and anxiety often stood in the way of ideal infant care. Although he urged breastfeeding for nine to twelve months, and assured mothers that their milk supply would be ample for at least that long, he acknowledged the environmental forces that hampered prolonged nursing. Breastfeeding "is often difficult," he sympathized, "especially in the hot, illy [sic] ventilated homes in the factory districts in summer for many mothers must do hard outside work, which adds to the anxiety of life among the working classes." Is it any wonder, he mused, that baby's irrelevant or temporary ailments might cause these mothers to fear something was wrong with their milk "and so they begin to feed." Keyes and many others assured Chicago's mothers, publicly and privately, that human milk almost never disagreed with infants while "other food than that which Nature provided" virtually guaranteed "bowel disturbance."[34] But mothers continued to insist that they could not sustain their babies on breast milk alone.

Mothers working outside the home had no choice but to ask a caretaker to give their babies artificial food in their absence. Observers sympathized with the plight of these women. Mrs. George Moulton, a member of the CMC's executive committee, pitied the women who fed their babies CMC milk, characterizing them as mothers who "go out early in the morning and work all day to get the bread for their helpless families, and leave the new born babe to the tender mercies of children but little older."[35] One Yiddish-language newspaper described the desperation of Jewish mothers forced to work: "You may rest assured that . . . [they] do not engage in other activities for the sake of pleasure or happiness. Want, privation, and hunger drive them to do other things than housekeeping. Many are employed in other work because their husbands are handicapped and earn too little."[36] One Chicago mother explained to the U.S. Children's Bureau that she attempted to breast-feed her baby, but because her husband "refused to provide for us," she had to work. Unable to nurse her infant except in the morning and evening, she had so little milk within one month that her baby was left "without the fountain nature had provided."[37]

Expressed breast milk would have been of little use to these mothers' babies; without ice boxes mothers had no place to safely store the milk. Even the manufacturers and promoters of breast pumps, which were available through the Sears Catalog and other venues by the early 1900s, did not recommend that pumped milk be stored and given to babies later. Rather, they advised mothers to use breast pumps only to express milk for babies unable to suck at the breast, that is, premature infants or infants with harelips, and to use the milk immediately.[38]

The Chicago Department of Health reported in 1911 that poverty indeed increased infant mortality because it forced women to work outside the home to supplement family income and thus prevented them from breastfeeding.[39] Myriad studies corroborated the fact that babies whose mothers were "employed at heavy labor"—as opposed to babies whose mothers worked for pay in the home by taking in laundry or boarders or cooking meals for unmarried men—died much more frequently than other infants, probably because they were not breastfed.[40]

To allay just such predicaments, medical charities occasionally intervened to rescue babies about to be weaned because their mothers were going back to work. One woman, whose husband was a "habitual deserter," informed Infant Welfare Society (IWS) physicians shortly after her son Joe was born that she had to return to work immediately to support her four children. The superintendent of the IWS reported that "the doctor found that she had plenty of breast milk and explained to her how much better it would be to keep Joe on the breast. . . . the necessary relief was given so she would not have to worry."[41]

This mother was unusually lucky; most in similar situations had little choice but to leave their babies in the care of their older children while they worked. As the IWS reported in 1912, "How frequently a little girl of eight or ten is met carrying the baby, and usually she knows more about the baby than her mother."[42] The dilemma of working mothers was so widespread that, beginning in 1912, the Chicago Department of Health offered infant-care classes—dubbed "Little Mothers' Clubs"—to school-age girls with infant siblings. Health department nurses taught the weekly classes in thirty-one public schools from 3:15 to 4:30 P.M., attracting a thousand girls in 1912 alone. Girls learned about the importance of fresh air and hygiene for babies and how to bathe and dress infants. They also learned, perfunctorily, the importance of breastfeeding and, in laborious detail, how to purchase, pasteurize, and modify cows' milk and how to clean and sterilize a baby's bottle.[43]

The curricular emphasis made sense. These girls cared for their infant siblings, not offspring, and comprehensive breastfeeding instruction was irrelevant to them. The myriad lessons on safe bottle use, on the other hand, were essential. Yet the lessons likely influenced the way these Little Mothers eventually cared for their own children and probably had an immediate impact on their own mothers as well. Immigrant mothers were particularly susceptible to the messages their daughters brought home. As social workers at the largest medical dispensary in Chicago observed, Italians "living as a homogenous group and religiously adhering to their native language and customs" were immune to advice from doctors and nurses and staunchly "antagonistic to health, hygiene or diet regulations." But, dispensary employees found, a woman's American-born children were "the faithful allies of the social worker, her spokesmen and disciplinarians. . . . Mother, particularly, must do as 'teacher' says."[44] So even as the medical community bombarded immigrant mothers with demands to breastfeed, their daughters learned—from nurses at school no less—how to use bottles safely.

Ignorance Is Not Bliss

Although all mothers did not necessarily share the same economic pressures, they did share experiences that influenced their infant-feeding practices, among them the opportunity, or, by the late nineteenth century, the lack of opportunity, to observe laboring and lactating women. As medical historian Judith Walzer Leavitt has argued, birth in eighteenth- and early nineteenth-century America was a social event attended by female friends, family, and neighbors of the laboring woman. Indeed, historians have dubbed the births of that era "social births." Birth attendants aided and comforted the parturient woman during labor and delivery and continued to care for her, as well as her home and family, as she recovered. The recipient of this generosity eventually reciprocated, probably many times over, when her benefactors were in similar need.[45]

Women's cooperative networks were not limited to births but extended to breastfeeding as well. When Lucy Towne fell ill a week after giving birth in 1789, her milk supply deteriorated. Two neighbors took turns nursing her baby until Towne (and her milk supply) recovered. Similarly, when Hannah Craig died less than two weeks after giving birth in 1790, her baby was not left to suffer and likely die owing to lack of mother's milk. Rather, "neighbors came by turns to 'give the infant suck.'"[46]

The constant mutual aid of this era allowed women to observe birth and breastfeeding often. Because attending births and nursing each other's babies were part of the social fabric, women gained a degree of familiarity with birth and lactation that subsequent generations did not. As birth became less a social event and more a medical one attended by few, if any, intimates, women found themselves in a peculiar position. The first birth they ever attended was, more often than not, the birth of their own first baby. For these women, birth and breastfeeding were shrouded in mystery.

As opportunities to observe what had once been quasi-public female biological functions diminished, it became more and more the sole responsibility of mothers to inform their daughters of what to expect from menstruation, sex, pregnancy, birth, and lactation. Mothers might have been an adequate substitute for experience, as women's letters and diaries attest to the intimacy of mother-daughter friendships in the nineteenth and early twentieth centuries. "I think I am in love with my beautiful mother," wrote one woman in the 1850s. "It seemed impossible to find a better stronger friend than my mother," wrote another woman a few decades later.[47]

Despite the obvious affection and intimacy between mothers and daughters, however, women were increasingly reluctant to discuss any aspect of reproduction with their daughters as the nineteenth century progressed, just as daughters needed such counsel most. In 1852 physician Edward John Tilt reported that 25 percent of American girls were wholly ignorant of menstruation when they had their first period. Consequently, they were terrified at menarche, fearing that they had been wounded. Such ignorance spread over time. In an 1895 study of Boston high school girls, 60 percent admitted that they had not known what menstruation was at the time of menarche. Marion Harland, a popular *Ladies' Home Journal* columnist, scolded mothers in her best-selling 1882 advice book, *Eve's Daughters; Or Common Sense for Maid, Wife, and Mother,* for the "criminal reserve" and "pseudo-delicacy" that prevented them from discussing menstruation with their daughters. Few women were chastened by Harland's advice, however. As historian Joan Jacobs Brumberg has documented, "my mother never told me" continued to be a pervasive American complaint.[48]

By the end of the nineteenth century, the traditional mediums that had informed girls of reproduction and their reproductive systems—observing births or learning from an older woman, customarily their mother—had vanished. Knowledge of labor, delivery, and lactation, and how to manage those bodily functions, ceased to be a continuous spool of knowledge passed seamlessly from one generation to the next. Instead, there appeared disparate threads of information, each the length of one woman's lifetime. Knowledge and traditional practice were lost. Who was a woman to go to for answers when she ran into difficulty breastfeeding?

Intimate Marriages

As birth and breastfeeding became privatized, marriages did too. Traditionally, the purpose of sex within marriage was reproduction—a social responsibility. Yet as the fertility rate for white women of childbearing age fell from 7.04 per capita in 1800 to 4.24 in 1880 to 3.56 in 1900, the seemingly inseparable link between sex and procreation loosened.[49] Birth control gave sex meaning beyond reproduction. Sex came to be largely an expression of intimacy and only occasionally a way to reproduce. Marriage consequently became associated with romance and companionship.[50]

Courtship intensified during this period. When Lester Ward wooed

Lizzie Vought in the 1860s, their romance went "from handholding and kisses on the face to kisses on the mouth and on 'her sweet breasts.'" Ward wrote in his diary, "she received me in her arms of tenderness and pressed me to her form of honey, and our lips touched and our souls entered paradise together. . . . That evening and that night we experienced the joys of love and tasted the felicity which belongs to married life alone."[51] Similarly, as the romance between Frederick Gookin and Marie Sieboth progressed in Chicago in 1897, Gookin wrote an adoring letter to Sieboth. "From early manhood I . . . felt the need of a woman's love, but, as the years went by I began . . . to doubt my ability . . . to inspire it. . . . Beloved, I doubt no longer, for I know the infinite sweetness of a passionate love which takes entire possession of my soul." Nor did their romance wane after marriage. In a letter to Marie while on a business trip in 1901 Frederick wrote, "Tomorrow will be St. Valentine's day and I want you to have this bit of a note in the morning just to tell you once more that I love you. I know that you don't need to be told, but I feel that I must say it for my heart is saying it all the time."[52]

As the expectation of romance and companionship within marriage altered views of sex, attitudes toward breastfeeding changed. With less emphasis on procreation as the purpose of sex, the feeding of infants likewise became estranged from reproduction. Lactation was no longer the last (and longest) stage of a viable pregnancy. Breasts acquired meaning beyond feeding a newborn. A woman's breasts now "belonged" to her husband at least as much as, if not more than, to her infant. Men and women alike began to define the breast less in physiological terms and more in sexual ones.

Advertisements for breast developers—creams, mechanical devices, and pills—were one indication of the sexualization of breasts. A half-page ad in the 1902 Sears catalog heralded The Princess Bust Developer and Bust Cream or Food—"the only treatment that will actually, permanently . . . cause [women's breasts] to fill out to nature's full proportions, give that swelling, rounded, firm white bosom, that queenly bearing, so attractive to the opposite sex."[53] Manufacturers of the Madame Mozelle Compound Bust Developing Treatment warned: "It is a matter of statistics that the great majority of neglected wives and old maids are . . . flat-chested. . . . Don't be one of the gray cohorts of hopeless femininty [sic] when it is so easy to attain that physical perfection that will turn you into an enchanting creature of many allurements."[54] Pauline Turner, "Originator of a Scientific Four-Part Treatment for the Rapid Development and Restoration of the Bust," offered to assist women and girls "in whom development has never taken place" and "mothers who have lost their development by nursing."[55]

Women's increasing discomfort with their breasts' dual physiological and sexual functions enhanced their unwillingness to breastfeed and made it easier to ignore the objections to artificial food. As one woman wrote to a magazine in 1886 on behalf of her pregnant daughter: "she wants to be more of a companion for her husband than she could be if she should nurse Baby; and . . . we wonder if it would not be best for all that the little one be fed." Other women worried that breastfeeding made their breasts unattractive. A Chicago woman complained, "Why, upon my weaning my boy, did my breasts, which always were round and full, become (to use a slangy phrase) 'flat as a pancake'? . . . Mine became flat and have remained so, greatly to my annoyance."[56]

The Food, Fly, and Foul Air Scare

As new sexual mores took firm hold by the end of the nineteenth century, public health departments around the country introduced the germ theory of disease to the masses. Campaigns featured a clear and disquieting message—illness was caused not by fate, divine retribution, inherited weakness, or a vague miasma, as previously believed, but by dangerous, unseen organisms omnipresent in food, water, milk, homes, public buildings, work sites, and streets. Babies, the smallest and weakest members of society, seemed most susceptible to the invisible threat. Consequently, newspapers, magazines, medical charities, municipal health departments, and infant welfare reformers directed pointed propaganda about germs to mothers.[57]

Public health crusades put women on the front line of the never ending battle against the invisible, life-threatening creatures that menaced everyone. Municipalities, like sergeants commanding platoons, ordered mothers to be on guard against flies, dirt, spoiled food, contaminated cows' milk, and impure air. Only meticulously cleaning a house, appropriately storing food, properly cooking meals, and scientifically caring for children would ward off the omnipresent danger. A mother's momentary carelessness or ignorance might inflict illness on innocent family members, particularly the most vulnerable in a mother's care, her infant.

The public and private health responsibilities of mothers abounded. "What Must We Do To Be Saved?" screamed the crowd of babies illustrating one 1911 Chicago Department of Health pamphlet. "The slaughter of little babies in the City of Chicago amounts to 6800 yearly," mothers learned, and "at least 3500 of these deaths are avoidable." Another poster illustrated "The Preventable Perils Surrounding The Child." This "Ring of Trouble" included "dirty milk," "diarrheal diseases," "ignorance," and "poor care."[58]

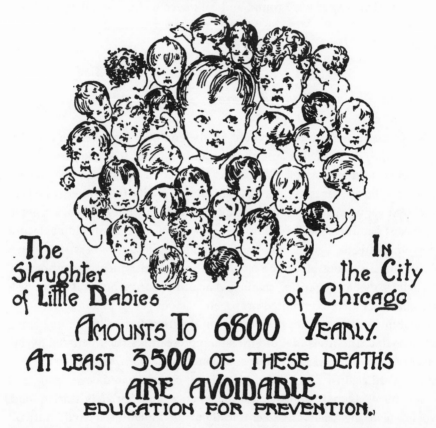

WHAT MUST WE DO TO BE SAVED ?

The Slaughter of Little Babies

In the City of Chicago

Amounts To 6800 Yearly.

At least 3500 of these deaths are avoidable.

EDUCATION FOR PREVENTION.

Figure 2 The public and private responsibilities of mothers abounded. This 1911 Chicago Department of Health poster, drawn by Katherine Field White, reminds women that more than 50 percent of infant deaths are preventable. *Source: Bulletin Chicago School of Sanitary Instruction,* 22 July 1911, 216.

To use a phrase of historian Nancy Tomes's, "antisepticonscious America" was being born. Women shouldered the burden of protecting everyone, but especially babies, from illness. Mothers' skill, knowledge, and "scientific" practices—not happenstance or physicians or public health infrastructure—were now the primary architects of babies' health.[59] Mothers learned from the literature at their disposal that their own skill and consci-

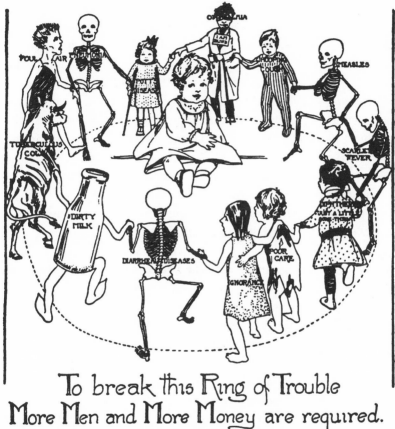

THE PREVENTABLE PERILS SURROUNDING THE CHILD
*One baby out of every five dies before
reaching the age of two years.
About 80 percent of these deaths are from
preventable diseases.*

To break this Ring of Trouble
More Men and More Money are required.
Department of Health—Chicago. Educational Series No. 99.

Figure 3 The Chicago Department of Health hung this 4′ x 5′ poster in Chicago's neighborhoods to remind mothers of all the preventable hazards that threatened their children. *Source: Bulletin Chicago School of Sanitary Instruction, 18 May 1912, 80.*

entiousness would determine whether or not their baby survived infancy. The extraordinarily influential Women's Christian Temperance Union (WCTU) urged, "Study the science of motherhood. . . . Ignorance will not be a sufficient excuse for our mistakes in this day when so much is written on child-nature, child-culture and child-training."[60]

Sole reliance on the ability of one's mammary glands to sustain an infant for six to nine months became more than a little daunting in this atmosphere. Women's anxiety was palpable, as "what am I doing wrong?" became their refrain. Mothers' descriptions of babies' maladies, real and imagined, dominated women's advice columns. These desperate letters frequently ended with a plea asking, in essence, "Could the problem be my milk?"

The most telling letters were from mothers with healthy babies and an excellent supply of milk, for even they fretted. One nursing mother reported that her two week old had gained eight ounces since birth, slept four to seven hours at a time, had not "cried an hour altogether since he came into the world," and appeared to be "a healthy, hearty little fellow." But, she explained, "The one trouble seems to be with his bowels, as he has not had a digested passage since his birth. My physician . . . has analyzed my milk and pronounced it satisfactory in quality and sufficient in quantity. Is this trouble likely to wear away, or will it, as I fear, result in loss of flesh and strength to the child if allowed to continue?" The magazine's response was reassuring. Whatever mother meant by "undigested passages," a more important symptom was baby's apparent health. The infant's mother learned, "A baby of fifteen days old who is as comfortable, in spite of the imperfect digestion of his food, as the one described does not seem to us to need much medicine."[61]

Whether that particular mother took comfort in those words is unknown, but few physicians or magazine editors could allay the anxiety of most women. Another mother complained that all three of her babies "for the first few months of their lives, had a severe gastro intestinal disturbance, due, possibly, to some peculiarity of the [breast] milk." How this stomach upset manifested itself is not clear, however, as the woman also reported, "Nutrition and growth did not seem to suffer." A doctor assured the woman that her first baby's "plump, rosy cheeks" were a sign that he "was growing nicely." Nevertheless, she insisted on bringing the infant to the physician for an examination every few days. She reported to friends, "The pictures, which I conjured up in my mind of him, suffering from malnutrition, rickets, possibly hydrocephalus were frightful. I allowed myself to be tormented by such thoughts till I was reduced to a state of melancholia."[62] Another mother of a breastfed baby who "was so large and strong . . . he gained a pound a week" complained that he digested her breast milk "imperfectly." Worse, she reported that her second baby, "not so strong," was unable to tolerate her milk at all. Artificial food was no better. "Nothing seemed to nourish him." Eventually she gave up on artificial food altogether and "by dieting, quiet, and massage" at last produced milk that put her baby "in perfect health."[63]

Given the ubiquitous pressure on women in post–germ theory America and the consequent high anxiety level among mothers, it is hardly surprising that queries to women's magazines about infant feeding remained legion for some time. Molly Ladd-Taylor discovered that, in a random sampling of 1,362 letters written by mothers to the U.S. Children's Bureau between 1914 and 1928, more than half the letters were about feeding children—either about nursing, weaning, the use of formulas, or an older child's diet.[64]

The infant-feeding advice relayed by experts to these anxious mothers remained static for almost three decades into the twentieth century. Chicago's public health workers, for example, repeated similar messages to women year after year, explaining in essence, "When mothers realize that there is less work, less inconvenience, less expense and less danger in breastfeeding, there will be less cow-feeding, and as a consequence, *there will be fewer sick babies.*"[65] Yet the number of babies whose mothers weaned them early, supplemented their breast milk with cows' milk, or, increasingly, did not breastfeed at all kept growing.

Mixed Messages

Why didn't the resolute advice reverse or at least temper what was becoming an inexorable move to artificial food? Because there were at the same time equally dramatic directives that contradicted the assurances that breastfeeding was the healthiest, safest, and simplest way to feed a baby. One physician, for example, instructed lactating women to analyze their own breast milk regularly. If they did not, he warned, their "nursing babies may be starving in spite of an abundant secretion of breast milk. The fluid may be abundant in quantity but poor in quality." He recommended that lactating women express their milk and let it stand in a test tube overnight. "Normal milk," he advised, formed a 3 to 4 percent layer of cream on top. "Very bad milk," on the other hand, produced a layer of less than 1 percent cream.[66]

Similarly, when F. W. Reilly, the Chicago Assistant Commissioner of Health, told mothers in no uncertain terms in 1895 to nurse their babies, he coupled his plea with an equally stern caveat. Under certain conditions, Reilly warned, "even breast milk" caused babies severe digestive distress. If a mother is overheated, he explained, she should always express a teaspoon of milk before breastfeeding, implying that the milk nearest the surface of her body could easily sour—exactly like cows' milk left standing on a kitchen counter on a hot summer day. He cautioned mothers who had not nursed their babies for more than two hours to do the same, insinuating that milk left sitting in the body for a time might spoil—just like cows' milk traveling for days in a stifling railroad car. "And if the mother has been badly frightened or very angry or excited," he claimed in a terrifying denouement, "it is not safe to give the breast at all; it should be drawn and the milk thrown away." Lest mothers foolishly ignore his advice, he added, "[M]ore than half the babies and young children that die in Chicago every year could be saved by following the advice here given."[67] Despite physicians' constant glorification of breast milk, they increasingly equated it with cows' milk. Doctors began to portray both substances as potentially dangerous if placed in careless hands or produced by faulty bodies.

Not Enough Milk

The reason women themselves gave most often for not breastfeeding had nothing to do with contradictory messages, economics, changing attitudes toward sex and marriage, or anxiety borne of public health campaigns. Rather, mothers reported with dismay that they simply did not have enough quality milk to successfully breastfeed.[68] Medical journals and women's magazines documented this pervasive problem beginning in the 1880s until well into the twentieth century. As late as 1924 physicians at Chicago's infant welfare stations noted that a majority of the mothers who stopped breastfeeding their babies at or before three months of age gave "no milk" or "lack of quantity" of milk as the reason for early weaning.[69]

One mother reported insufficient milk and her solution to the problem in *Babyhood* magazine in 1886. "In the light of my own experience I can truthfully say that the bottle was like food from heaven to the poor, starved, little beings, who were weary and well-nigh spent with the struggle to sustain life on the meager and innutritious milk which nature had unkindly provided." She disagreed with the oft-heard admonition "the only safe method of feeding is the natural one," and suggested instead that mothers with inadequate milk rely on the "placid and tranquil and free from nerves" cow rather than their own nerve-wracked bodies. Her only caveat about artificial feeding, in keeping with the "gospel of germs," was that mothers provide their babies with "sweet and *clean*" bottles.[70]

Physicians studied lactation failure and offered explanations for the phenomenon. Some argued that as the physical demand on women lessened, that is, as they led more "civilized" lives, their "power of endurance" diminished and their ability to breastfeed ebbed accordingly.[71] Assorted explanations for women's seeming inability to breastfeed continued well into the twentieth century. Isaac Abt contended in a 1904 Domestic Science column in the *Chicago Tribune* that two-thirds of mothers "found it impossible" to breast-feed and warned that the problem would worsen. "Women tend to inherit from their mothers the disability to nurse their offspring," he explained, "from which it will be seen that the race will eventually suffer from this incapacity, and the nursing function is destined gradually to disappear."[72] By 1910, women's insistence that their bodies could not produce enough quality milk to feed their babies was so widespread that delegates at child-welfare conferences were discussing the likelihood that the inability to lactate was the next step in human evolution.[73]

To many mothers their seeming inability to breastfeed was a source of great sorrow. One woman wrote a letter to *Babyhood* magazine in 1887 defending the women who appeared to be physically incapable of nursing their infants:

> I cannot here refrain from a protest against the injustice done to the mothers of this generation in the way in which they are constantly accused of refusing to nurse their children either from selfishness or laziness, whereas in all of the cases I have known (and they are many) it has invariably been the mother's misfortune and not her fault. Why it should be so no one knows, but in all these instances everything has been done, every effort honestly made, but without success, or success only to slight degree.[74]

Inadequate breast milk was such a pervasive problem among women that ads for galactogogues—substances to increase and enhance mothers' milk—became common in women's magazines. One 1902 advertisement for Nutrolactis promised to increase the quantity of a mother's milk, "greatly improve" its quality, and energize any woman "debilitated by nursing." The ad explained, "Nutrolactis acts chiefly by strengthening and building up the mother's system; it does not *force* mothers to yield good milk copiously, it *enables* them to do so." One bewildered physician wrote to the *Journal of the American Medical Association* seeking information about Nutrolactis because so many of his patients insisted they could not breastfeed without it.[75]

Feeding Schedules: "Teaching the Child . . . Self-Control, or the Contrary"

Few in the medical community connected mothers' complaints of insufficient milk, and their growing dependence on galactogogues, with a new and widespread devotion to infant-feeding schedules. As scheduling became vital to the management of factories and railroads, many suggested the innovation would also improve domestic life and infants' health. One Chicago physician advised, "I care not whether the child be given mother's milk, or a wet nurse's milk, or one cows' milk or a hundred; if not given at absolutely regular intervals . . . that child cannot under any circumstances thrive." Infant-care advice columnist Helen Moody lauded this wisdom: "Women have fed babies from time immemorial, but it remained for the trained observation of men to discover that a baby should be fed only at certain times, like any other rational human being, and not every time it cried."[76]

Traditionally, advice on when to feed an infant had been vague. In the seventeenth and eighteenth centuries women learned to feed babies according to hunger cues: "As to the time and hour it needs no limits, for it may be at any time, night or day, when he hath a mind." By the nineteenth century advice was only slightly more explicit. "The younger the baby, the shorter should be the interval from one feeding time to another" was typical. Or, feed a newborn "as often as twelve times in twenty-four hours" and allow the baby "to continue nursing until it voluntarily ceases." By the end of the nineteenth century, however, prevailing wisdom was strikingly different. As one writer suggested, babies on precise schedules "will . . . become a creature of habit, and consequently will be less troublesome to care for and will be far more comfortable and happy." This latter advice stuck for decades. Mothers learned from the Chicago Department of Health in 1926 that "a clock in the baby's room is as important to the mother and baby as a good watch is to a railroad engineer. . . . Spoiling the baby often begins in the first few days. *Doing things by the clock* develops the habit of doing things on time and at the same time makes a baby with good habits."[77]

Advice on how to schedule feedings became quite explicit. Never nurse baby for more than twenty minutes. Nursing intervals should never be less than four hours.[78] In 1911 the Chicago Department of Health berated women, "never feed the baby oftener than every three hours; four hours is better still. If the baby 'won't go three or four hours,' it's your fault, not his."[79] By 1916 the Chicago Department of Health suggested nursing a baby every six hours for the first two days of life and every three hours after that until a baby was four months old. Those rules, however, only applied to daytime. Public health officials recommended only one feeding at night until the baby was four months old, when mothers were to halt the lone night feeding.[80] Other experts cautioned mothers never to feed a baby at night because mothers needed uninterrupted sleep.[81] One physician reported ominously, "Healthy babies do not require night feedings" and warned women that night feedings "exhaust the milk supply."[82]

Although mothers did not recognize it at the time, these increasingly strict feeding schedules violated the sole rule of milk maintenance: the more a baby sucks on her mother, the more milk the mother's body will produce. The schedules were one likely cause, if not the primary cause, of the epidemic of lactation failure. If a baby wants to suck significantly longer and more often on its mother—which mothers and many physicians interpreted as proof of "not enough milk" and hence the need for a bottle—it is indeed because the milk quantity is not meeting the baby's current needs. But frequent and prolonged sucking, if allowed according to a baby's cues, almost immediately increases the supply.[83] Women's turn-of-the-century observation that they did not have enough milk was likely accurate, but the low milk supplies had cultural, not physical, origins.[84]

There were a few physicians who recognized the source of the problem. One doctor warned colleagues at a Chicago Medical Society meeting in 1892 that a mother who offered her baby cows' milk to supplement her own allegedly insufficient milk would not only sicken her baby but reduce her own milk supply even further. Complete weaning from the breast would soon follow. "Diminished demand," he explained, "soon leads to diminished supply."[85]

Yet feeding schedules rapidly became the norm as mothers found these schedules inherently attractive. Indeed, women seem to have taken the lead in instituting them, for an array of reasons. Given the changing attitude toward marriage, parents now wanted chunks of predictable time alone with their spouses and feeding schedules promised just such opportunities. In one fictionalized 1889 account of life with a newborn, a new mother enjoyed a leisurely breakfast with her husband while their baby slumbered. She triumphed, "Now Jack, you see how little trouble a baby really is—if you only know how to manage him." Convenience was becoming a watchword. As one doctor urged, "First, we must teach regularity, the cultivation of accurate habits in the baby; make a machine of the little one. Teach it to employ its various functions at fixed and convenient times."[86]

Feeding schedules—in combination with occasional bottle use—also granted mothers large blocks of predictable time away from the baby. As such, schedules became one of physicians' ploys to make breastfeeding more palatable to women. One physician proposed that caretakers give babies a bottle at 3 P.M. each day (only after the babies' first month, when a mother's milk supply was well established) so mothers could leave the house from noon to 6 P.M. He explained, "[T]his gives the mother a chance to get out and see her friends, and to get away from the baby for a while, which may be just what she needs." Another physician maintained that a four-hour feeding schedule "does better for the mother, as she can go out to social functions, and have a comfortable day with five feedings; she sleeps all night, and the whole family is contented." In 1934 Clifford Grulee, a Chicago pediatrician and longtime editor of the *American Journal of Diseases of Children,* likewise urged long intervals between nursings, "within limits," because "it allows the mother time when she may seek recreation and if possible get away from the cares of the child; an all important factor." Katharine Kerr Moore was one of many women who occasionally took advantage of bottles and scheduling. When her third son was five months old she wrote to her mother, "am breaking away from home this Wednesday from 12 to 6. Helen Frank will look after my family and administer a bottle feeding to Marvin in the middle of the afternoon. I have ordered a pint bottle of baby milk from the milkman and will prepare the feeding before I go, so all she will have to do is heat it up."[87]

The desire to toilet train babies quickly in order to reduce the pile of laundry, arguably the era's most loathsome household task, also made scheduled feedings attractive. Dirty diapers could be easily and quickly eliminated, infant care experts suggested, if mothers fed their babies at precisely the same time each day, teaching them to "gradually acquire habits of regularity." Mothers learned they could predict exactly when to hold their babies over the chamber pot by the time their babies were nine or ten months (and some experts contended as early as six weeks) of age.[88] Belief in early toilet training stuck for decades. When her son was six weeks old in 1921, Moore wrote to her mother, "Am beginning to train him. Started yesterday and saved 3 diapers." (Moore remained persistent but not soon successful. When her son was twenty-two months old she reported, "He is awful hard to train—guess I will have to spank.)[89]

The WCTU, from its headquarters in the Chicago suburb of Evanston, also endorsed feeding infants on a strict schedule lest a baby become an alcoholic or drug addict. Mary Wood-Allen, physician and editor of *New Crusade,* the WCTU's popular national women's magazine, reminded women that they were not merely physically sustaining their babies when they fed them but also "teaching the child temperance, regular habits, self-control, or the contrary." Intemperance, she explained, stemmed not from "grief and destitution" but from "vicious feeding." She warned that a baby fed every time it cried for food would, as an adult, "probably . . . turn to the pleasures of sense [that is, "the narcotics of alcohol, tobacco, opium or kindred drugs"] to allay physical or mental uneasiness."[90]

Similarly, the conviction that paying too much attention to babies would spoil them strengthened women's adherence to scheduled feeding.[91] As one mother told other mothers, smart women inculcated "good habits" in their infants immediately after birth, teaching babies to get through the day "without being constantly held and cared for."[92] The Chicago Department of Health suggested that mothers regulate their baby's habits "in a proper way by day and night" and warned women that a baby fed or held every time it cried became a "resisting, angry and contrary tyrant."[93]

Some physicians encouraged mothers' preoccupation with infant-feeding schedules with unwitting misinformation. Although a few physicians insisted, correctly, that short intervals between nursings provide the frequent nipple stimulation necessary to produce sufficient milk, many other physicians, including Grulee, believed that waiting at least four hours between nursings gave mothers' breasts time to fill up.[94] A New York doctor similarly suggested that supplementing a breastfed baby's diet with artificial food, "often tends to build up the breast milk rather than to decrease it."[95] Equally confusing to mothers, a single piece of infant-feeding advice literature was often rife with internal contradiction. One article written for Chicago's mothers warned correctly, "You can dry up a mother's milk by putting the baby to her breast only at long intervals, say morning and evening or only at night. Such habits will spoil the best wet nurse ever created." But the same article also recommended that "an ordinary baby" would do best on seven feedings a day during the first three months "and often will do as well or better on six feedings." So in a single article mothers were told to breastfeed often, but to be sure to limit the frequency of feedings.[96]

The women who breastfed their babies successfully seem to have ignored all the exhortations to schedule and simply nursed their babies whenever and for as long as the infants wished. When Katharine Kerr Moore's baby was seven weeks old in 1917 she wrote to her mother, "One thing that makes it much easier is that Babins [her pet name for her infant son, Malcolm] nurses much better than he did—gets right down to business and doesn't suck his lip or waste any time so that instead of keeping him at the breast an hour or more as I had to at first, he is generally through in half an hour or twenty minutes." When her third son, Marvin, was born in 1921 she reported, "He is the best baby yet. Nursed so well right from the start that my milk came Monday evening. He nurses every 3 hours and usually wakes of his own accord, right on the dot." She apparently was not fanatic about timing Marvin's feedings, listening instead to his cues, as she wrote on another occasion, "Must be time for Marvin to nurse—hear him stirring around." Moore also reported that her friends modified physician-ordered feeding schedules to suit their babies' needs. She told her mother about one friend, a first-time mother whose doctor "started the baby on a rather unusual feeding schedule—every 4 hours straight through the 24—day and night." Within three weeks, however, the new mother changed the "unusual" timetable to every three hours, "as every 4 hrs. was too long."[97]

Many mothers learned, however, that if they wholly ignored feeding schedules they might make the most serious mistake of all and "overfeed" their baby. The Chicago Department of Health cautioned mothers in 1907 that nothing was more detrimental to an infant's health than overeating. "In the young the administration of an excessive amount of food leads slowly yet surely . . . often without any evidence of gastrointestinal disorder, to a serious injury of the body—that invites a general infection."[98] The IWS joined the chorus in 1911. Their pamphlet "How to Keep the Baby Well," given to each mother on her first visit to an infant welfare station, explained to women the benefits of breastfeeding: "The greatest good you can do your children is to nurse them during the first year. . . . Ten bottle fed babies die to one that is breast-fed." The booklet also warned, however, that even breast milk had to be administered judiciously. Mothers learned, from the only two sentences in the entire pamphlet highlighted with italic type and underscored: "_Do not feed the baby oftener than every four hours. The stomach must have a chance to rest or the baby will get sick._"[99] The Chicago Department of Health continued to remind mothers of the perils of overfeeding with pithy slogans. In 1912: "Overfeeding kills hundreds of babies." In 1913: "Remember, overfeeding kills thousands of babies where underfeeding kills one." By 1919 the health department had toned down the admonitions. "Be careful about overfeeding" was the extent of their warning.[100]

Fear of overfeeding was likely fueled by the contemporary obsession with intestinal regularity. Many philosophies stemmed from this preoccupation, among them the theory of autointoxication which contended that all illness stemmed from self-poisoning, not a spurious assumption in an era of unregulated milk, water, and food.[101] Before the laying of sewers in cities, before routine garbage pickup, before the 1906 federal Pure Food and Drugs Act, and before scattered municipal laws to control the purity of milk and water, milk-, water-, and food-borne illnesses struck human gastrointestinal tracts regularly. Horrifying symptoms included the violent diarrhea of cholera infantum, the agonizing cramps of cholera, and the anorexia of typhoid fever.[102] Concern over babies' precise food intake thus constituted a logical, even healthy, fascination.

The caveats, however, not only prompted the use of premeasured food to avoid the dire consequences of overfeeding, but also persuaded some mothers to fret that they could not leave an involuntary function like babies' digestion to its own devices any more than they could the production of breast milk. Chicago pediatrician Frank Walls warned that even a food "as wholesome . . . as breast milk," when "administered irregularly, may soon exhaust the powers of the child to utilize foods." If mothers stuck to strict scheduling, however, they did not have to worry. One physician explained that when a mother fed her baby at precisely the same time each day, the stomach learned to anticipate the arrival of food and provided gastric juice expectantly. "When food is ingested when the stomach is not so supplied," he cautioned, "the food must remain in the organ—warm, moist, already with ferments in it, being rolled about and generating unwanted and unwonted chemical products."[103] Here was another specter to haunt mothers if they failed to schedule infants' feedings.

By the 1920s medical wisdom had reversed and many physicians rescinded their admonitions governing scheduled feeding and overfeeding. Joseph Brennemann noted in 1928 that he had been one of the first doctors twenty years earlier to recommend feeding babies at four-hour intervals but that he had "long ago abandoned it as a fixed rule." Now he advised that "while the majority of babies can perhaps be fed successfully every four hours, it is to me still an unwise and harmful thing to foist such an interval upon the weak, the premature, the vomiting, and especially the lazy baby." A baby could be fed as often as a mother liked with no ill effect, he now counseled—every three hours, every two hours, every one hour, "and sometimes oftener." Another physician, also in 1928, assured mothers that overfeeding a baby did not constitute a serious health threat. "All of us used to think it a terrible thing to overfeed a nursing baby—though no one could state exactly what would happen to him if we did! . . . Underfeding [*sic*] causes colic; overfeeding never does. In fact overfeeding is practically impossible, because in the vast majority of instances, a baby will not take too great a quantity of food."[104]

By the 1920s physicians were dismissing women's complaints of "not enough milk" and questioning the convictions concerning women's physical inability to breastfeed formed a short generation before. Now mothers learned from women's magazines that "the cases where a mother really cannot nurse her child are so rare as to be curiosities,—the cases in which a woman thinks that she cannot fulfill her duty are, sad to say, far commoner."[105] One physician, studying the relationship between breastfeeding and infant mortality, did not give "the bogey"—milk insufficiency—any credence after he observed a thousand consecutive mothers leave Minneapolis hospitals breastfeeding their newborns.[106] Julius Hess argued in 1925 that it is "now well-known" that almost all mothers are physically capable of breastfeeding.

Contemporary women, he explained, are "more vigorous," "more nearly normal individuals" than their counterparts had been fifteen or twenty years before. Hess blamed both lack of knowledge and lack of encouragement for mothers' failures at breastfeeding, not physical maladies.[107] The Chicago Department of Health informed mothers in 1929 that "nearly every mother can nurse her baby if she only has patience to keep on trying."[108] Even Abt, who in 1904 asserted authoritatively in a *Chicago Tribune* column that women would be physically unable to breastfeed in ever increasing numbers owing to the inheritability of lactation failure, remembered the phenomenon quite differently in his 1944 autobiography. Some women, he wrote, "apparently lacked the will to nurse . . . others were unable to do so. It was difficult to determine the exact reason for this, but I often felt that a woman could nurse her baby if she honestly wanted to, and I tried to urge upon her the necessity for doing so."[109]

Physicians began to recognize feeding schedules as a possible cause of diminished milk supplies. One Chicago physician told colleagues in 1922, "We should have the baby suck until he gets all he can or wants for these infants have an intuitive sense, if you please, of how much they need. I am getting to the point at which I advise mothers to turn the clocks to the wall when they are suckling their babies." In 1925 Julius Hess told Chicago's mothers, "Regular, repeated nursing is the normal stimulant to produce and maintain an adequate supply of milk. The supply is regulated by the demand."[110]

The "Contagion of Example"

But for mothers the good news that physiological impediments to breastfeeding were rare came too late. Women had already accepted the fact that breastfeeding was a task likely to end in failure, and fewer mothers each year even made the attempt. As early as 1887 mothers defended bottle-feeding as a necessity. As one woman begged, "Please let me put in a plea for the poor bottle baby whose case seems to excite so much commiseration. . . . I do not deny that nature's food is the best in a majority of cases, but I do deny, most emphatically, that the bottle-baby does not stand as good a chance for its life (other things being equal) as the breast-fed baby, and the one way is no more trouble than the other."[111]

Even in the 1880s mothers reassured each other that feeding a baby something other than breast milk was not a death sentence. "The trend of a large majority of the articles seems to be toward the conclusion that a bottle-fed baby is the most pitiable, and his mother the most blamable, of mortals," scolded one mother who got sick a few weeks after her son's birth and could no longer nurse him. Her inability to breastfeed "was not only a disappointment, but a source of anxiety to me," she explained. "With utter perverseness," however, her baby "refused to consider himself 'wretched,' as a bottle baby should, and throve right merrily," even calling his bottle "Mr. Mellin" after Mellin's Food, a popular brand of commercial infant food. She echoed what was becoming an increasingly popular belief—that human milk could be at least as deficient as artificial food. "I confidently believe that it is far better to feed a child, carefully and intelligently, on artificial food, than to give it mother's milk which is poor in quality or deficient in quantity, or which, good in itself, is given at the expense of the mother's vitality." She conceded that mothers who "selfishly withhold from their offspring the nourishment which they could as well give" had no excuse for their action, but "to those who stand, as I myself have stood, dreading the obnoxious bottle for the dear baby, I will say one earnest word, I wish it might be of comfort. Regard the bottle as your baby's friend, not his foe."[112]

As mothers observed other mothers using bottles, that too hastened the use of artificial food. *Babyhood* magazine warned women away from this "contagion of example" in 1902. "Nowadays there is no privacy of life," *Babyhood* explained. "Once a woman could suckle her infant with pleasure or wean it with regret in the secrecy of her household." No more, they lamented. Now "if the fashionable Mrs. A. or the rich Mrs. B. cannot or does not suckle her child, it unconsciously acts upon many persons of that type whose ailments are always modified by those of some distinguished sufferer."[113]

The giving of unsolicited advice became as common as the mimicking of other's infant care. A minister's wife, who was breastfeeding her seven-month-old daughter and wished to continue doing so, complained in 1906 that members of her husband's congregation insisted upon showering her with unwanted guidance. The entire congregation, she protested, "seem[ed] to think it very strange not to feed it." In 1914 another mother found it increasingly difficult to follow her own instincts and ignore the admonitions of friends and neighbors. "I find it is not always easy to do with your own baby just as you think best and sometimes it takes quite a little courage to stand out against your best friends and not let them feed baby things she should not have, but I guess it pays in the end."[114]

Grulee, cognizant of how easily bottle use could spread, tried in vain to warn women away from the practice in 1914, telling them that just because one baby in their neighborhood thrived on a particular food did not mean that another baby would. He especially feared that mothers were unwilling to admit to feeding mistakes that caused a baby's illness or death and, consequently, were not wholly honest about the ramifications of their infant-feeding practices. He counseled women to ignore the feeding advice of other mothers: "Mothers, for reason of affection . . . never tell of the countless . . . little ones past recall as the result of unreasonable nutrition." In 1925 the Chicago Department of Health cautioned women "not [to] take the advice of well-meaning relatives, friends or neighbors, as no two babies can be fed just alike."[115]

Despite the ongoing warnings about artificial food, by the 1920s and 1930s most women never even attempted breastfeeding, or they abandoned the practice after a few days or weeks. After giving birth to her first child in 1932, Dorothy Smith Dushkin complained that her breasts felt uncomfortable, "but even so I adored the sensation of the tiny face snuggling & snorting against me blindly hunting for the nipple." Nevertheless, Dushkin gave up nursing her daughter within days "& put her on the bottle—a much more satisfactory arrangement."[116] That sentiment, that artificial food was "much more satisfactory" than human milk, was by then so prevalent as to be unquestioned.

♦

During the last quarter of the nineteenth century, women—prompted by economic and class considerations and changing views of sex, marriage, medicine, health, time, efficiency, and self-control—began to "hand feed" their babies in increasing numbers. Physicians consequently studied "the most vexing problem"[117] of infant feeding.

Women, of course, never set out to sacrifice their infants' health to contemporary fashion. Yet marriages based on romance and companionship placed new emphasis on relations between husband and wife and deemphasized relations between mother and child. The popular belief that men found their breasts attractive made it easier for some women to forget about their breasts' biological importance to their babies. New, less social birthing practices and mothers' reticence to discuss bodily functions with their daughters meant one generation no longer passed breastfeeding information on to the next. Knowledge of disease causation and the persistent suggestion that only meticulous, well-trained mothers could keep their babies well created anxiety among women and a concomitant distrust of breast milk. Feeding schedules—efficient, disciplined, utilitarian, and, most important, convenient—diminished mothers' milk supplies and led to the use of even more artificial food. Increasingly, mothers who could afford servants often left their infants to be bottle-fed or wet-nursed. Working-class mothers forced to return to work left infants with older children and bottles. Bottle use snowballed; mothers who observed other mothers using bottles decided to try it themselves.

Physicians responded to the crisis with mixed messages that undoubtedly confused the issue. Because they treated so many babies dying from the side effects of artificial food, doctors urged mothers to breastfeed. The effectiveness of their calls to breastfeed was undermined, however, by caveats that encouraged bottle-feeding. They warned women in overwrought tones not to "overfeed" their babies, thus encouraging either the use of premeasured artificial food or strict breastfeeding schedules. As more and more women complained that they had no milk, doctors responded with explanations for the phenomenon—urbanization, heredity, human evolution—that made lactation failure seem inevitable. In an era of medical advances and scientific motherhood, the fact that physicians were associated with artificial feeding, however warily, seemed to sanctify it.[118]

For physicians, the contradictions inherent in a service profession were eventually too much to bear. Breastfeeding may have been the best for babies, but doctors had to respond to the activities and complaints of their patients' mothers too. Physicians reluctantly, and with reservations that lingered for years, became mired in the infant food arena—altering cows' milk in the hope that a few ingredients added or subtracted or "modified" would make it as good for babies as human milk. Although their efforts continued to fall short, the notion that bottle-feeding was more modern and thus more effective nonetheless prevailed. Grulee complained in 1934, that "now one is regarded as rather old-fashioned if he attempts to persuade a mother that for her own sake and for the good of the baby nursing it is by long odds the best choice."[119]

For women, bottle versus breast became not a matter of illness versus health, as physicians urged, but a matter of science versus ignorance, efficiency versus inefficiency, and propriety versus vulgarity. Abt reminisced in 1944 that in his early twentieth-century pediatric practice "progress had not [yet] dispensed with breast milk."[120] As women's needs, anxieties, attitudes, and self-images—not physicians' agendas—ensured the predominance of artificial food, "progress" managed to do just that.

2

"Slaughter of the Innocents": Infant Mortality and the Urban Milk Supply

As mothers ceased breastfeeding in the traditional sense, their myriad individual decisions signaled many changes. The increased use of artificial food meant most women now interacted with their babies in a fundamentally different way than they had previously. Wealthy mothers who fed their babies artificially placed their children in the care of servants for longer periods. Middle-class mothers learned to care for their babies according to the clock. Some immigrant mothers fed their babies cows' milk as a sign of acculturation. In the most immediate, concrete sense, however, the use of less human milk meant, simply, that more babies consumed more cows' milk.

In big cities like Chicago this change in diet posed a grave threat to infants' health. The late nineteenth-century urban milk supply was dreadful. Cows' milk—stored in huge uncovered vats, shipped in unrefrigerated railroad cars, and often produced by miserably sick animals—was dirty, spoiled, easily adulterated, and loaded with pathogens. The medical community declared babies' consumption of the stuff an alarming medical problem.

Infant mortality statistics legitimated the worry. During the last few years of the nineteenth century, public health departments correlated age at death with cause of death for the first time in their annual vital statistics. One of the clearest findings of this new tally was that the majority of babies who died before their first birthday died of gastrointestinal ailments.

Physicians trumpeted the meaning of this finding. At a 1909 conference on the cause and prevention of infant mortality in the United States, one physician, observing that most dead infants had been artificially fed, remarked dryly, "Obviously Nature's normal nutriment does not predispose to death." Another doctor at the same conference admonished colleagues, "That physician, or that mother, who, except for cogent reasons, omits . . .

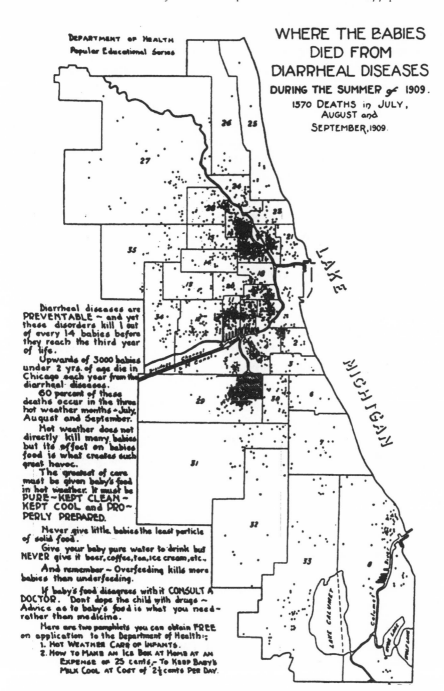

WHERE THE BABIES
DIED FROM
DIARRHEAL DISEASES
DURING THE SUMMER of 1909.
1570 DEATHS in JULY,
AUGUST and
SEPTEMBER, 1909.

DEPARTMENT of HEALTH
Popular Educational Series

Diarrheal diseases are
PREVENTABLE ~ and yet
these disorders kill 1 out
of every 14 babies before
they reach the third year
of life.

Upwards of 3000 babies
under 2 yrs. of age die in
Chicago each year from the
diarrheal diseases.

60 percent of these
deaths occur in the three
hot weather months ~ July,
August and September.

Hot weather does not
directly kill many babies,
but its effect on babies
food is what creates such
great havoc.

The greatest of care
must be given baby's food
in hot weather. It must be
PURE ~ KEPT CLEAN ~
KEPT COOL and PRO~
PERLY PREPARED.

Never give little babies the least particle
of solid food.

Give your baby pure water to drink but
NEVER give it beer, coffee, tea, ice cream, etc.

And remember ~ Overfeeding kills more
babies than underfeeding.

If baby's food disagrees with it CONSULT A
DOCTOR. Dont dope the child with drugs ~
Advice as to baby's food is what you need ~
rather than medicine.

Here are two pamphlets you can obtain FREE
on application to the Department of Health:
1. HOT WEATHER CARE OF INFANTS.
2. HOW TO MAKE AN ICE BOX AT HOME AT AN
EXPENSE OF 25 CENTS ~ TO KEEP BABY'S
MILK COOL AT COST of 2¼ cents PER DAY.

Figure 4 In 1909 Chicago health department workers began to map each infant death from diarrhea. The Department of Health and assorted medical charities located their infant welfare stations in the neighborhoods with the highest death rates and deployed visiting nurses to talk to mothers in these areas about the importance of breastfeeding. *Source: Report of the Department of Health of the City of Chicago for the Years 1907, 1908, 1909, 1910, 174.*

breast-feeding thereby deprives the infant of the most powerful agency of the conservation of life and health." The injustice of such a situation was obvious, he reminded his audience: "The punishment falls not upon the offender, but upon the helpless victim."[1]

The medical community responded to the two-part problem of diminished breastfeeding rates and the appalling state of cows' milk with a two-part solution. Public health authorities and medical charities publicly urged mothers to breastfeed their babies. These same health officials, however, conceded that if mothers did not embrace prolonged, exclusive breastfeeding, then cows' milk—the most widely used human milk substitute—needed immediate and vast improvement. Consequently, even as they orchestrated breastfeeding campaigns, municipalities, medical charities, and, at least in Chicago, newspapers, also engaged in prolonged battles with dairies in an effort to clean up the urban milk supply.

The milk crusades were long-lived and controversial. Dairy farmers, dairies, railroads, and milk dealers vigorously resisted changing the way they produced, stored, shipped, and sold milk. Consumers often opposed change as well. Many were leery of pasteurization. Despite the milk crusaders' efforts to educate consumers, money-strapped housewives preferred cheap milk, which was much more likely to be spoiled and adulterated, and avoided buying the expensive ice that would have kept pure milk fresh. Given this reluctance to institute safer manufacturing, shipping, storage, and purchasing practices, it took more than thirty years—from 1892 to 1926 in Chicago—before the dairy industry sealed (1904), bottled (1912), and pasteurized milk (1916), kept milk cold during shipping (1920), and tested cows for bovine tuberculosis (1926).

Reformers equated the clean-milk campaigns with saving babies, so it was not just the histrionics of late nineteenth-century journalism that generated years of emotional newspaper editorials demanding milk reform. The *Chicago Tribune* said of adulterated milk in 1892, "It is worse than fraud, it is murder. The infant mortality in Chicago is very large. How much of it is due to the poisonous germs swallowed in this alleged milk it is hard to determine, but it must play no small part in this colossal crime of infanticide."[2]

The lingo was not the only radical aspect of the milk wars—the conviction that infant death could be prevented at all was a revolutionary concept. In Chicago, health department officials admitted sheepishly in 1910 that they had long dismissed infant deaths from diarrhea as unavoidable. "We calmly accepted the annual harvest of death as if it were as inevitable as the weather; as if indeed a part of the weather. 'Hot weather, babies die,' was our unconscious thought."[3]

These deaths became increasingly disturbing, however, as the perception of adult illness and death changed. When the first major cholera epidemic hit the United States in 1832, for example, the public regarded the disease as a "scourge of the sinful." The largely poverty-stricken immigrant victims of the swift and dramatic killer were said to deserve their fate. But by 1866, when the country limped through its last significant cholera epidemic, the majority of Americans had come to view cholera as a predictable consequence of poor sanitation.[4]

Sanitary reforms accompanied this change in view. Between 1880 and 1900, cities built water and sewer systems and established methods to collect garbage. By 1900 most municipalities had passed laws forbidding chickens, pigs, and cows within city limits. The establishment of electric train lines largely eliminated horses from city streets.[5] The absence of urban livestock not only cut down on animal waste, a source of illness commonly spread by flies, but eliminated a primary source of infectious disease as well.[6]

When urban reformers first tried to measure the success of these assorted Herculean efforts, they used the crude death rate as a yardstick. They quickly discarded that gauge, however, because it was too easily affected by variables having nothing to do with sanitation, like age. The infant death rate, deemed most likely to be affected by the environment, subsequently became the principal way of assessing societal well-being. As the weakest members of society, infants were most sensitive to improvements or problems in their physical surroundings, went the rationale.[7] Babies thus became the country's early warning system, the canaries in the coal mine for the urban populace. This use of the infant death rate soon aroused interest in the myriad causes of high infant morbidity and mortality. International, national, and local campaigns to lower infant mortality abounded.[8]

Richard Meckel divides the efforts to lower infant mortality in the United States into three overlapping stages. From roughly 1850 to 1880 (dates varied depending on locale) activities focused on cleaning up the environment. In the second stage, from about 1880 to 1920, reformers concentrated their efforts on purifying cows' milk, the food most often consumed by infants who were not breastfed.[9] Then, from roughly 1910 to 1930, municipalities and philanthropic organizations enhanced their earlier baby-saving work by teaching mothers how better to care for themselves during pregnancy and their children in infancy.[10] This final endeavor included explicit information on the importance of breastfeeding. By the late 1920s these three diverse, albeit interconnected, efforts had dramatically lowered infant death, especially from diarrhea. Yet government officials, physicians, and reformers gave the bulk of the credit for improving infant health to only one phase of the reform efforts: the pure milk campaigns.[11]

In Chicago the milk campaigns were the subject of unrelenting publicity for more than thirty years. During that time no reformer touted pure cows' milk as the best solution to the high infant morbidity and mortality. Quite the contrary: given the "attendant evils" of cows' milk in urban areas, the nation's mothers learned that "the sovereign prevention [of infant death] is for a mother to nurse her own child; or if she is unable to do so, to get a healthy woman to nurse it for her." The Chicago Department of Health warned mothers in 1907, when Chicago's pure milk campaign was in full swing, that "no form of baby feeding is ever more than a substitute for breast milk."[12]

After years of the extraordinarily visible warnings to mothers of the importance of clean milk for babies, however, mothers and physicians alike came to think of dirty cows' milk as a far greater threat to infant health than the irreconcilable differences between human and cows' milk. As early as 1892, one Chicago doctor advised, "I suspect it is the experience of a great many physicians that we need not be afraid of the chemical difference between cows' milk and mother's milk, if cows' milk is taken from a healthy animal, is undiluted and unskimmed and properly sterilized."[13] By the time Chicago's reformers won every milk battle in 1926, this thought predominated. The primary reason for the milk crusades—physicians' dismay at fewer and fewer breastfed babies—was long forgotten. Although physicians continued to recommend human milk over cows' milk for babies throughout the milk campaigns, the unrelenting publicity generated by the clean-milk crusades touted pasteurized, sealed, and bottled cows' milk as safe, palatable sustenance for babies. Soon it was the preferable sustenance as well.

◆

Chicago was the quintessential unplanned urban mess for much of the nineteenth century. In 1833, the year Chicago was incorporated as a town, the site on which Chicago would eventually sit was manageable enough: only 150 people lived there. Less than seventy years later, however, the city included two million people, the country's railroad hub, and many of the nation's largest and most influential businesses. In 1900 more than one-third of the city's population was foreign born; by 1914 that number had grown to 69 percent. This rapid growth in industry, transportation, population, and immigrants took its toll. Sidewalks, paved streets, and sewers were lacking; poverty, inadequate housing, unsanitary drinking water, filth, and flies were legion; and the infant mortality rate was alarmingly high.[14]

The problems were so painfully obvious that by the end of the nine-teenth century the city was tackling its most serious health threats in earnest and with some success. The chronic flooding of streets and buildings, and the disease it caused, dissipated when innovative entrepreneurs—soon-to-be railroad car magnate George Pullman among them—began in late 1855 to raise all the streets and buildings adjacent to Lake Michigan and the Chicago River four to seven feet. By 1889 Chicago's police and fire protection and its sewer and water system were so efficient and appealing that residents of a 120-square-mile area surrounding the city voted to be annexed. The year 1889 turned out to be a particularly propitious one for the city. In addition to the annexation, the Illinois legislature authorized construction of the twenty-five-mile-long Sanitary and Ship Canal to drain the city's waste away from Lake Michigan, the city's water supply. Workers began building the canal in 1892. Samuel Preston and Michael Haines argue that the over-whelming public acceptance of this extraordinarily expensive venture was testimony to citizens' awareness of disease causation and their fervent desire for disease prevention.[15]

Even as Chicago's residents cleaned up their environment, however, the city's infant death rate remained stubbornly high, symptomatic of the city's poor housing, the poverty of so many of its citizens, and, especially, its steady stream of bacteria-ridden, dirty, spoiled, and adulterated cows' milk.[16] The feeding of bovine rather than human milk to babies was the proximate cause of most infant deaths, physicians agreed, because the majority of babies who died before their first birthday were artificially fed and succumbed to diar-rhea. "When Nature devised milk . . . she intended it to be the food of suck-lings only," one New York physician explained to mothers in an 1885 issue of *Babyhood* magazine, "and never meant that it should be exposed to the air at all; otherwise so ingenious a worker would have made of it an article of food less easily affected by such exposure."[17] Another physician, speaking before the American Association for the Study and Prevention of Infant Mor-tality in 1910, charged angrily, "It is not a feature of natural selection that babies' milk should be adulterated or contaminated with germs. Nature gave infants as their birthright their mothers' milk . . . without a chance for con-tamination, without 100 miles intervening for the milk man to bring it." The connection between efforts to lower infant mortality and clean up the urban milk supply was an intimate one according to this physician. "The movement for the prevention of infant mortality amounts in the end simply to this," he explained, "to give back to the baby what is the baby's natural birthright, namely, pure milk."[18]

Infant Diarrhea: Complex Nomenclature, One Dread Disease

The concerted late nineteenth-century efforts to halt infants' diarrheal deaths were a long time coming. As early as 1773, physician Benjamin Rush described infant diarrhea, dubbed "cholera infantum" by Rush and his contemporaries. Each summer, long before urban reformers blamed the problem on the urban milk supply, the illness was epidemic, "the dread of parents and the opprobrium of physicians."[19] Yet even then, cows' milk was the likely culprit. In 1829 Deborah Fiske, suffering from tuberculosis, was so "fatigued and feverish" after the birth of her first child that her doctor persuaded her that it was "unsafe" for her to breastfeed her baby. A friend agreed to take the child into her home while Fiske recuperated and, lacking breast milk, she fed the baby cows' milk. Within a month David Vinal Fiske was dead of "bowel complaint."[20] In 1849 Mary Poor began to feed cows' milk to her three-month-old baby. She wrote to her mother, "It is much more common here to bring up babies by hand than in any place I was ever in before [she was in Maine] and they seem to do as well as those who nurse." Within six months her baby was dead of cholera infantum.[21]

Frustrated physicians and grieving families felt there was little they could do to prevent such tragedies. Infants' "natural weakness and sensibility" seemed to make their deaths unavoidable. Given this prevailing wisdom, one physician noted in 1833, cholera infantum "excited less public sympathy, and . . . attracted less professional attention than any disease so pernicious." Years later, Chicago Department of Health annual reports reflected that attitude. In 1872, when 3,441 infant deaths were reported—1,469 from cholera infantum—the health department did not discuss cholera infantum in its annual report, choosing instead to run lengthy articles on cholera and smallpox, diseases which killed far fewer individuals.[22]

Over the years the Chicago Department of Health gave many labels to infant diarrhea. Physicians understood so little about the cause of babies' gastrointestinal ailments that they considered the tiniest nuances in symptoms—color and texture of stools, severity of abdominal pain, amount of flatulence, and the presence or absence of vomiting, for example—to be significant to diagnosis and treatment, hence the myriad names for the disease.[23] As Isaac Abt explained in his memoir, "Doctors everywhere were attempting to classify the gastrointestinal disorders [of infancy] in order to get a clear understanding of them."[24] In Chicago, infant diarrhea, depending on its subtle set of symptoms, was called cholera infantum, infantile diarrhea, diarrhea, inanition, convulsions, marasmus, intestinal inflammation, dysentery, enteritis, gastritis, gastroenteritis, or diarrhea and enteritis. In other areas of the country infant diarrhea was also called "summer complaint" or "summer diarrhea" because of its prevalence in summer when food spoiled quickly. The ostensibly different illnesses had marked similarities. One nineteenth-century physician described their customary course: severe vomiting, rapid pulse, abdominal cramps, and "violent" diarrhea that was "frequent, and often enormous, wetting the child's clothing and everything near it." Debilitating bouts of diarrhea were followed by a feeble pulse; shriveled, cold skin; sunken eyes; stupor; and coma. Death usually occurred within three to four days, but sometimes within twenty-four hours of initial symptoms.[25]

Before 1907, when the Chicago Department of Health placed infant diarrhea under a single ailment—"diarrhea & enteritis" (see appendix B.2)—physicians underreported infant diarrhea due to the varied and, as it turned out, meaningless, nomenclature. In 1893, for example, four years before the department of health began correlating cause of death with age at death, 1,623 babies died of cholera infantum. An additional 378 died of infantile marasmus. But that same year there were also 389 deaths from enterocolitis, 651 from inanition, 564 from enteritis, and 790 from gastroenteritis—2,394 potential additional infant deaths caused by diarrhea.[26]

Babies' deaths from diarrhea likely were missing from the mortality rolls in other ways as well. Each year, for decades, the Department of Health attributed hundreds of infant deaths to "infantile convulsions," often under the rubric "diseases due largely to faulty or imperfect nutrition." In 1908 the health department announced that virtually all deaths from "infantile convulsions" were attributable to dehydration from diarrhea. That same year, deaths from "marasmus and other ill-defined causes" were moved to the diarrheal disease category as well. Even the majority of infant deaths due to pneumonia, the health department explained, were probably precipitated by diarrhea because babies weakened by diarrhea often eventually died of opportunistic respiratory infections.[27]

Although the cause of infant diarrhea remained a mystery for some time, prolonged breastfeeding appeared to prevent the illness, and physicians consequently warned mothers not to wean their infants until after "two or even three summers." The medical community, however, did not understand until the end of the nineteenth century that feeding babies something other than human milk might *cause* cholera infantum. Once physicians made this connection, they implored women to breastfeed and avoid artificial food. When frightened mothers brought sick babies to doctors for care, doctors scrutinized the babies' diets. "The greatest mortalities at all times and among all nations," charged Charles Warrington Earle, a Chicago physician, "is due to the lack of mother's milk." Earle called human milk "the food par excellence for a baby" and urged parents to procure a wet nurse if mother's milk was unavailable. Only if "nature's best food can not be obtained for affection or gold" did Earle recommend a "properly sterilized" artificial diet.[28]

"They Water and Color the Milk"

What exactly constituted a safe and beneficial artificial diet, however, became the medical community's oft-debated "feeding question." Clean milk, doctors agreed, was key to any infant nourishment. Chicago physician E. J. Doering noted simply that "given pure air, pure water and pure milk . . . the so-called summer complaints of children become of interest only by reason of their rare occurrence."[29] But in Chicago, clean milk was not an easy commodity to come by, and so the clean-milk question was soon indivisible from the feeding question. What methods could be put in place to keep milk pure as it traveled from rural enclave to urban baby?

The threat that cows' milk posed to infants' health was no secret in Chicago. The city's newspapers, medical community, and even a few conscientious dairies had broadcast its dangers for years. As one reputable Chicago milk distributor—who aimed not "to sell cheap milk, but good milk"—noted in 1885, "There is no business, profession or calling in life, without its human hawks and conscienceless spiders, who fatten and feast upon the ignorant and poor; the milk business is no exception."[30]

Watering milk was an especially common phenomenon in Chicago, and the exposure of this practice in 1892 was the first of many milk scandals reported by Chicago's newspapers. Journalists deplored all the babies who had "gone to a premature grave because . . . [their] cry for milk was unwittingly answered by a supply of a weak, unnutritious [sic] mixture of milk and water. Could a proper death certificate be made out many an entry of 'cholera infantum' would be changed to starvation from being fed on watered milk." The *Chicago Tribune* accused milk dealers of selling whole milk to the rich, skimmed milk to the middle class, and "so-called milk, which is three-fourths water if not something worse" to the poor.[31]

The problem appeared straightforward enough, but there were no easy solutions. Every proposed remedy generated controversy. In 1885, when a chemist working for the Chicago Department of Health found watered milk to be the norm rather than the exception, he urged the commissioner of health to work for passage of a state law mandating that only "pure milk" be sold in the state.[32] But what was pure milk? Massachusetts required 13 percent solids in its milk. Chicago's largest dairies worried that imposing the 13 percent standard would be unfair "as the milk produced on the western prairies is not as rich as that produced on eastern farms, where the grasses are richer."[33] So even as reformers proposed solutions, inaction prevailed.

Although watered milk long remained a problem, water was probably the most benign substance added to Chicago's milk. When Chicago physician W. S. Christopher analyzed milk samples in 1892, he expected to find evidence of spoiled and adulterated milk only in the city's poorest neighborhoods. He was startled and dismayed when he found it everywhere. One of his discoveries was the ubiquitous use of a "milk expander" composed of soda, ammonia, salt, and water. When two gallons of expander were mixed with one gallon of milk it required "a very experienced palate to detect anything in the three gallons but pure milk." The blend, Christopher noted sarcastically, was "a nice mixture to give a weak infant!"[34]

Dye was another common additive. Milk dealers favored yellow dye because it fooled consumers into thinking that the milk they purchased was rich with cream, even after the milk had been skimmed. Chalk was also a common additive, used to whiten dirty milk.[35] Milk coloring, on sale everywhere and advertised for that purpose, was made of patent butter, burnt sugar, and aniline dyes.[36]

The Milk of Toothless, Stump-Tailed, Besotted Cows

"Swill milk," milk produced by cows fed distillery waste, was another ubiquitous problem.[37] Urban dairy farmers often purchased the by-products of breweries—and there were many in Chicago and nearby Milwaukee—to use as cow feed. Farmers used distillery slops as cow feed because, at four to six dollars a ton, it was far cheaper than twenty-dollar-a-ton grain.[38] Farmers also found distillery waste alluring because it overstimulated cows' mammary glands, creating an enormous milk flow.[39]

The cows offered brewery waste as feed initially disdained it. Eventually near starvation, they not only ate it, they became addicted to their daily fare. The cows living on distillery waste—"conglomerated stuff, all fermenting and bubbling with carbonic gas, reeking with an intolerable stench"—soon lost their teeth. Their skin ulcerated. Large, running sores covered their bodies. Their tails decayed and dropped off. One physician, outraged by the common consumption of swill milk by babies, demanded, "Would any of us tolerate a sot as a wetnurse for our offspring?"[40]

Swill milk was an old story in Chicago. In 1876 one horrified Department of Health sanitary inspector notified the sanitary superintendent that many dairy farmers fed their cows brewery slops and fermented grains. The inspector warned, "The extent to which milk of this kind is consumed in these wards most densely populated, is very great, the effects of which upon the health and mortality of infants and young children during the summer months must prove exceedingly deleterious. . . . I have repeatedly witnessed the injurious effects of its use." He proposed passage of a tame law prohibiting the sale of swill milk only during the summer (when infant death was highest), to no avail.[41] In 1885 the secretary of the Chicago Medical Society charged that swill milk, still a best-selling commodity, was "a poison." He suggested that only inspected milk be labeled safe for infants' consumption, also to no avail.[42]

In September 1892 city officials finally confronted the swill milk problem when they notified all dairy farmers "that after this . . . date you will be prosecuted to the full extent of the law if found feeding swill or slops to milch cows within the city limits." To catch offenders, the Department of Health stationed inspectors at the city's distillery and vinegar factory entrances.[43]

Despite the effort, the swill milk trade remained. Almost one-quarter of the 2,857 dairies inspected in 1904 fed distillery slops to their cows. By 1907, as consumers were becoming aware of the advantages of pasteurized milk, with some even learning how to pasteurize milk at home, many continued to purchase swill milk. The Department of Health had to warn the public, "no amount of pasteurizing can make . . . [swill milk] wholesome." In 1910 the Chicago Department of Health reported that several malt and brewery factories had advertised falsely in rural newspapers that Chicago now permitted dairy farmers to feed wet malt to cows. Consequently city dairy inspectors quickly discovered forty-four farms in Wisconsin and Illinois that had purchased the waste. Inspectors notified authorities at the city's ports of entry to refuse to allow milk from those farms into the city.[44]

Despite its obvious dangers, swill milk sold for half the price of "country milk," and the desire for cheap feed by farmers and cheap milk by consumers ensured its ongoing popularity. The medical community warned the public that "good milk cannot be low-priced milk. If we demand a low price we must be willing to accept anything that can dodge the milk inspector's vigilance." The health department advised consumers, "The price per quart paid by the consumer is generally the best test as to quality."[45]

One milk peddler blamed unscrupulous milk dealers for tempting poverty-stricken consumers with cheap, adulterated fare. He argued, "The very poor are not always the very ignorant, but the very ignorant are generally the very poor. To them milk is milk. . . . [E]ven should the baby die, they would patronize the milkman. . . . Like spiders, they weave their webs, to catch the . . . ignorant." Abt puzzled over the "strange economy" practiced by all—not just poor—mothers who objected to paying a few cents more for a quart of milk even though the extra cost guaranteed quality. He charged, "Those who buy their hats in Paris, who eat strawberries in January and pay the highest prices for various articles of food, are satisfied with an inferior quality of milk."[46]

The problem remained serious enough that in 1914 the Department of Health engineered another in a long line of campaigns denouncing cheap milk, this time appealing to temperance sympathizers. Health officials argued that quality milk at eight cents a quart was far cheaper than beer at twenty cents a quart, soda water at forty cents a quart, and whisky, "if it can be called a beverage," at one to three dollars a quart. "Surely the head of the house," health officials scolded, "who indulges in the use of beer, soda, wine or liquor of any kind, even in the most moderate way, has no good reason to kick at having to pay 8 cents a quart for clean, wholesome milk." Cheap milk nevertheless remained a threat to babies' health. As late as 1921 the Department of Health continued to remind mothers, "If you have a baby in the home that is being artificially fed, don't buy cheap milk. Get the best."[47]

Dairy, Dirt, and Disease

Dirt in even the best milk was yet another hazard. In 1912 Department of Health officials publicized a tale told to them by "a prominent opponent of pasteurization" who was contemplating a change of stance. While touring a dairy farm, he was appalled to see a young boy nonchalantly prop his bare and filthy feet on the milk bucket as he milked a cow. The milk squirted "directly upon . . . first . . . one foot, then . . . the other . . . flow[ing] from his feet into the milk pail." The outraged man berated the boy, explaining that his childish act could kill. The boy responded, "What do you care, you ain't goin' to drink this milk; we ship it to the city."[48]

Stories like this one prompted the Department of Health to order random testing of milk for foreign matter beginning in 1912. That year, workers filtered 16,122 samples of milk through cotton to catch visible dirt. They judged 3,400 of the samples "absolutely filthy," 7,015 samples "more or less dirty," and only 5,707 samples "clean." Department of Health officials concluded, "Much of the city's milk-supply is better adapted to fertilizing purposes than to feeding purposes. Yet that's the kind of milk so many poor babies get."[49]

The health department's method for finding dirt in milk became so well known that health officials were forced to explain to consumers that straining milk through cotton did not solve the milk problem; that while straining removed "gross dirt" from milk, it did not remove bacteria.[50] Milk-borne illness, in fact, so threatened the public health that one of the earliest laws governing milk production required that any milk handler report immediately to the health department any member of his family with a contagious disease. The health department would then shut down the business until they could verify that all employees were well. The law was difficult to enforce, however. When the children of one milk depot owner died within two days of each other in the summer of 1895, one reportedly of diphtheria and the other of croup, the physician who examined both children was unaware that they even lived at a milk depot. In their father's words, "not to have any card on the house, and not to stop selling milk" he moved his children to his brother's house before summoning the doctor.[51]

The threat of milk-borne illness was not eliminated even if milk arrived in the city unadulterated and bacteria-free. Milk could still fall into the hands of careless merchants. Before 1912 Chicago milkmen delivered milk to grocers in uncovered eight-gallon vats. Dairies regularly defended this practice, arguing that bottling and sealing milk in individual containers was "the worst possible contrivance" to ensure cleanliness because "milk, in large cans, more or less exposed to the air . . . improves it."[52] Merchants ladled milk from the large, open vat into small containers provided by customers. Before purchase, customers commonly sampled the milk by plunging a finger in the vat to taste. Occasionally they used a communal dipper. When milkmen delivered milk directly to homes, distribution was equally dangerous. Milkmen customarily took an empty, dirty bottle from one house, ladled milk into it, and immediately delivered it to another customer.[53] In this manner tuberculosis, diphtheria, typhoid, scarlet fever, and other communicable diseases were spread, the illnesses arising from merchants' practices, not farmers'. The Chicago Department of Health begged consumers to report dirty milk bottles, dirty milk cans, dirty milk wagons, dirty milk depots, dirty milkmen, and milkmen's dirty habits to health authorities.[54]

Demand for "Inspectors Who Inspect"

Chicago issued a series of weak municipal ordinances over many years, ostensibly to solve these problems. Beginning in 1877 the city required milk deal-

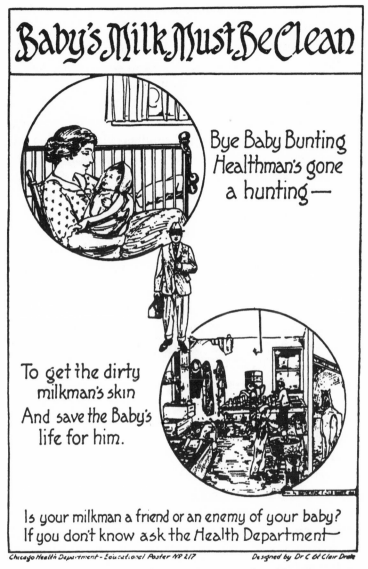

Baby's Milk Must Be Clean

Bye Baby Bunting
Healthman's gone
a hunting—

To get the dirty
milkman's skin
And save the Baby's
life for him.

Is your milkman a friend or an enemy of your baby?
If you don't know ask the Health Department

Chicago Health Department - Educational Poster Nº 217   Designed by Dr C St Clair Drake

Figure 5   This is one of the many Chicago Department of Health posters inspired by the milk crusades. Note the last lines enlisting mothers' help to identify and punish "bad" milkmen. *Source: Bulletin Chicago School of Sanitary Instruction,* 25 April 1914.

ers to obtain licenses. That same year, Chicago's first milk inspector procured random samples of milk for the Department of Health's chemist to examine. Between September 1, 1877, and January 1, 1878, the milk inspector brought twenty-nine suits against milk dealers for selling "unwholesome milk" to the public. With 430 licensed milk dealers in the city, however, and more than fifteen million gallons of milk sold in 1877, twenty-nine suits did little to improve the city's milk.[55]

These initial inspection and enforcement activities quickly disintegrated. Milk was not in the public eye again in any prolonged or effective way until 1892 when, with great fanfare, Chicago's Health Commissioner attributed the city's high infant and child death rate to the city's milk. He called for a widespread system of regular milk inspection and a legal standard for milk purity to lower infant and child morbidity and mortality.[56]

Much of the ensuing clamor was due to Chicago's designation as host to the World Columbian Exposition to be held in 1893. Health officials feared epidemic disease, and worried that some of it might be milk-borne, among the hundreds of thousands of anticipated tourists. One physician fumed that in "this World's Fair city, a city which boasts of its energy and progressive character, there is absolutely no inspection whatever of the milk furnished in vast quantities to its citizens." The Chicago Medical Society likewise called for action after releasing a report accusing a majority of the city's milk dealers of adulterating milk "both with water and injurious preparations." One Board of Health physician, exasperated with ominous studies and no remedies, noted that Chicago was the only large city in the world without a milk inspection ordinance. The *Chicago Inter Ocean* demanded an independent health department with "inspectors who . . . inspect" and argued that "its chief should be chief in fact as well as in name."[57]

The Board of Aldermen bowed to the pressure. The city's first pure milk ordinance with any teeth became effective January 1, 1893, just in time to protect Columbian Exposition tourists. The ordinance established a Bureau of Milk Inspection staffed by two chemists and a "microscopist."[58] Their mandate was to save the lives of babies who suffered "so much from disease and premature death caused by an impure, unfit and adulterated article."[59] During its first year, the Bureau of Milk Inspection operated out of the back room of a drugstore where staff tested milk labeled "whole country milk" for signs of skimming.[60]

During its first month of operation Dr. E. B. Stuart, the bureau's chief, declared "Chicago's milk supply . . . not in the worst possible condition." He attributed the adulteration of milk less to dairymen's and merchants' greed or indifference than to a combination of "sharp competition . . . and the unwillingness of many thousands of citizens to pay a decent price for good milk." Accordingly, he ordered bureau workers to be lenient with violators. In September 1893 the *Chicago Herald* complained, "It is a regrettable fact to note that this municipal law, strict and explicit as it is, is not enforced with that vigor and energy which is so desirable in the case of an evil that had grown of such enormous proportions and had wrought so much harm to life and health in this city." Stuart's policy of leniency was a failure, charged the *Herald*. Only vigorous enforcement would "stamp out the evil and . . . compel the knavish members of the milk-selling fraternity to mend their ways or go out of business."[61]

Stuart's leniency was not the only impediment to enforcement of the milk ordinance. Inspectors could not discern who adulterated the samples they collected—inspectors suspected the merchants, merchants blamed farmers, and farmers accused shippers. Not until more than a decade later, in 1904, when the city council passed an ordinance forbidding the shipment of milk in open vats and ordered that any milk delivered unsealed be returned to the shipper, did the finger-pointing end. Sealed milk containers made it easier for inspectors to pinpoint who had the opportunity to adulterate the milk, so it became less likely that anyone would add to, or take anything from, the milk being sold.[62]

The 1893 ordinance also proved ineffective because it provided only five inspectors to cover an awesome terrain. In 1892, 3,000 dairymen owned the 75,000 cows that supplied the city with milk. Workers unloaded that milk—12,000 to 15,000 cans daily—at twenty different railway stations. One of Chicago's principal ports of entry was in the city of Elgin, forty miles away. And those numbers represented only the milk produced outside the city. Hundreds of urban dairy farmers produced their ware within city limits. Three thousand horse-drawn milk wagons distributed the milk to consumers.[63]

The city assigned one district to each of the five harried inspectors. Beginning at 4 A.M. each day they obtained samples directly from milkmen's horse-drawn wagons and from the milk unloaded at railroad depots. In this way they procured and analyzed more than 10,000 milk samples that first year. The samples, however, represented only an average 3.3 examinations of each of Chicago's more than 3,000 milk dealers.[64]

Even more obstructive to the effort was the fact that milk inspectors had the power to punish only offending dairy farmers who housed their cows within city limits. In 1895 Health Commissioner William R. Kerr appealed to the Illinois State Board of Health for help in remedying that situation. Responding quickly, the State Board of Health agreed in September 1895 that "for the benefit of municipalities whose milk supply is obtained . . . from localities beyond their respective jurisdictions" the State Board would supply the inspectors needed to enforce milk regulations, as long as Chicago agreed to pay for them.[65]

Chicago's newspapers aided the effort to catch unscrupulous and careless milk dealers. The *Chicago Herald* printed the names of milk dealers fined for selling impure, watered, or skimmed milk.[66] The city's other newspapers and the Department of Health's weekly bulletin soon followed the *Herald*'s lead. The tactic proved so successful that milk dealers, to prevent publication of their names, began bringing their milk in voluntarily for testing.[67] Consumers did the same, bringing samples of the milk they purchased to the Bureau of Milk Inspection laboratory. The health department encouraged women in particular to police milk dealers because "when a housewife confronts her milkman with the pink slip of the Department, showing 'below grade' milk or cream, the lesson is not soon forgotten."[68]

After the city brought the Bureau of Milk Inspection under the immediate supervision of the Commissioner of Health in 1894, reformers hoped for a new era of strict inspection and enforcement.[69] Yet Dr. Cass L. Kennicott, the bureau's chemist, reported that two practices—coloring milk, and skimming it and labeling it whole—remained common. Worse, adding preservatives—formaldehyde, salicylic acid, borax, boracic acid, and carbonate of soda—to prevent milk from spoiling likewise continued unabated. One Department of Health bacteriologist warned, "Milk containing preservatives is valueless as a food, and a baby fed on such milk, while apparently getting a large amount of food, really starves."[70]

Health department officials admitted in 1906 that quality milk remained an elusive commodity. Declaring that only a "campaign of education and enlightenment among the dairymen" would ensure wholesome milk, the Department of Health instituted regular and thorough surprise inspections of all the dairies that supplied Chicago.[71] City milk inspectors arrived at milking time to investigate farms. Although inspectors still had no authority to demand that dairies outside the city alter any practices, inspectors could revoke the license of any Chicago milk dealer who purchased milk from a substandard dairy. Similarly, inspectors now had the power to issue "shut off" orders against specific dairies as well—that is, instruct workers at Chicago's ports of entry to confiscate the milk of a substandard dairy.[72] The Department of Health also began systematic bacteriologic examinations of milk in an effort to halt the spread of tuberculosis, scarlet fever, typhoid fever, diphtheria, and, of course, cholera infantum.[73]

The tactics had an impact. Despite initial recalcitrance, dairy farmers began to recognize that Chicago's laws might benefit them. The city, for example, ordered shippers to return empty milking cans sterile and dry to farmers within forty-eight hours or face severe penalties. Some dairymen were so grateful that they began to cooperate with Chicago's inspectors voluntarily.[74] By 1909, 60 percent of the city's milk was pasteurized, and the sanitary handling of milk was an everyday occurrence. Despite an unusually hot summer that year, Chicago's infant death rate was lower than in 1908. The Department of Health attributed the good news to a better milk supply.[75]

"The Dumping Ground for Tubercular Cows"

Yet barriers to wholesome milk still loomed. A good portion of Chicago's milk remained unpasteurized and few dairy farmers tested their cows for bovine tuberculosis. Tuberculosis first became a pure milk issue in 1901 when the Laboratory of the State Livestock Sanitary Board of Pennsylvania found bovine tuberculosis bacilli in the body of a child who had died of TB. "We can not afford to trifle with this question," warned one Wisconsin physician who urged that all dairy cattle be tested for the disease to prevent its spread to humans. "We have the most abundant scientific evidence on which to take our stand." Farmers, however, objected to the cost of TB testing and feared that the tests would cause "great injury" to their herds, halting milk flow and killing cows. John Cook, the first president of the Chicago Pediatric Society, pointed out that even conscientious dairy farmers hesitated to call a veterinarian when a cow sickened, because when a vet discovered a cow with tuberculosis he killed the animal immediately.[76]

The 1908 Evans Pasteurization Ordinance was the first law in Chicago to require the testing of dairy cows for tuberculosis. Milwaukee inspired the ordinance when it forbade the selling of milk from tubercular cows within its city limits. Soon, many Wisconsin farmers were selling their sick cows to the farms in more lenient Illinois. Declaring that "Chicago does not want it if it is not good enough for Milwaukee," Health Commissioner W. A. Evans pushed for passage of the ordinance that bore his name.[77]

Yet the ordinance had three fatal flaws. The first was Chicago's perennial problem—the city had legal authority to require testing only of the relatively few cows housed by dairy farmers within city limits. Second, despite the ordinance's name, pasteurization was neither a primary nor a permanent aim of the law. The law stipulated that milk be pasteurized only until the city established TB testing procedures for urban dairy cattle. Finally, the ordinance did not define pasteurization, leaving the safety of even pasteurized milk in doubt.[78]

Absent universal pasteurization and the testing of cows for tuberculosis, the milk crusades were far from over. Department of Health officials, exasperated over the ongoing battles with the dairy industry, wrote in 1910, "Are not the rights of 50,000 babies greater than the rights of these . . . [milk] dealers?" And in 1911 health officials hoped that "the time is not far away when it will be as much of a crime to palm off on the people dirty, dangerous milk as it now is to sell diseased, infected meat. . . . [T]he consumer's milk bill will be a little higher, but his doctors' bills will be less."[79]

The bitterness between Chicagoans and the rural farmers who supplied their milk reached its apex in 1912. The partisans in the conflict—led by municipal government on one side and state government on the other—simply had different concerns. Chicago's health officials recognized the urgent need to regulate milk in an urban environment while the rest of Illinois, largely rural farmers with cows in their backyard, did not.[80] Although the Chicago Department of Health begged farmers to behave as if they were "the mother of every little baby who feeds upon the milk which comes from your farm," dairymen largely ignored the emotional plea. When Chicago passed an ordinance in 1912 declaring that all milk sold in the city had to be either pasteurized or produced by cows guaranteed free from tuberculosis, outraged dairy farmers turned to the state for redress.[81]

The Illinois legislature, housed far from Chicago and made up largely of downstate, rural residents, quickly passed a law declaring that no city or town in Illinois could require that dairy cattle be tested for TB. When Chicago's legal department declared that this new state law invalidated the city's entire milk ordinance, including the requirement that milk from cows not tested for tuberculosis be pasteurized, Chicago's milk supply was left with less protection than it had had in years.[82] The bacterial count in Chicago's milk reflected the disaster, averaging 4,759,255 per cubic centimeter in July 1912 as compared with 2,559,610 in July 1911, despite a much cooler summer in 1912. More babies died in July 1912 than in July 1911. The Department of Health blamed cows' milk.[83]

For months, the Department of Health called upon citizens to lobby their aldermen to support legislation that the state legislature would have a harder time nullifying. "This is a poor man's fight. The well-to-do have ways to protect their children's milk, but the great mass of the people must rely on the Health Department to guard its little ones. We will do what we can for you. Get busy and do what you can for us." On July 31, 1912, shortly before the vote on the newly proposed ordinance, the Chicago City Council's Committee on Health held a public meeting to rouse support for the measure. In "A CALL TO CITIZENS OF CHICAGO" members of the committee announced,

"Chicago's milk supply is without protection at its source, the farm. There is no ordinance barring disease-laden milk from the city. Thousands of infants are in danger." The Department of Health joined the chorus: "A fight for pure milk is a fight for life. The man who places profits above considerations for conserving child-life, is the most loathsome enemy of the race. Be guilty of wilfully [sic] serving dirty milk and you become guilty of destroying child-life—in other words, MURDER."[84]

The city council passed the new milk ordinance in August. For the first time, all milk sold in Chicago had to be in sealed bottles and the seals had to be stamped with the milking date. The new law also permitted only two kinds of milk to be sold in the city: inspected milk and pasteurized milk. The city defined inspected milk as milk that came from dairies adhering to standards set by the health department. Standards included clean barns, clean cows certified tuberculosis-free by veterinarians, and milk kept at a temperature no higher than 60° until it reached the consumer. Inspected milk could have no more than 75,000 bacteria per c.c. from October 1 to May 1 and 125,000 bacteria per c.c. from May 2 to September 30.

Any milk not labeled "Inspected" had to be pasteurized. Procedures for pasteurization were quite specific—milk had to be heated either at 140° for 20 minutes, 150° for 15 minutes, 155° for 5 minutes, 160° for 1½ minutes, or 165° for 1 minute.[85] The health department heavily publicized the new ordinance, imploring women in particular to keep milk dealers in line by buying only milk labeled "Inspected" or "Pasteurized."[86]

Milk dealers responded to the new law with a lawsuit charging that the new milk ordinance was "unreasonable, unjust and oppressive." The suit wended its way to the U.S. Supreme Court where, in 1914, justices declared the law constitutional, agreeing with the city that because milk could imperil public health, milk could and should be regulated.[87]

Members of the medical community remained dissatisfied, however. They still wanted all cows tested for tuberculosis. Just before passage of the new milk ordinance, the Chicago Department of Health hung a large poster in city neighborhoods depicting, on the top half, a policeman shooting a rabid dog. The caption read, "Everybody holds a mad dog in deadly fear—all rush for safety." On the poster's bottom half was a bucolic portrait of a mother and child watching a cow being milked under a tree. That caption read, "Few people have any fear for the deadly tuberculous cow. The tuberculous cow kills thousands where the mad dog kills one."[88]

In 1914 the still-frustrated Department of Health hung another broadside throughout the city. This one was a map of the Midwest: Illinois in the

A CONTRAST

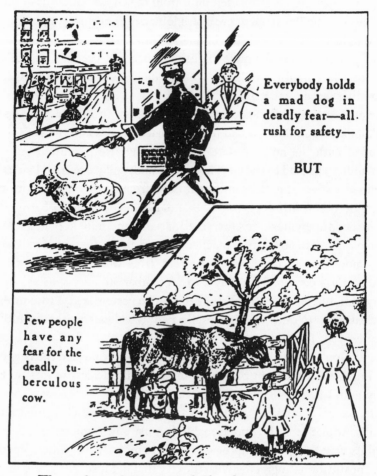

The tuberculous cow kills thousands where the mad dog kills one.

DEPARTMENT OF HEALTH—EDUCATIONAL POSTER SERIES.

Figure 6 This poster was part of the Chicago Department of Health's long campaign to require dairy farmers to test their cows for bovine tuberculosis. *Source: Bulletin Chicago School of Sanitary Instruction,* 25 May 1912, 84.

center surrounded by Wisconsin, Iowa, Missouri, Kentucky, Indiana, and Michigan. Stumbling into Illinois from these surrounding states were dozens of emaciated cows. The poster demanded that Illinois pass a tuberculin test law for dairy cattle and explained that until the governor of Illinois stopped the "infamous traffic" in tubercular cows in 1913, Illinois, as the only midwestern state without a tuberculin test law, had been a "dumping ground" for tubercular cows. As the poster warned, the sick cows shipped to Illinois before 1913 remained in the state producing milk. Health officials protested, "This is a positive menace to the public health."[89]

Chicago did not obtain all its milk from cows certified tuberculosis-free until 1926 when the Chicago City Council passed its Pure Milk Ordinance.

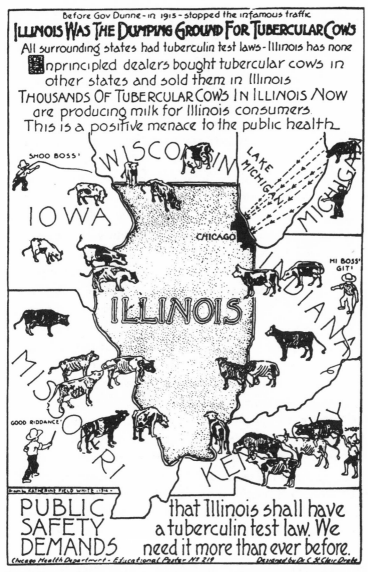

Figure 7 In 1914 frustrated Chicago health department officials hung this broadside in city neighborhoods to graphically demonstrate to Chicago's citizens the ramifications of no tuberculin test law when surrounding states had one. *Source: Bulletin Chicago School of Sanitary Instruction,* 2 May 1914, 78.

Even then the legal maneuvers were not over. The courts granted dairymen a temporary injunction preventing Chicago Health Commissioner Herman Bundesen from putting the law into effect. An enraged Bundesen responded, "If it is within my power I'm going to see that every drop of milk that my six children and the milk that other children drink in the City of Chicago is safe and pure if I have to go to jail to do it."[90] The courts lifted the injunction later that year. Public health reformers had finally prevailed in the bovine tuberculosis controversy.

Pasteurization: Preventer or Promoter of Putrefication?

The question of whether to pasteurize milk proved even more contentious than testing cows for tuberculosis, arousing the wrath of dairies, milk dealers, the public, and even some in the medical community. The issue was so controversial that the first dairy in New York to pasteurize its milk did so secretly, to avoid hurting business.[91] As late as 1907 Chicago Department of Health officials contended that inspected milk was preferable to pasteurized milk for infants.[92] Dairies used the same argument to avoid pasteurization that they had used a few years earlier to escape bottling and sealing milk, insisting that the additional cost would put them out of business.[93]

Arguments against pasteurization abounded. Some argued that nature had not designed milk to be pasteurized. Others worried that pasteurization might encourage carelessness because it concealed dairymen's egregious mistakes. The list of objections continued to grow: pasteurization made milk difficult to digest; caused scurvy, rickets, and malnutrition; killed most bacteria in milk but not all and so might encourage the growth of super-toxic bacteria; destroyed the taste of milk; preserved milk inefficiently.[94]

Given the protests, the initial emphasis of the clean-milk campaigns was on sanitary dairy practices, not on pasteurization. It seemed to make more sense to maintain milk's purity throughout the production process rather than kill the germs in tainted milk.[95] Henry Coit, the inventor of inspected (he called it "certified") milk, worried that milk could be pasteurized too much, destroying its nutritive value. He recalled a personal experience to prove the superiority of raw, certified milk. One day his cook heated some certified milk for an unusually long time, thinking, Coit joked, that superheating would make the milk "a little better than Certified." Then the cook cooled the milk and offered it to Coit's cat. The cat refused even to taste it, choosing to lap up raw, certified milk instead.[96]

The supporters of pasteurization mustered counterattacks. One physician, after hearing Coit's story about the cat, wondered "if he had offered a mouse to that cat of his, the cat would have jumped at it. I would, therefore, ask if he thinks that he ought to have fed the baby a mouse?"[97] By 1910 Chicago Health Department officials, finally convinced of the efficacy of pasteurization, tried to persuade wary milk dealers that the cost would be negligible. Any dealer, health officials contended, could install an efficient pasteurizer for $150 and quickly recoup the expense. Because pasteurization delayed milk spoilage, they explained, small milk dealers would actually save fifty to one hundred dollars a year on a typical two-can (sixteen gallons) per day route. The real cost of pasteurizing one quart of milk, they argued, amounted to only between $\frac{1}{20}$ and $\frac{1}{3}$ of a cent.[98]

Convincing consumers to support the universal pasteurization of milk became another focus of the health department's public education campaigns. Officials explained to nervous citizens that getting milk from cow to consumer was a complex process, prone to error at every step. Clean milk meant dozens of perfectly orchestrated activities: healthy cows living in pristine barns milked by healthy farmers with sterile hands, which allowed the milk to flow into disinfected cans, pails, and bottles. If farmers failed to cool fresh milk immediately, if shippers did not keep it on ice during transit, if milkmen did not deliver it promptly once it arrived in the city, and if mothers did not care for it properly in the home, someone, usually a baby, could get very sick. Pasteurization, health officials told their wary audience, ensured that no misstep would be fatal. "Pasteurization," they assured the public, "is the poor man's hope for [safe] cheap milk."[99]

Despite the loud and long ruckus, the requirement to pasteurize milk in Chicago was only indirectly the result of demands from citizens, physicians, and public health officials. Elected officials never even had the opportunity to vote on the issue. In 1916, anticipating a polio epidemic and fearing the disease might spread through contaminated milk, Chicago's Commissioner of Health issued an emergency executive order declaring all milk sold in the city be pasteurized. From that date on it was. In 1915, only 65 percent of the milk sold in Chicago was pasteurized. After the decree, 98 percent was pasteurized. The likelihood of a milk-borne outbreak of communicable disease became negligible.[100] Infant deaths from diarrhea began to decrease. (See appendixes A.1 and B.1.)

Keeping Milk Cold

Pasteurization did not end the milk crusades. There was still the problem of keeping milk cold in warm weather. In 1902 a New York study confirmed what many physicians had long suspected: cows' milk left unrefrigerated during the summer was the primary cause of infants' digestive ailments. The study revealed that during the winter, 93 percent of babies appeared to thrive on cows' milk and only 7 percent sickened. In the summer 69 percent did well while 31 percent did poorly.[101]

Unfortunately, how to keep milk cold as it traveled between cow and consumer was an enigma. In 1918 only 41 percent of the milk transported to the city from distant rural dairies arrived in refrigerated railcars. Like the dairymen before them who balked at inspecting, sealing, bottling, testing, and pasteurizing, most railroads called the municipal requests to keep milk cool during transit unreasonable. Railroad managers contended that because they received most milk warm, they should not be expected to shoulder the burden of cooling it. They argued that railroad stations were too close together and railcar doors opened too frequently to maintain a cold temperature. They insisted that there was too little time between the last milk shipment loaded in the country and the first milk shipment unloaded on the outskirts of the city to allow time for cooling.[102]

After passage of the milk ordinance of August 1912, which required among other things that all milk sent to Chicago be kept at or below 60° during shipping, the railroads remained obstinate. The city eventually won a lawsuit against the Chicago and North Western Railroad in 1915 for noncompliance with the 1912 ordinance. The Illinois Supreme Court, however, reversed the decision in October 1916. The Supreme Court agreed with the Chicago and North Western Railroad that it was impossible to both keep milk sealed at all times (another requirement of the 1912 ordinance) *and* ascertain its temperature within the container.[103] Not until August 1920 could railroad platform inspectors legally refuse milk warmer than 60°.[104]

In the unlikely event that milk arrived at a consumer's door fresh, clean, and cold, milk spoilage still remained a threat. As late as 1925 the Chicago Department of Public Welfare reported a "tendency in foreign quarters to adhere to their native customs" and shun the use of ice.[105] One 1925 door-to-door survey of Chicago's near west side—where housing was described as "very low grade"—determined that 23 percent of all families never purchased ice and 30 percent of African American households with children did not use ice. Opinions about the necessity of keeping milk and other foodstuff cold varied widely among these families, from those who considered it vital to health, to those who considered it "an unnecessary trouble and expense." In general, those who never purchased ice gave two reasons. Because ice was such a troublesome commodity, consumers normally shopped for food in small quantities several times a day and ate it shortly thereafter, rendering ice unnecessary. Second, its cost was prohibitive. Sixty-eight percent of the families who purchased ice spent an average sixty cents a week on it.[106] Even more frustrating to health officials, use of ice in the home did not necessarily maintain milk's freshness anyway. One physician discovered in 1915 that most iceboxes "of the ordinary construction" maintained a temperature of between 60 to 65° during the summer.[107]

Educating Mothers

Knowing so few citizens purchased ice regularly and so few iceboxes kept food cold, the city's health officials—in addition to battling dairy farmers, milk dealers, and railroads—turned their attention to educating mothers. "If the producer and dealer will do their duty," explained the Department of Health in 1909, "there will be left daily at the consumer's door a bottle of clean, cold, unadulterated milk. It will then be up to the housewife to see that the milk is kept clean and wholesome."[108] Health department posters instructed mothers in the arts of pasteurizing, storing, and preparing milk, and keeping it cold.

Municipalities were not alone in this venture. Women's magazines, which proliferated in the 1890s and pitched all their editorial and advertising messages to white, middle-class women, whom the periodicals defined as "average" American women, had long reminded mothers of their sacred duty in this arena.[109] Articles instructed women how to care for, recognize, and "humanize" clean cows' milk,[110] even as these same articles reminded women that human, and not cows', milk was the preferred aliment for babies.

Instructing mothers how to care for milk in the home was as complex a task as teaching the public about germs. Before 1912, when milkmen finally left milk on doorsteps bottled and sealed, women normally left open jars outside their doors each day to receive the milk ladled from the milkman's eight-gallon can. In the summer—when heat, flies, dust, and small, thirsty mammals abounded—this was a particularly dangerous practice.[111] The Department of Health taught women to cover milk receptacles and place them in the shade in a bucket of ice. Health officials repeated their care-of-milk-in-the-home instructions so often they became mothers' mantra. "Keep baby's milk clean and cool. Use only good bottled milk. Keep the cap on the bottle. Keep the bottle in a clean, cool place. Never allow flies near milk."[112]

Before 1916 Chicago mothers also learned—via the free Chicago Department of Health weekly bulletin, assorted newspaper articles, and women's

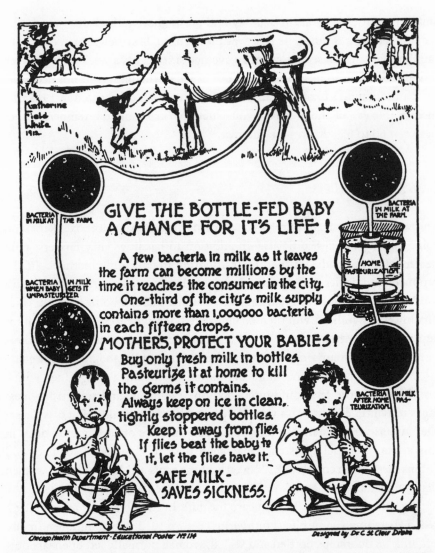

Figure 8 The purpose of this 1912 Chicago Department of Health poster was twofold: to urge mothers to buy only top-quality, bottled milk and to pasteurize the milk and store it properly at home. *Source: Bulletin Chicago School of Sanitary Instruction,* 31 August 1912.

magazines—how to sterilize and pasteurize milk at home in order to "render milk almost absolutely free from any germ."[113] Women learned to place a quart bottle of milk with the stopper still in it on a plate in a two-quart boiler, fill the boiler with cold water, and place it over a fire. When the water began to boil, they removed the boiler from the fire and, with the milk bottle still in it, set it aside to cool.[114] In 1912 the health department continued to explain that germs multiply rapidly in unpasteurized, unrefrigerated milk. "If you drink . . . milk raw, you take into your body millions of *live,* disease-producing germs. The only way that you can make . . . milk reasonably safe is to pasteurize it before using."[115]

The Chicago Department of Health was unceasing in its efforts to educate mothers. On July 21–22, 1915, health department workers placed 500,000 tags on milk bottles. The tags advised purchasers that the milk had been "carefully supervised" from cow to consumer. Now it was up to mothers to keep the milk cold and guard it from flies, dirt, and germs "until you prepare it for your baby's stomach." The tags urged knowledgeable women to share their sanitary training with a neighbor so "that her baby may be as healthy as yours."[116]

The memory of thousands of babies dying from diarrhea every summer was still vivid, and given the relentless publicity, keeping cows' milk safe became an understandable obsession for many women. If they were to prepare milk according to experts' recommendations, the mothers who fed their babies artificially had to devote considerable time, energy, and knowledge to the process. As one woman explained in 1889, "It is conceivable that . . . [a mother] may study carefully into the question of what kind of food will best meet her baby's needs; that she will procure the best attainable quality of food; that she will prepare and administer it herself; that long tubes, ragged nipples, cold slops and sour bottles may be articles foreign to her creed and practice; in short, that she will devote really more time and trouble to the baby than if she nursed it."[117] Some mothers were so preoccupied with the purchase and preparation of cows' milk that they could quote the exact bacterial count in the milk that they provided their children. One troubled woman explained to *Hygeia,* a magazine published by the American Medical Association for a lay audience, that she had ordered an analysis of the pasteurized milk consumed by her children only to find that it had a bacterial count of 57,000. Now she gave her children raw milk, which, she found, had a bacterial count of between 14,000 and 25,000. After receiving the alarming analyses, she even forbade her daughter to drink the pasteurized available at school.[118] Mothers used litmus paper to test for strongly alkaline milk (indicating "possibly the animal is diseased") or strongly acid milk (indicating "the milk has been contaminated, from long exposure to the air, or from impure dishes which have held it").[119] They cleaned babies' bottles with coarse sand, baking soda, and water, then rinsed and scalded them.[120] Mothers made iceboxes using a soapbox or fruit packing case, sawdust, tin pail, newspaper, and ice.[121] In 1919 Chicago's milk dealers passed out cards on "Clean Milk Day" instructing mothers:

Don't put milk on window ledge to save ice.

Don't place milk in open, unclean vessels exposed to air and flies.

Don't use milk over 24 hours old for the baby.

Don't mix old and new milk.

Don't have janitor take in milk unless he puts it into an ice box. . . .

Don't economize on ice. Ice is cheaper than milk.

Don't fail to keep milk cold.

Don't forget that good milk is good food.[122]

Although by 1922 the summer deaths of infants from diarrhea had been waning for years, the warnings did not stop. The Chicago Department of Health continued to remind mothers that "hot weather spoils the milk and spoiled milk makes babies sick and this increases the baby death rate during the hot weather months."[123] The reminder was likely mere habit. Mothers had been demonstrating devotion to the care of milk for years.

"The Original Food"

The seasonal incidence of diarrhea among babies had disappeared completely in Chicago by 1928, thanks to clean, pasteurized milk and wider access to home refrigeration (see appendix A.1).[124] By then the dairy industry, having fought every innovation from pasteurization to bottling to keeping milk cold, was using the negative publicity generated by the milk crusades to their advantage. Now they could exploit the public's awareness of the dairy industry's foibles to tout the industry's new practices and the consequent wholesomeness of milk. Shortly before Chicago passed its Pure Milk Ordinance in 1926, "progressive-minded" farmers in the Chicago milk shed—the vast area including Wisconsin, Iowa, Ohio, Michigan, Minnesota, and Indiana that provided Chicago with milk—formed the Pure Milk Association. Their slogan—"We intend to produce good milk for Chicagoland, not because we have to, but because we *want* to"—demonstrated how far both consumers and dairy farmers had come.[125]

The dairy industry now extolled the many benefits of their product and, like the milk reformers before them had done, pitched their messages directly at mothers. In the 1920s, Chicago's Bowman Dairy advertised its milk as "BEST FOR BABIES. . . . Perfect pasteurization makes it so."[126] This was quite a change from just a few years earlier when mothers learned that cows' milk was to be given to babies only when human milk was wholly unavailable and even then to regard cows' milk as, at best, an unsatisfactory substitute for mother's milk. Now, as one magazine noted in 1918, baby "has [cows'] milk for breakfast, [cows'] milk for lunch, [cows'] milk for dinner, [cows'] milk for 'tea' and [cows'] milk for supper. Considering the fact that he grows so fast there must be some magic quality in [cows'] milk as a food."[127] Now human milk *and* cows' milk were equally miraculous, both were the "original food."[128]

In 1927 Chicago Commissioner of Health Arnold Kegel still told mothers, "Nature intended that the human mother should furnish nourishment to her offspring during the first year of life. A baby raised on breast milk has a far better chance of thriving and surviving than one fed on other kinds of milk or artificial foods." But he coupled that caveat with a reassurance not uttered by Chicago health officials in previous years. Cows' milk was a perfectly adequate substitute for human milk. Kegel assured mothers, "So extensive is the use of cows' milk as a substitute for breast milk that the cow has been appropriately called 'the foster mother of the human race.'"[129]

City officials assured mothers in 1925 that thanks to milk reform, cows' milk was not just safer than before but 100 percent safe. "From the cow to the consumer," wrote Chicago Commissioner of Health Herman Bundesen, "Chicago's milk is kept as pure and fresh as human ability can make it." The victory in Chicago was so complete, and milk had become such an important part of consumers' consciousness, that the city even started using cows' milk in its pitches touting Chicago as an ideal family vacation spot. Cows' milk, Bundesen explained in 1925, is "something to think about in contemplating a vacation in which the 'Kiddies' are taken along. . . . Spending a vacation in Chicago eliminates the necessity of worrying about the milk supply."[130]

Over the more than thirty years that Chicago struggled to clean up its milk supply, reformers fought state government, dairy farmers, railroads, dairies, delivery men, small grocers, public ignorance, and even some in the medical community. The city won every battle. Enforcement of the laws regulating the production and shipment of milk became so rigorous that between 1915 and 1918 milk inspectors closed more than half the milk dealers in Chicago, greatly simplifying inspection and enforcement.[131] By 1921 victory was so complete that even the Michigan dairy district felt the "good-sized reach" of the Chicago Department of Health. A vacationing food inspector, investigating an offensive odor, found a creamery dumping its waste into an open field. The inspector was helpless at the time, but when the creamery applied to sell its product in Chicago the city denied the business a license.[132] In 1929 Chicago obtained its milk from 400,000 cows on 35,000 farms in seven states. Chicago milk inspectors visited these farms regularly and rarely found irregularities. Dairy farmers did not balk at the visits.[133]

Chicagoans now enjoyed the luxury of taking clean cows' milk for granted. Milk, the food that sustained human babies, had become cows' milk. Human milk was now on the periphery of public consciousness, at best. Clean cows' milk had become the hard-won solution to the problem of sick and dead babies caused by the decline in breastfeeding.

♦

Chicago's decades-long milk reform movement had two unintended consequences. First, it allowed the dairy industry, long the bitter enemy of milk reform, to become a respected citizen. In 1924 the National Dairy Council celebrated "three great advancements in the milk industry": the delivery of milk to the customer in individual bottles rather than via the dipper method, the implementation and enforcement of sanitary measures governing milk, and the pasteurization of all milk. The Dairy Council never even hinted that the dairy industry had fought each "great advancement" at every turn. Long the targets of reformers' dire warnings, mothers now wholly embraced this newly sanctified product. In 1919 one expert estimated that two-thirds of American children under the age of one consumed cows' milk. Even breastfed babies ingested a "considerable" amount.[134]

The second consequence of the fight for pure milk was subtler, and more significant. The milk crusades had taken place on a public stage and the ubiquitous pleas for clean milk to save babies gave mothers the impression that cows' milk was an indispensable baby food. This further discouraged them from exclusive breastfeeding. Workers at Chicago Milk Commission milk stations, who provided certified milk to mothers beginning in 1903, complained that women regarded inspected cows' milk as a magic bullet of sorts to perk up the baby.[135] Some physicians' rhetoric enhanced that notion. One doctor attending the annual conference of the American Association of Medical Milk Commissions in 1917 urged that inspected milk be viewed in a class by itself, "as a medicine." Only one physician at the conference rose to disagree. He admonished the audience, "I think we ought to get over the idea that Certified Milk is a medicine and . . . regard it as a food. I still belong to the group that I suppose is small now, who believed the Almighty knew what he was doing when he provided for the natural order of things."[136]

This physician's perception that breastfeeding advocates were outnumbered was right. By the 1920s and 1930s the vast majority of mothers and physicians alike deemed the champions of human milk old-fashioned. As the Bowman Dairy claimed in its ads, bovine, and not human, milk was now "Best For Babies."[137] While the milk crusades undeniably improved infants' health, the very visible campaigns also guaranteed that no mother would ever again think of human milk as a necessity if she wanted her baby to survive infancy. The battle for pure milk predisposed more mothers than ever before to think of cows' milk as all they needed to provide a pure, safe, and wholesome diet for their babies.

By the 1920s everyone—mothers, physicians, public health authorities, and city officials—seemed to have forgotten that the milk reform movement was prompted by more than the failures of the dairy industry. As one physician reminded the public in 1923, diarrhea in infants was caused primarily by mothers' failure to breastfeed and only secondarily by bad cows' milk.[138] Yet palatable cows' milk made the dearth of human milk seem to be no problem at all.

3

"They Cannot Transform Cows' Milk into Woman's Milk":
Physicians and Infant Feeding

Inherent in every milk reform effort was a question that physicians often debated among themselves: what is the best food for babies with no access to human milk? This question set the pediatric community in frenetic motion as they theorized the cause of what appeared to be imminent universal lactation failure and proposed solutions to the problem. The need for an answer was urgent, as babies' lives were in the balance. Physicians consequently began their long search for what most in the medical community considered an oxymoron: the perfect artificial food.

Indeed, nothing attracted the attention of that first generation of American pediatricians like the "feeding question"—not traditional childhood diseases, not respiratory ailments, not premature birth, not stillbirth. They became so embroiled in artificial food formulation, to the exclusion of other medical services, that one physician, on a visit to Chicago in the late 1930s, observed that the "pediatrician is a dying race" because artificial food no longer caused high infant morbidity and mortality. Consequently, this physician prophesied, there would be little left in the future for pediatricians to do.[1]

The ostensibly insoluble problems associated with lactation failure and the dearth of human milk were new developments in medicine. Physicians did not consider infant feeding a problem, medical or otherwise, until the last quarter of the nineteenth century. Historically, the medical and lay communities alike assumed that a mother would and could breastfeed her baby.[2] If she did not, her family hired a wet nurse.[3] If human milk was wholly unavailable, the baby almost always died. Society deemed such a death tragic but unavoidable. Most viewed human milk as the only conceivable antidote to an infant's hunger.

Late nineteenth-century infant mortality statistics eradicated this complacency over babies' food. The figures revealed not only the high infant mortality rate but also the numerous infant deaths from diarrhea. Clearly, many babies consumed something other than human milk, and this "something" was vastly inferior to the sustenance produced by mothers' bodies. It appeared to the medical community that a baby's food—preferably human milk but perhaps, given women's growing propensity to bottle-feed, some undiscovered food that mimicked human milk—was the key to lowered infant mortality. The editor of *Babyhood* magazine explained the new philosophy in 1902: "Formerly, if a child was at the breast, there was . . . the end of it; he throve or not. . . . Now it is not the end of it. . . . [I]f a child does not thrive, questions are asked and changes made."[4]

Originally intended to benefit only the babies "so unfortunate as to be deprived of their natural sustenance,"[5] artificial food soon seemed a potential necessity for every infant. Few physicians realized, most likely because of their ongoing glorification of human milk, that their heated debate and formulation of artificial food dissuaded even more mothers from breastfeeding or breastfeeding for long.

♦

In a paper he presented at the inaugural meeting of the American Pediatric Society in 1889, pediatrician Arthur Meigs acknowledged the "great disagreement among physicians with regard to how infants should be fed." His allusion, however, was not to some doctors' preference for human milk and others' partiality for artificial food. On that question there was unanimity. Human milk, Meigs noted matter-of-factly, "we all know to be the most perfect food for infants."[6] His colleagues agreed. The "great disagreement" arose, not over the importance of human milk to human health, but over how to feed an infant deprived of mothers' milk.

Questions abounded. What was the best way to alter cows' milk to make it suitable for a baby's consumption? What ingredients in cows' milk were most harmful to babies' immature digestive systems? What ingredients were most beneficial? In what amounts? Should the percentages vary as a baby grew? If percentages varied, should they vary simultaneously or in turn? When milk was modified should it be sterilized, pasteurized, or certified first? Were commercial infant foods useful alternatives to human milk? If yes, were they best mixed with cows' milk or water or both? Were complementary or supplementary feedings of artificial food ever appropriate for breast-fed babies?[7] Should mothers err on the side of overfeeding or underfeeding babies? Each question engendered interminable discussion.

Physicians had yet to enjoy anything approaching consistent success with any artificial food, hence the contentious debate. In 1908, as one promising claim after another disintegrated, one physician protested, "No medical man is now willing to claim that he can by deft manipulation of cows' milk duplicate breast milk any more than he is willing to claim that he can, by clipping its tail and ears, so modify a calf that it can be substituted for a baby."[8] "Cows' milk, doctors advised, might be a second best alternative to breast milk, but as one physician lectured, "I say 'best,' but in this connection the word is almost meaningless, for the difference between mother's milk and cows' milk is abysmal. The first is at once a perfect food and an efficient medicine, while the second is a very unsatisfactory food and no medicine at all."[9] In the 1914 edition of his popular tome on infant care, the renowned pediatrician L. Emmett Holt told a vast audience what he and his colleagues had been telling individual women privately for decades: "[T]here is no perfect substitute for good breast-feeding."[10]

Artificial food remained, at best, an unsatisfactory alternative to mother's milk. At worst, it was a deadly one. Hence, no physician recommended bottle-feeding lightly. Charles Warrington Earle, one-time president of the Chicago Medical Society, spoke for virtually all physicians in the 1890s when he put infant foods in a preferred order. First came mother's milk, "always when possible"; second, the milk of a wet nurse; third, "mixed food," that is, part breast and part bottle. Only "when all other resources have failed" did he advise putting a baby on "a sterilized artificial diet."[11]

Physicians of that era exalted human milk. Chicago pediatrician Joseph Brennemann was typical in that he went to great lengths to provide human milk to every baby in his care, if only for a few weeks after birth. He found that the value of such a practice could "hardly be overestimated."[12] Physicians heralded human milk because babies digested it easily. Late nineteenth- and early twentieth-century doctors also knew that breast milk protected babies from infectious disease.[13] Physicians based their knowledge of the immunizing properties of breast milk both on observations garnered in their medical practices and on several studies that demonstrated that baby mammals fed exclusively by their mothers rarely became seriously ill. Henry L. Coit, the inventor of certified milk, fed the milk of one species to the offspring of another and found that such a practice invariably portended health problems. He discovered that puppies fed human milk, for example, "remained alive, but were in a very miserable condition." In his study, all the newborn animals fed the milk of another species "were inferior to the breast-fed animals, both at the time of the experiment and afterwards."[14] In another report examining 1,943 infants who died of "degenerative disturbances," researchers noted that only 3 percent were breastfed. In yet another study, this one of 718 babies who succumbed to diarrhea, only 30 were breastfed. Experiments with mice demonstrated that the offspring of a mouse not resistant to a particular disease acquired resistance after suckling a mouse with immunity.[15]

The studies came as no surprise to physicians who had observed that few breastfed infants fell ill as long as they were nursing and seemed heartier than bottle-fed babies even when they ceased breastfeeding. As one doctor said of human milk in 1909, "When I say medicine, I speak literally, for mother's milk gives to the baby some measure of her own acquired power of resistance to disease. There is, indeed good ground for the old saying that, so long as a child is at the breast, the blood of its mother continues to flow through its veins." When Chicago pediatrician Frank Walls examined critically ill, artificially fed babies, he found that "human milk even in very small amount seems to act as a curative measure and without it some of these cases are hopeless." Julius Hess reminded mothers in 1923 that on the few occasions breastfed babies did succumb to a bacteria or virus, they were always less sick and recovered more quickly than artificially fed babies.[16]

Until the late 1920s, physicians attributed the vast majority of infant deaths to lack of mother's milk and were never at a loss for a dramatic tale to prove it. Particularly harrowing were the stories told by doctors who worked in foundling homes where, because of the perpetual dearth of wet nurses, caretakers usually fed babies artificially. In 1870 Abraham Jacobi, eventually renowned as the father of American pediatrics, worked for the Nursery and Child's Hospital, a medical charity in New York City. Every infant admitted to the hospital and kept there for more than three months, he reported years later, died.[17] Pediatrician Henry Dwight Chapin concurred that institutionalized, bottle-fed babies were invariably hopeless cases. "I have had the best hospital wards, roof gardens, convalescent homes especially for these cases," he explained, "and yet it was the same thing; every baby under one year of age did badly if kept long."[18]

Physicians in private practice saw babies in nearly as dire straits. Frank Spooner Churchill examined a baby boy in 1896 who did well on artificial food for the first three months of his life. Suddenly, and unsurprisingly to Churchill, who had seen it many times before, "putrid diarrhea, hot weather and unhygienic surroundings resulted in his death." Isaac Abt described what customarily happened to a baby whose mother used artificial food in lieu of breast milk. Frequently the baby suffered from diarrhea and his frightened mother usually responded to the crisis by substituting barley water for the artificial food, as was the custom. When the baby seemed better, after a day or so according to Abt, mother put baby back on artificial food. The diarrhea was likely to return, and if it did, out came the barley water again. After this vicious cycle had gone on for some time, the distraught mother invariably came to Abt. "I saw many of these babies in a condition bordering on starvation," Abt lamented, "suffering from rickets or scurvy, with ulcers of the cornea and other serious symptoms."[19]

Given the consequences that could arise from the use of artificial food, the medical community was initially wary of it. Jacobi argued that even clean, pure cows' milk, when used as an infant food, could "lay a gradual foundation for future ailing." He charged that animal milk could no more stand in for human milk than animal blood could substitute for human blood.[20] Yet these same physicians were quick to ask, what were they to offer the innocent babe whom, for whatever reason, had no access to human milk?

The Great Debate

Perhaps it was inevitable that the ensuing experimentation with artificial food formulation produced, not unanimity of purpose or dynamic cooperative endeavor, but disagreement and disgust. George Acker, president of the American Pediatric Society, complained in 1915, "There has never been a time in the history of modern medicine when more unsubstantiated theories were before us for consideration. Everything new is seized with avidity and has its period of popularity, only to be relegated to its proper sphere of usefulness, or more often to oblivion." He decried the lack of unanimity surrounding the infant-feeding question in particular which, he charged, often resulted in the "normal infant [being] deprived of breast milk." Given the rancorous debate, he lamented, the majority of medical students left medical school "confused as [to] the most important subject in the whole realm of pediatrics."[21] Another disgusted doctor saw in the entire business "a little too much of the cry of the nostrum vendor."[22]

Physicians failed to agree even on precisely which ingredients in cows' milk sickened babies.[23] Jacobi was of the too-much-fat-is-a-problem school, reminding his colleagues that "fat feeding has been a fad in America for some time. The worst cases of destructive indigestion I meet are those of overgenerous fat-feeding doctors."[24] Abt likewise blamed fat as "by far the most toxic ingredient" in cows' milk. He found, however, that too much starch in a baby's food was equally injurious.[25] Frank Walls, who divided a baby's "food intolerance" into four deteriorating stages—balance disturbance, dyspepsia, disintegration, and intoxication—also blamed fat for artificially fed babies' downward spirals.[26] Another Chicago doctor insisted that milk sugar caused the most acute gastrointestinal disturbances.[27] Thomas Rotch, a Harvard University pediatrician, worried about protein.[28]

Physicians coupled the disagreement over the most offensive ingredient in cows' milk with another debate. Did artificially fed babies chronically consume too much or too little food? Brennemann feared overfeeding. James Warren Van Derslice, another Chicago physician, feared the opposite—that bottle-fed babies slowly starved on diluted condensed milk. Abt declared overfeeding and underfeeding equally disastrous.[29]

Doctors also differed on the efficacy of supplemental feedings. Did offering breastfed babies occasional bottles of cows' milk benefit breastfeeding or undermine it? One physician argued that supplementation protected babies from the dangers of weaning. He contended that "no matter how scant" a mother's milk, human milk made artificial food palatable to babies. He argued that as long as a mother with "deficient breasts" provided her baby with just one skimpy daily nursing, she would never have an ailing infant in need of a wet nurse. The debate long continued. In 1917 Minneapolis pediatrician Julius Sedgwick roundly denounced supplemental feeding, charging that it was "one of the most frequent causes of the breast drying up and the loss of milk. The breast is not stimulated; it is, in fact, the best method of weaning the infant." Abt argued that supplemental feedings were usually unnecessary, urged by physicians who misunderstood the crucial difference between complementary and supplementary feedings. He explained that a mother gave a complemental feeding to her baby immediately after nursing if the baby was still hungry. A supplemental feeding wholly replaced a nursing. Abt contended that complemental feedings encouraged nervous mothers to continue breastfeeding, while supplemental feedings led inexorably to weaning.[30]

Although some in the medical community understood milk's supply-and-demand principle, many physicians had simply come to believe that supplementing breast milk with artificial food was necessary during virtually every child's infancy. Hess, for example, urged mothers to breastfeed for nine months "or even longer, if possible" but worried that many women would run low on milk long before their babies reached nine months. Convinced that bottle-feeding was almost always inevitable, he suggested it was "usually wise" to give the baby one bottle a day by its third to fourth month "in order to relieve the mother and train the baby in bottle feeding."[31]

Mimicking Mother's Milk

One of the few points of agreement among these dueling doctors was that artificial food had to mimic human milk. "Our only hope," Arthur Meigs wrote
in 1885, "is that by carefully studying the composition of human milk, and
seeking to imitate it, can we do anything to save the hundreds of thousands
of infants who are, year after year, sacrificed to our want of knowledge."[32]

Meigs suggested that there were two ways to find the most satisfactory
food for a baby who "must be hand-fed." The most common, and most dangerous, was trial and error.[33] Some physicians justified this course, arguing,
"It is impossible to say in a given case that one, or that another, kind of food
will prove best; have as admirable theories as you please in the selection and
combination of ingredients; the final test is in experiment."[34] Meigs condemned this process—the emotional cost to parents and the physical cost to
infants were simply too great. He suggested instead that doctors try to imitate human milk. "Justice has never been done to this method as an understanding of the composition of human milk has always been wanting," he
wrote in 1884.[35]

Mothers soon learned of Meigs's work: his *Milk Analysis and Infant Feeding: A Practical Treatise on the Examination of Human and Cows' Milk,
Cream, Condensed Milk, Etc., and Directions As to the Diet of Young Infants*
was recommended reading in an 1886 issue of *Babyhood* magazine. Although
women's magazines (*Babyhood* included) continued to remind their readers
that breastfeeding was the best way to feed an infant—"all medical men agree
that no artificial food can possibly be so good for an infant as its mother's
milk"[36]—*Babyhood*'s endorsement of Meigs's tome sent a mixed message. If
mother's milk could be quasi-duplicated, *Babyhood* editors implied with their
recommendation, perhaps infant-feeding woes would soon be over. In a magazine intended for their eyes alone, mothers witnessed the first stirrings of
the legitimization of artificial food as physicians reinforced mothers' doubts
about human milk by devoting themselves to infant-food formulation.

Meigs led the charge, tackling one daunting obstacle after another. Most
troubling was how to transform the protein in cows' milk to resemble the
protein in human milk because, Meigs discovered, "the caseins of the two
milks are essentially, and in their nature, unlike." Chapin made a similar pro-
nouncement in 1903, arguing that the protein in the two milks differed so
radically that "no known method of procedure will convert cows' milk into
human milk."[37]

The quantitative differences between the two milks were as troubling as the qualitative ones. Various chemists handed Meigs widely divergent analyses of human milk. How was he to mimic mother's milk when no one could agree on the amounts of its ingredients? Meigs was especially perturbed about the disagreement over the amount of casein in human milk, since he considered casein the key to breast milk's digestibility.[38] The disparate analyses likely stemmed in part from the fact that human milk, indeed all mammals' milk, varies in content from week to week and month to month according to an infant's changing needs.[39] Even more vexing for Meigs's purpose, mammals' milk varies dramatically during a single feeding. What is now called "fore milk," the substance excreted by the human mammary gland when an infant begins to nurse, is highest in protein, while "hind milk," which is produced later in a feeding, is highest in fat.[40] Meigs knew of this phenomenon and to solve the conundrum he analyzed mother's milk "at all sorts of times . . . for it is a well-known fact that in cows, the first milk drawn from the animal is much poorer in fat than that which comes last in the milking . . . and that it holds good with regard to women as well as cows, is beyond dispute."[41]

After years of study and experimentation, Meigs concluded that to approximate human milk physicians or mothers needed to dilute cows' milk with lime water to diminish its casein, add cream to enhance its fat, and add commercial milk-sugar because human milk is so much sweeter than bovine milk.[42] Meigs tested this mix "extensively" and announced in his *Milk Analysis and Infant Feeding* that the brew was "wonderfully useful and easily digested." This was likely enormously tantalizing news to the women who followed *Babyhood*'s advice and waded through Meigs's book. Although Meigs continued to caution, "Of course, no food has been found, or ever will be found so good as the nourishment which a healthy mother is able to give her child, and the food recommended will sometimes fail, as all things fail," he also noted optimistically, "in the opinion of the author, it is much more nearly what is wanted than anything previously recommended."[43] Assorted physicians, medical institutions, and mothers used the concoction, known as the "Meigs Mixture," for at least the next twenty years.[44]

By 1889 Meigs was even more pleased with his formulation, recommending it enthusiastically both to the mothers of the infants he saw in private practice and to the caretakers of institutionalized foundlings. The Meigs Mixture, he assured them, was likely to produce an outcome "better than my most sanguine hopes had led me to expect." If a baby did sicken on the mix, Meigs blamed mothers' ignorance or impatience. "If I have had intelligent people to deal with . . . the result has almost uniformly been success" he explained. "[O]n the other hand, if people are foolish, and try a succession of different foods . . . failure often attends one's most strenuous efforts." He suggested that physicians guard against the tendency of mothers "to be constantly trying different foods in such rapid succession that not one of them is given an adequate trial." He advised colleagues to stand firm in the face of a distraught parent's opposition "until there arises some real and definite reason to think he [the physician] is in error." When a foundling sickened—and Meigs had the opportunity to use his formulation on all the infants at the Sheltering Arms of Philadelphia—he similarly blamed the nurses' "bad regimen."[45] While doctors, including Meigs, still preferred human milk for babies, and breastfeeding remained, for the time being, the purview of mothers, physicians now claimed sole expertise in the artificial food arena.

The "Terrifying" Mathematics and "Higher Astronomy" of Infant Feeding

Thomas Rotch's work at Harvard on what he dubbed "percentage feeding" benefited greatly from Meigs's discoveries and became the most closely watched and widely discussed method of artificial feeding from the 1890s until the early 1910s, when its popularity eventually waned. Rotch theorized that "to copy nature closely" physicians had to prepare food "not only for the many but for the individual, and when introducing new methods for preparing a substitute food we must recognize the necessity for providing for many prescription possibilities."[46] Rotch and his adherents employed an endless array of mathematical formulas—which is where the word "formula" in relation to infant feeding originated—to indicate how much the percentage of each significant ingredient in cows' milk needed to be weakened or strengthened given the condition of a particular baby.

To fill his prescriptions, Rotch pushed for the establishment of milk laboratories, quasi pharmacies whose chemists created the infinite cows' milk permutations for the precise needs of a particular infant. Key to Rotch's philosophy was the belief that "even slight changes" in the percentages of fat, sugar, and protein in cows' milk "are of real value in the management of the digestion and nutrition of the infant, and that these changes are often necessary day by day as well as month by month."[47] Many physicians soon embraced Rotch's theory that babies would weather artificial feeding with ease if doctors responded instantly to the slightest change in an infant's health or behavior with an appropriate prescription to be filled at the nearest milk laboratory.

Rotch based percentage feeding on the theory that each mammalian species produced milk with vastly different percentages of similar ingredients. Unlike Meigs, Rotch did not consider the casein in cows' milk to be different from the casein in human milk. "The product of the mammary glands of all mammals is essentially the same," he contended. "It is composed of elements which in an individual milk resemble the corresponding elements in all the others." Abt disagreed with Rotch and sided with Meigs on this issue, telling members of the Chicago Medical Society in 1897 that differences between the casein in human and cows' milk were "impossible to overcome." Rotch moved slightly closer to Meigs's and Abt's view a few years later when he admitted that the best chemist at Harvard had not been able to tell him if the albuminoids in cows' milk were identical to those in mother's milk. Nevertheless, he still argued "that is no reason why we should not make use of the percentage method." Eventually Rotch complicated percentage feeding even further by reversing his stance, even differentiating between the types of fat found in the milk of Jersey versus Holstein cows.[48]

Physicians on the East Coast were most devoted to percentage feeding, but the method was known to, and used by, physicians all over the country, including nationally renowned Chicago pediatricians. Rotch's modified milk formulas even inspired urban medical charities to formulate and give away generic formulas to the poor at philanthropic milk stations.[49] For a time the kudos were ubiquitous. Percentage feeding, imperiously dubbed the "American Method," "received such universal and unqualified approval among our pediatricians that it seems almost like heresy to doubt its tenets," Brennemann noted in 1908.[50] Frank Spooner Churchill described milk modified by the American Method as "being more like the average human breast milk than any other known preparation."[51] One of Rotch's Boston colleagues argued, "It is . . . of unquestioned advantage to think and write in percentages for in this way only may we express scientifically the manner in which the problems of infant feeding are to be worked out."[52] Percentage feeding, another physician contended, permitted doctors to forget the evils of cows' milk and thus "leave out the prejudice" and "fit the food to the individual baby."[53] Abt told his Chicago colleagues that the medical profession was indebted to Rotch. Not only did the American Method "modify the milk so as to approach as near as possible . . . human milk," but the milk laboratories that filled physicians' math-laden prescriptions used only inspected milk, thus introducing a system for the supervision of dairies eventually copied by municipalities and medical charities.[54] The assorted clean-milk movements around the country clearly influenced Rotch. Their genesis was virtually simultaneous with that of percentage feeding, and Rotch's milk laboratories employed inspection and pasteurization systems second to none.

Rotch was as concerned about modifying cows' milk with "the most exact precision" as he was with strict adherence to sanitary measures.[55] His mathematical formulas dictated the precise degree of milk modification and were based on a number of variables, including an infant's age, weight, height, appearance, and overall health. Physicians also considered the condition of an infant's stools and assorted illnesses the infant might have suffered. Diagnoses varied: "duodenal jaundice," "proteid digestion weak," and "sugar digestion weak" were only three of dozens. Rotch recommended that formulas err on the side of weak, rather than strong, percentages. Only if a baby did well on a particular formula did he slowly increase all percentages together as a baby grew. In later years he recommended raising the percentage of each element in turn. That way, if an increase disagreed with an infant, a physician immediately could discern the offending element.[56]

As complicated as Rotch's initial formulas were, percentage feeding was destined to become even more complex. Physicians began to break down milk, not just into its customary protein/sugar/fat/ash components, but into components of the components. One group of doctors, for example, published the percentage of each of the six elements of ash in human and cows' milk.[57] This expanded the ongoing debate. Were the varying amounts of these subcomponents also important factors to consider?

In the same vein, one physician called for a closer look at what constituted the protein in cows' milk. Chemists, he pointed out, now believed that the protein in cows' milk consisted of one-fifth "soluble whey proteid" and four-fifths "caseinogen." Human milk, on the other hand, was made up of two-thirds soluble whey proteid and only one-third "curd-forming caseinogen." He suggested modifying the relative percentages of these two components of protein in order to imitate human milk more precisely. Another doctor insisted that the amount of starch in barley water—commonly used to dilute cows' milk—be considered when writing a modified milk prescription. "No one will question the fact," he wrote, "that it may make a great difference to a very young infant whether it receives .51 per cent. starch or 4.8 per cent. starch in its food."[58]

The calorie question brought still more elements into play.[59] Van Derslice, one-time president of the Chicago Pediatric Society, argued in 1907 that in order for cows' milk to supply an infant with sufficient nutrients, it needed an "energy quotient" equal to mother's milk. To equalize the "energy quotient" of the two substances, he suggested that physicians add citrate of soda to cows' milk. Citrate of soda had an additional benefit, Van Derslice explained, as it made cows' milk curds physically resemble human milk curds.[60] Thomas Allen, another Chicago pediatrician, defined the "energy quotient" as "a proper amount of energy for the baby" or the amount of food needed "to furnish the required energy."[61] To calculate the amount of energy (*E*), milk (*M*), proteid (*P*), and sugar (*S*) in a particular formula (where baby's weight is *W*, ratio is *R*, and the ratio of food used is *r*) Allen employed the following equation:

$$E = PR$$
$$M = WP/4$$
$$S = WP(R - r)$$
$$\text{Water} = 2 \text{ to } 3 \ W - M$$

He offered the following example to colleagues:

W 12, P 5, R $7\frac{1}{4}$, whole milk $r = 4\frac{1}{4}$
$E = 5 \times 7\frac{1}{4} = 36\frac{1}{4}$
Milk $= 12 \times 5/4 = 15$ oz.
Sugar $= 12 \times 5 \times 3 = 1.8$ oz.
Water $= 12 \times 2.5 - 15 = 15$ oz.[62]

Brennemann was one of many who worried that Rotch's system was becoming so "peculiarly complicated" that the formulas were bound to produce "a wide range of error."[63] As his system came under burgeoning criticism, Rotch continued to defend it, explaining in 1908, "I am simply taking up what I think is an advance in infant feeding, namely, why it is that some foods agree with babies better than others."[64] His defense fell on increasingly deaf ears. One doctor likened the work of artificial food pioneers to that of alchemists; they failed dismally yet discovered some principles that might one day lead to a viable product.[65] Jacobi foreshadowed the abandonment of percentage feeding when he said in 1908, "Feeding can not be regulated by mathematics as well as by brains, and by the wants of the individual baby."[66] But he refused to openly criticize Rotch, telling colleagues, "There is not a man in the profession in America that has done more original work on . . . the study of the chemistry and biology of milk, than our friend Dr. Rotch."[67]

Brennemann eventually wrote the epitaph for the American Method in a brief history of infant feeding presented to American Pediatric Society members on the organization's fiftieth anniversary in 1938. "It became increasingly more complicated and involved as ever . . . so-called 'simpler' methods of calculation appeared until . . . some of the articles seemed terrifyingly like treatises on mathematics or higher astronomy." Brennemann recalled that long ago one of his former medical students, after having practiced medicine for several years, returned to the hospital diet kitchen where he had failed to understand percentage feeding as a student. After years of agonizing over his failure, he told the attending nurse, he finally was prepared to master the complex computations. The nurse stunned the poor fellow by telling him that percentage feeding was now wholly out of fashion. Nobody used it anymore. "It all gradually became a headache to most of us," explained an amused Brennemann. "The whole edifice finally collapsed because the superstructure was top heavy and the foundations weak, and because really simpler ideas came into play."[68]

Monitoring Mothers

Yet the legacy of percentage feeding lingered as the American Method paved the way for the monitoring of mothers and babies by physicians. Like Meigs, Rotch deplored artificial feeding if it manifested itself as a series of mother's experiments. He rued the day when women who did not breastfeed "dominated the physicians" and "food stuffs of all kinds were made use of." He wanted his years of carefully honed medical knowledge to replace mothers' impetuous actions. Peers across the country agreed that while Rotch's theory would benefit babies, mothers needed the constant guidance of physicians to institute percentage feeding. In 1909 Frank Walls issued what was by then a familiar warning: "The infant who is so unfortunate that it must be fed artificially should command the greatest watchfulness in order to avoid the almost inevitable food disorders in infancy."[69] Medically monitoring artificially fed babies, an apparent necessity given their death rate, was soon the pediatric philosophy governing the care of all babies.

Likewise "scientific motherhood"—the notion that while women retained primary responsibility for their children, they could not hope to raise them without physicians' omnipresent guidance—became a guiding principle of motherhood. Mothers' use of artificial food for babies, their fanatic dedication to cleaning their homes and their children's bodies, annual medical examinations for healthy children, and the wholesale belief in the necessity of vitamin supplements for children are only a few manifestations of this philosophy.[70] That these practices were vital to children's health and that women needed training and guidance from the medical community to implement then sustain these activities became cultural axioms.

Fear for the health of artificially fed babies was so great that early manifestations of mother-monitoring by physicians were extreme. Thomas Allen, for example, recommended that a doctor's "eternal vigilance [when caring for an artificially fed infant] will usually make the difference between success and failure." He insisted that physicians could not be too "fussy or over-particular," because until the doctor "has the baby well started he can not be too cautious." Allen recommended that physicians visit each artificially fed baby in their care every two or three days during the first three weeks of life to examine the baby's stools and urine and to record the baby's weight. He explained that the visits also permitted physicians to ensure "that the baby is being properly trained in regular habits of feeding, sleeping, evacuation of the bowels and urination." If all appeared well after three weeks, Allen suggested that doctors cut their visits to weekly ones if mothers agreed to supplement the weekly examinations with written reports delivered daily to the doctor. Mothers' reports described their infant's crying, sleeping, feeding, bladder, and bowel habits, and the "quantity, color, odor, amount of mucus and size of curds" of any vomit. After two weekly visits and fourteen daily reports, Allen advised that mothers send information to physicians weekly and that physicians curtail the prescheduled home visits. Mothers then expanded the weekly reports to also include the number, color, odor, and consistency of baby's stools and any additional observations that a mother considered noteworthy.[71]

The kind of medical surveillance urged by Allen, and soon institutionalized to a degree, did not simply prompt a microscopic examination of the habits and care of artificially fed babies. It also inspired doctors' and mothers' concerns with nuances in breastfed babies' behavior. Physicians began to recommend that breastfed babies be weighed before and after each nursing to make sure they ingested enough milk and that mothers' milk be examined, either microscopically or chemically, for potential irregularities.[72]

The medical community did not wholly embrace these activities, however. One doctor charged that physicians who insisted on weighing babies and examining mothers' milk were bound to find trouble where none existed and were to blame for the steadily decreasing breastfeeding rates.[73] Now, at the first imagined sign of trouble, a mother with sufficient money could turn to a physician for breast milk analysis. More often than not the physician, predisposed by a mother's distress, saw irregularities in her milk and advised an immediate switch from breast milk to artificial food.[74]

Creating Lactation Pathology

The public conversation among women bemoaning their breastfeeding problems and the ensuing debate among physicians suggesting assorted reasons
for women's complaints created an "information environment" detrimental
to breastfeeding.[75] The discussion was everywhere. Mothers wrote letters to
women's and infant-care magazines. Physicians published articles in the same
magazines as well as in newspapers and medical journals. The talk popular-
ized the assumption that women's breasts tended to founder when called
upon to perform their primary function, and prompted the medical community and mothers to anticipate lactation failure, if not immediately after a
baby's birth then surely within a few months of the birth.

Two late nineteenth-century populations—mothers who avidly read
magazines in their quest to keep their babies well and pediatricians seeking
acceptance of their new medical specialty—first formulated the notion that
breastfeeding mothers were likely to fail in their attempts to sustain their
babies on human milk alone. These mothers and doctors, albeit for different
reasons, proved unusually susceptible to the persistent suggestion that
lactation is a precarious body function.

Mothers were particularly sensitive to the fears generated by the germ
theory of disease. In order to keep germs at bay, women learned to perform
the complex activities that composed "scientific housekeeping." Now that
they believed in the necessity of antiseptic practices in all walks of life (see
chapter 1), women began to distrust their mammary glands' ability to sustain infants without scientific and medical aid. Simultaneously, pediatricians
found themselves in a vulnerable position. As new specialists in the 1890s,
they struggled to convince mothers of the need for pediatricians even as colleagues derisively labeled them "baby doctors." Fighting for public respect
and concomitantly attempting to carve a role for themselves in the medical
community, pediatricians, prompted by mothers' complaints of lactation
failure, embraced the need for medical expertise in infant feeding. Mothers'
fears in light of their new attitude toward housework, infant care, and germs
converged with pediatricians' insecurities about status within the medical
community to lower breastfeeding rates and popularize artificial food.
Women and physicians alike came to believe that most mothers were unable
to feed their babies without the scientific food and medical management
available exclusively from pediatricians.[76] The "infant-feeding question"
posed by mothers to doctors thus became a reliable entrée for pediatricians
into the world of mothers and their babies.

Aspiring pediatricians needed the hook, as the difficulties they encountered when trying to build a practice were numerous. Isaac Abt's experience was typical. When he was in medical school, older physicians urged him to abandon his interest in children's medicine. They assured him that the care of children was and always would be the domain of the general practitioner. Abt ignored the admonitions and, after graduating from medical school in 1891, traveled to Europe for extended pediatric training. When he returned to Chicago to open a pediatric practice, however, it appeared his medical school advisers had been right. Only relatives brought their children to him for treatment. Abt reminisced years later that at the time people judged doctors by their ability to treat adults. If they did not treat adults, the consumer had no way to measure their competence.[77]

The infant-feeding guidance that pediatricians offered to mothers became an important justification for pediatricians' existence. Now physicians could argue that artificial feeding, at long last under the aegis of medicine, was a considerably safer activity thanks to the efforts of pediatricians. Although pediatricians continued to urge mothers to breastfeed, they were equally vested in believing that human milk could be less than optimal. The medical modification of cows' milk for infant consumption was instrumental, in the words of the president of the Chicago Pediatric Society, in bringing "American paediatrists so well to the fore."[78]

Mother-pediatrician interaction did not provide the only impetus for the creation of lactation-failure theories. Eugenics—the influential early twentieth-century movement that fought for improvement of the human gene pool through natural selection, sterilization, segregation, and euthanasia—provided a context for the alleged tendency of women's mammary glands to fail.[79] That women—the bearers, nursers, and raisers of children—seemed sapped of their ability to breastfeed, a phenomenon unknown to previous generations, seemed almost logical in light of the new concern over "race suicide." Dr. John Kellogg argued, in typical eugenicist lingo, that "the increasing number of infants that cannot enjoy the advantages of breastfeeding because of the drying up of the maternal fount" was clear evidence of "race degeneracy" in "all civilized lands."[80]

Among the most influential eugenic theories were the notions that disease bolstered the human stock by killing off "degenerates" and that public health innovations ultimately diminished humanity by allowing the "unfit" to survive.[81] Theories like these were used to explain lactation failure. Under the influence of eugenics, popular health theories romanticized "primitive" lifestyles—that is, lifestyles ostensibly governed by natural selection—and damned soft, "civilized" urban lifestyles that allowed even the weak, the immoral, the immigrant, and the poverty-stricken to survive. Physicians pointed to "civilized" women's demands for anesthesia in childbirth as one bit of evidence that that branch of the human race was weakening. Doctors likewise pointed to the tendency of "overcivilized" women to have meager milk supplies as further proof of civilization's debilitating impact on humanity.

Abt told colleagues that "the progress of civilization and the stress of modern life" impeded lactation. Eminent pediatrician L. Emmett Holt encouraged all mothers to "lead a simple natural life" free from the worry and anxiety that "more than anything else" caused "the failure of the modern mother as a nurse." One physician theorized that women who lived in cities were akin to "hot-house plant[s]" forced to "conform to definite rules," as opposed to rural women who led stress-free, "natural lives" and who, consequently, had no trouble breastfeeding. Mary Wood-Allen, physician-editor of the Women's Christian Temperance Union's magazine *New Crusade,* assured one worried mother that because she "live[d] out of doors all that is possible" breastfeeding would not be a problem for her. Living a natural life, Wood-Allen assured her, her body would have little trouble with natural functions.[82]

This notion that "primitive," "natural" lifestyles strengthened bodies and "civilized" lifestyles weakened them permeated public consciousness. One mother, for example, complained to *Babyhood* magazine that "civilization, which has brought so many blessings," also caused debilitating anxiety. She protested, "Placid existence which is absolutely necessary to a nursing mother is impossible. Nerves are rampant; neuralgia, the worst of enemies, acts like a thunder-storm in the dog-days on the mother's milk." A Chicago father, on a cruise of Caribbean islands in 1912, observed enviously, "Raising children does not seem difficult here. The mother is food supply for the year until the next one comes."[83]

These "natural lives" espoused by doctors and romanticized by the public were devoid of the entertainment opportunities available in big cities. Writing about tantalizing urban amusements, one physician warned, "All this activity costs and as each person has a limit beyond which she or he cannot go, nature must retrench somewhere. Many functions of the body may suffer."[84] Girls were especially susceptible to harm because their bodies, the theory went, developed in one exhausting burst, while boys' bodies developed slowly and steadily throughout adolescence.[85] As Chicago doctor Henry Parker Newman put it, modern-day schools taxed young girls' brains "to the utmost" at precisely the time that "nature is concentrating all her energies upon the development of the generative organs and the establishment of their physiological functions." Newman and others worried that schoolgirls' brains would snatch the energy their growing reproductive organs needed. He acknowledged that girls needed an education but argued that their education should not be overly taxing, should not rob the women that these girls would become of their "natural privileges."[86]

Underlying all the theories of lactation failure were the notions that life in a "natural" environment, namely, the countryside, was good for one's health and good for girls' growing bodies, while an "artificial" environment, namely, the city, was detrimental. Life in cities, physicians contended, created a necessity for all kinds of unnatural accoutrements, artificial food for babies among them. The presumption in both the medical and lay communities that urbanization weakened the human body added further credence to the notion that substandard breast milk was largely unavoidable. After all, women who lived in cities could not altogether avoid the traffic, shopping, entertainment, and schooling that allegedly doomed their procreative abilities.[87]

The contradictory beliefs that human milk was both ideal *and* faulty were voiced by many, in overt as well as subtle ways. Churchill, for example, contended that artificial food "should simulate as closely as possible good average breast-milk."[88] As Churchill's tribute to "good average breast-milk" implied, however, bad, substandard breast milk existed as well. When physicians spoke of the superiority of human milk they no longer meant *any* human milk, only *average* human milk.[89] Anything more or less than this middle-of-the-road milk might harm.

Rotch explained how breast milk might veer from average. The human mammary gland, he contended, was not just a "normal" secretory organ but an "abnormal" excretory one as well. Abnormal excretions were most pronounced at three times: immediately after birth, several months after birth "when normal metabolism is interfered with," and just before weaning. Thus danger always lurked: when mothers started lactating, when lactation was well established, and when babies were about to wean. At any or all of these times a mother's breasts might "lack . . . equipoise" and become part secretory, part excretory, and the more excretory they became "the more abnormal . . . the finished product."[90]

Breast milk quality was thought to be most precarious right after birth. Rotch argued that colostrum[91] indicated de facto an immaturity or disturbance in a mother's system.[92] To avoid this allegedly faulty milk, Rotch recommended that infants not breastfeed for the first twelve to thirty-six hours of their lives. If a baby appeared "restless and evidently hungry" during this time, he advised mothers to dissolve milk-sugar in sterile water. If a mother's breasts continued to produce colostrum thirty-six hours after a baby's birth, Rotch suggested filling a prescription at the nearest milk laboratory containing 1 percent fat, 5 percent sugar and .75 percent protein.[93] Jacobi also feared colostrum, which he called "not normal milk."[94]

By the early twentieth century some physicians did recognize the enormous value of colostrum. Chicago obstetrician Effa Davis insisted that "the early secretion from the mother's breasts is useful in sustaining the child, and babies should be encouraged to nurse from the first day of life in every case possible." Colostrum's scanty quantity, however, continued to distress many and contributed to human milk pathology theories. Davis reassured women, "Do not think it [the baby] will starve the first three days while the mother's milk is 'coming in.' Nature knows her own business best and would have provided a larger helping of food for that period if it were needed." In 1922 another doctor called colostrum "essential" to babies and advised, "A dram of colostrum is worth a quart of water." Yet doubt remained. In 1928 Brennemann cautioned that, given its meager quantity, colostrum alone was an inadequate food for babies during the first few days of life. He suggested that although mother's milk was obviously the desirable diet for babies—"if one could get an ample and unexceptionable product by merely turning the faucet"—it was insufficient during the first few days of life.[95]

The artificial food debates became an intellectual tug-of-war, even within individual minds. A baby's natural food might be the ideal, but nature takes many disastrous turns. Thus, even as physicians continued to pay homage to human milk, they emphasized its tenuous quality. Because nature was precarious, they argued, mothers and physicians had to prepare for the worst. By the late 1920s, the majority of doctors no longer believed that successful breastfeeding was the inevitable outcome of a full-term pregnancy. And women learned from physicians' widely publicized theories that "few functions with which we have to deal are so variable and uncertain as the production of breast milk."[96]

"Bad Milk" Diagnoses

Long before famed Chicago obstetrician Joseph DeLee referred to birth in 1920 as "a decidedly pathological process," a significant number of physicians feared breastfeeding could easily become a pathological process.[97] A mother's fear that her milk supply might be scanty, some physicians argued, indicated on its face that her milk was "usually a bad milk."[98] As women complained of breastfeeding failures and doctors responded that substandard human milk was an inevitable outgrowth of civilized society, human lactation seemed to cry out for medical scrutiny.

The microscopic and chemical examination of human milk became an increasingly common service beginning in the late 1890s, offered by physicians to the middle and upper class.[99] Many doctors took this analysis very seriously, basing diagnoses and therapies on its results. Unbeknownst to these physicians, however, human milk analysis was an inexact science at best during this era (see table 3.1, for example). The basic components of human milk are remarkably uniform in amount across cultures and varied diets. Even maternal nutritional status has little impact on the basic components of milk unless a mother is severely malnourished.[100] Yet the tests physicians performed in the late nineteenth and early twentieth centuries showed quite the opposite; human milk was highly and unpredictably variable. Few in the medical community questioned these findings. Quite the contrary, with the increasingly routine examination of human milk, physicians anticipated findings that indicated something was seriously wrong with the milk under examination.

Churchill analyzed the breast milk consumed by every infant he examined "regardless of the illness in question" and was not surprised to find many human milk samples dangerously "deficient in one or more . . . essential elements." Another Chicago doctor examined the milk of a mother in 1892 whose baby was "a very poor, scrawny child." He described the alarming sight of her milk under a microscope. "It looked as if some unseen person was playing billiards with it, there were so many micrococci, and so active that they would run up against a globule of fat and set it whirling." Before he could order the child weaned, the baby died. Jacobi described one emaciated baby with "an offensive diarrhea . . . [and] ammoniacal urine." An obstetrician who had analyzed the milk of the baby's mother and found it contained 7 percent fat congratulated the mother for having what he thought was above average milk. "She was consoled for a day or two," explained Jacobi, "the boy not at all. His riches disagreed with him more and more, until he recovered with temporary starvation and barley water."[101]

Yet even physicians who put stock in breast milk analysis admitted that babies seemed to thrive on a variety of breast milks. Rotch argued that the variation in "good" human milk could be great; fat varied between 3 and 4 percent, sugar between 6 and 7 percent, and protein between 1 and 2 percent. Churchill likewise observed that many babies blossomed on a "peculiar

Table 3.1   "Normal" Human Milk and "Bad" Human Milk Caused by Lack of Exercise

	Normal milk	Mother not exercising. Milk causing infant to vomit.	Mother walking 2 miles daily, but has blisters from French shoes. Infant still vomiting.	Mother walking 2 miles daily. Good shoes, no blisters. Infant doing well.
Fat	4.00	3.05	0.65	3.34
Sugar	7.00	6.10	5.25	6.30
Proteids	1.50	3.89	3.82	2.61
Ash	0.15	0.16	0.18	0.16
Total solids	12.65	13.20	9.90	12.41
Water	87.35	86.80	90.10	87.59
	100.00	100.00	100.00	100.00

Source: Thomas Morgan Rotch, *Pediatrics: The Hygienic and Medical Treatment of Children* (Philadelphia: J. B. Lippincott Company, 1896): 191.
Note: There is no contemporary evidence that the protein in human milk ever comes in the concentration described in columns 2–4. The analysis doctors based their medical decisions and treatment on was apparently faulty.

diet" that veered "considerably" from "average" breast milk. Likely alluding to Rotch's theory that artificial food should be individually designed for the special needs of each baby, he argued that nature provided "different qualities of milk for different individuals, according to the peculiar idiosyncrasies of each infant."[102]

Despite contentions that babies thrived on a wide variety of human milk, Churchill called the analysis of a mother's milk an "absolute necessity" if a baby's health "did not run as smoothly as we could wish." Like Rotch did at Harvard, he taught his students at Chicago's Rush Medical College that infants fed "average" breast milk gave physicians little trouble. However, a baby fed "not on such a breast milk, but on one too poor or too rich, does give considerable difficulty." Although he continued to urge "every attempt" to keep a baby at the breast, "so much superior is mother's milk," he feared that at times such persistence was dangerous.[103]

Julius Sedgwick, a Minneapolis physician and one of the nation's strongest proponents of breastfeeding, was one of the few physicians who roundly criticized breast milk analysis.[104] In 1909 Sedgwick encountered a sick baby who was being fed artificially because the baby's doctor had determined that the milk of the baby's mother contained an alarming 4 percent protein. The doctor immediately ordered the baby, who was thriving, off the breast. The infant quickly sickened on the bottle, and the baby's terrified mother went to Sedgwick. He examined two samples of the mother's milk, decided that her milk contained 1.4, not 4, percent protein and put the baby back on the breast. An angry Sedgwick charged that great harm was inflicted upon babies by "inaccurate examination [of human milk], and then basing our therapy on such examinations."[105] Yet few joined him in criticizing the routine—and imprecise—analysis making physicians and mothers so edgy about human milk.

The scrutiny did not stop with breast milk. Physicians examined babies' stools as well, a preoccupation that became an integral part of percentage feeding and another way to judge the quality of a mother's milk. Rotch argued that the unique color, consistency, and odor of bowel movements indicated to what degree babies were able to digest the fat, protein, and sugar in the milk they consumed.[106] Thus, not only did stool examination reveal how well a mother's milk suited her baby, it pointed physicians to appropriate percentage-feeding prescriptions.

Routine stool analysis seemed a potent tool, and physicians typically counted, smelled, dissected, chemically analyzed, weighed, and photographed babies' bowel movements. Some physicians concluded that masses in stools evidenced excessive fat in a baby's diet. Others argued that masses were a sign of too much protein. Abt was a proponent of the latter theory, explaining that even when he fed fat-free milk to babies suffering from what he presumed to be "fat indigestion," offending curds in the stools persisted. Other doctors dismissed all the fuss, insisting that any curds in an infant's stools were only normal "milk curds whose origin depends upon the formation of acid paracasein and that the inclusion of fat is but an inevitable mechanical accident."[107]

At first physicians examined only the stools of artificially fed babies. Some physicians, however, came to believe that the bowel movements of breastfed infants, too, would "show much light upon the conditions existing within the intestine." They contended that the peculiar characteristics of a baby's stools allowed them to pinpoint the exact location of any "systemic disturbance," as unique irregularities originated in "this or that portion of the digestive tract." One annoyed Chicago doctor complained in 1922 that there would be a lot more breastfed babies had physicians never studied babies' bowel movements. The practice long remained, however. Brennemann admitted in 1929 that he still belonged to "that ancient order of pediatricians who like to count, look at, mash, and smell a baby's stool and who feel that they get some useful information as to the baby's condition from each of these activities."[108]

By the 1890s physicians had lost sight of the original purpose of all the analysis: to ascertain the differences between bovine and human milk and to adjust cows' milk accordingly. Studying milk and babies' stools had instead become a means of judging human milk. Labels ran the gamut—"good," "bad," "average," "too rich," "poor"—but, increasingly, the judgments were negative. Few noticed that the routine examination of human milk and babies' stools was curtailing breastfeeding, the feeding method virtually every doctor still endorsed as a more reliable way to lower infant mortality than the use of "good" artificial food. Physicians had difficulty discerning cause and effect. Fewer women breastfeeding each year indicated to them that their efforts to formulate artificial food were more imperative than ever, not that these activities prompted ever greater numbers of women not to breastfeed.

Mothers' Missteps and Doctors' Declarations

With the general acceptance of routine milk and stool analysis, physicians, even those who championed breastfeeding, were less likely to encourage a mother to continue breastfeeding if she voiced doubt about her milk and more likely to accept the fact that something might be amiss. Indeed, many doctors became convinced that something could *easily* go wrong with human milk. Rotch's study of breast milk, vital to his work on percentage feeding, convinced him that unless a woman followed a prescribed regimen any one of a number of bad habits could spoil her milk. A mother's sedentary lifestyle, he told his students, decreased the water and increased the solids in her milk. Rich foods had the same effect. Meat increased the fat. He instructed mothers to walk an average one to two miles daily—"about what the average healthy woman in New England needs to reduce her albuminoid percentage"—in order to reduce the protein in "very bad" or "very rich" milk.[109] Although Rotch admitted that most babies seemed untroubled by human milk's apparent variety, he nevertheless warned that when mother's milk veered from the "normal average" babies might sicken.[110]

Now physicians handed mothers a laundry list of caveats. Mothers with "uncontrollable temperaments"; unhappy mothers; mothers deemed too old; mothers deemed too young; mothers who did not want to nurse; mothers "who are hurried in the detail of their life"; mothers with improper diet, rest, and exercise routines; mothers with a chronic disease; mothers with a disease that their infants could inherit all learned not to nurse their babies. Rotch cautioned, "Even if their milk happens to be sufficient in quantity, it will probably be so changeable in quality as to be a source of discomfort and even of danger rather than the best nutriment for their offspring." Rotch argued that although the mammary gland "in its perfect state" was a "beautifully adapted piece of mechanism constructed for the elaboration and secretion of an animal food," women's breasts could be corrupted by disease, nervousness, or "improper living." Rotch explained that women suffering from "nervous disturbances" and "uncontrolled emotions" produced milk with too much protein and, in some cases, reduced fat. He explained, "Women . . . when living in the midst of our modern civilization, so harmful for the production of good nursing, present an exaggerated example of disturbance of the equipoise of the mammary gland."[111]

Jacobi likewise contended that in the absence of ideal surroundings and a mother's serene outlook, breast milk could become an "alien food," as harmful to a baby as "the most badly prepared artificial food."[112] He noted that "many a mother raises at her own breast sickly, bloated, rachitical children, until finally one is born that she is quite unable to nurse; then, for the first time, appears in the family a noisy, ruddy, muscular baby."[113] Churchill observed, "You may find a nervous hysteric woman, worrying about her baby, easily upset by trifles, making 'mountains out of mole-hills,' utterly unfit to serve the purpose of a cow."[114] Hess suggested that artificial food could prove a temporary necessity if a mother suffered from "anger, fright, worry, shock, distress, sorrow, or if she witnessed an accident." He warned lactating women that "the mother should be temperate in all things" and argued that the key to successful nursing was "a tranquil mind."[115]

Yet even relaxed, happy, and healthy mothers could misstep. Women learned that momentary discomforts, minor annoyances, sudden frights, and fleeting upsets could, all or in turn, egregiously alter their breast milk. Churchill warned his medical students that if they did not "*insist*" on babies being breastfed with fanatic regularity, a "good milk" could become "poor." He explained that nursing a baby too frequently increased the solids in milk, while nursing too infrequently diluted milk. "Thus, in the one case, is produced a milk too concentrated in quality, overtaxing the digestive powers of the infant, and in the other case a milk too watery and insufficient for purposes of nutrition."[116]

Mother's milk was now on a par with artificial food, not necessarily normal, natural, safe, or beneficial at all. Clifford Grulee cautioned that although nutritional disturbances were "usually mild" in breastfed infants, they were also "of very frequent occurrence" and could "lead to serious consequences" if they became chronic. So potentially lethal was mother's milk that Rotch even warned his students that bad breast milk could make a baby sicker than inappropriate artificial food. He told the tale of a mother who weaned her baby without the knowledge of her baby's doctor. The infant was "suddenly deprived of the plentiful supply of breast-milk of its healthy mother," and fed oatmeal. "Vomiting and prostration immediately began." The horrified mother immediately returned her baby to breast milk with "a disastrous result, as her milk from nervous influences was so changed in its quality that it acted like a poison on the infant, who fell into a condition of collapse." By the time the baby's physician called Rotch in, the infant's "skin was gray and cold, the fontanelle sunken, and the eyes fixed."[117]

Some physicians went to enormous lengths to rescue babies from the milk of their excitable mothers. Churchill treated a two month old whose mother's milk had been spoiled by the mother's nervousness. He reported,

> After trying in vain to improve the quality of the milk [I] stopped it at once, and mindful of the baby's weak proteid digesting power put him on: fat 2, sugar 6, proteids 0.25. He stopped crying at once, gained slowly in weight, the fat being increased every third day the proteids kept at 0.25 till the tenth day, when he was given and took well: fat 3.50, sugar 6, proteids 0.75. A week later he was given: fat 4, sugar 6, proteids 1, with disastrous results, vomiting and colic starting up in two days. He was then put on: fat 3.50, sugar 6, alb 0.75, did well, and in a week was again tried on fat 4, sugar 6, alb 1, which he took well for a week, when again digestive disturbances forced us back to: Fat 3 per cent., sugar 6, proteids 0.50, upon which he throve for six weeks, when he was promoted to: Fat 4 per cent., sugar 7 per-cent, proteids 1 per cent., doing well on this for two weeks, when in hot weather a slight diarrhea necessitated a temporary return to: Fat 3.50, sugar 6, proteids 0.50. He has now been for three weeks on: Fat 4, sugar 7, proteids .75, weighs at seven months, 16 pounds, has two teeth . . . and notwithstanding the erratic course of his diet, his flesh is hard and firm and his general condition excellent.[118]

Paradoxically, through some forty years of exacting work on artificial food doctors continued to insist that human milk was preferable. Physicians' mantra remained, "When possible mother's milk."[119] But as time wore on, the emphasis was less on "mother's milk" and more on "when possible." As artificial food reached an expanding audience, the expectation that human milk would somehow fail infants became standard. Physicians' activities reinforced women's worry that no pair of mammary glands could be trusted to keep a baby alive. In the end, a product originally intended only for the least fortunate babies—those without access to their mother's milk—became the norm for all babies.

♦

In his 1944 autobiography, Isaac Abt reminisced that late nineteenth- and early twentieth-century pediatricians advised mothers about infant feeding only after mothers brought sick, artificially fed babies to them for examination.[120] This first generation of American pediatricians did not approve of artificial food, they did not tout artificial food, and they did not deliberately thrust artificial food on mothers. Even Thomas Rotch carefully explained to his students that breastfeeding "is so far superior to any other [method of feeding infants] which has ever been known that I shall assume that it is the best, and the one from which in almost every particular all others should be copied."[121] Jacobi likewise reminded colleagues, "No matter how beneficial boiling, or sterilization, or pasteurization may be they cannot transform cows' milk into woman's milk . . . it is a makeshift after all."[122]

Nevertheless, between 1900 and 1915 American Pediatric Society members presented ninety papers at annual meetings on assorted artificial-food topics.[123] Why did physicians find themselves intimately involved in the arduous work of perfecting artificial food, a feeding method they appeared to abhor? The initial efforts to formulate a safe human milk substitute were a largely futile attempt to reduce the mortality in asylums and hospitals where babies had no access to either their mothers or wet nurses.[124] Later, as mothers' breastfeeding problems seemed to reach epidemic proportions, the need for artificial food appeared far more urgent.

Although mothers initially introduced physicians to the "feeding question," physicians' subsequent activities likewise influenced mothers. Rotch's work in particular imbued artificial feeding with such an aura of complexity and sophistication, quite beyond the grasp of mere mothers, that it gave pediatrics just the boost in prestige that it needed. As milk laboratories professionalized infant feeding—putting it, in Rotch's words, "in the hands of educated, intelligent men"—the "science" of infant feeding professionalized pediatrics, making the specialty more acceptable, even necessary, to mothers.[125]

Yet the generation of physicians who toiled at making artificial food safer, all the while debating the merit of their work, never intended artificial food to wholly replace breast milk. The anxieties created by growing artificial food use, however, spread to breast milk. Cows' milk caused all kinds of dreaded ailments in babies; soon doctors feared human milk might be as faulty. Physicians examined and photographed the stools of artificially fed babies; they eventually scrutinized the stools of breastfed babies as well.

The many dangers associated with artificial food tainted mother's milk. Consequently, improved artificial food came to be viewed as not just a viable solution to the most serious problem of the orphaned infant but a potential necessity for any baby. Women and physicians alike anticipated that inadequate breast milk would prove the norm for most nursing mothers.

After years of near single-minded involvement, doctors eventually wearied of the intricacies of the infant-feeding business. When the Pediatric Section of the Medical Society of the State of Pennsylvania asked Grulee in 1930 to speak before them on infant feeding, he proposed other topics for a talk. He explained, "I am sort of fed up on these feeding problems since I think they have been exalted far beyond their real value. In other words, I think that common sense will feed a lot more babies than evaporated or acid milk mixtures, but I know no yard stick by which these can be judged and individual judgment is always biased."[126]

The impatience demonstrated by Grulee, plus the relative safety of artificial food that accompanied universal pasteurization, signaled an end to physicians' intense interest in breastfeeding. In 1932 Brennemann advised colleagues that "artificial feeding has become so simple and so safe that it is no longer put off to a dangerous period" but started at the first hint of trouble.[127]

But even as this type of optimism about artificial feeding became the norm, the generation of physicians who participated in the initial formulation of scientifically sanctioned artificial food never felt wholly comfortable with the innovation. Twenty years after Grulee promised mothers that artificial food could be made to "approximate [human milk] very closely," he regretted that possibility. "I think one of the most abused things in medicine today is the question of breastfeeding, abused by not being insisted upon," he told his Illinois colleagues in 1936. "We have gained the idea because we have learned something about the artificial feeding of children that we can go ahead and feed them artificially with impunity, get away with it and the children will be as well off as before."[128] Older physicians in particular continued to insist that "the finer shades of the argument are always in favor of human milk."[129] One Chicago doctor, describing conditions in the city at the end of the nineteenth century, wrote in 1927, "In those days everybody lived in houses and few babies were born in hospitals. Few mothers trusted their children to nurses, and bottle-feeding was looked upon as a family catastrophe, as it was and *is*" (emphasis added).[130] In 1936 another Chicago doctor, noting that physicians had dumped the complicated formulas popular at the beginning of the century and were "getting back to simplicity in formula preparation," wished in vain that mothers and physicians would revert to the "ultimate in simplicity—breast feeding."[131]

But by then it was too late. Few physicians had noticed that the activities associated with artificial food production—milk analysis and the like— not only discouraged mothers from breastfeeding but shook physicians' faith in human milk as well. A new generation of doctors now almost uniformly lauded artificial food and distrusted breast milk. One doctor warned women in 1934, "The fact that the fluid comes from the maternal mammary gland does not make it good. It may be nothing but water."[132]

Physicians saw only their task, not its side effects. The original aim of artificial food—to safely feed a baby who had no mother—was forever lost, to the chagrin of the first generation of pediatricians. These physicians never ceased acknowledging the superiority of breast milk and, likely for that very reason, never understood that they had helped engineer what was to become the near national abandonment of breastfeeding.

4

"Insist upon Breast Feeding": Public Health Organizations and Infant Feeding

While physicians in private practice treated individual patients, the doctors and nurses working for Chicago's medical charities and the Department of Health shouldered an additional, broader responsibility. It was their job to treat the urban masses as a single organism, and to prevent illness and death among them accordingly. Mass education became one important tool for fulfilling that task, and working-class mothers' practices directed the course of that education in much the same way that upper- and middle-class mothers' practices shaped private physicians' activities.[1]

Before the early twentieth century, medical charities, not the health department, disseminated the bulk of health maintenance information to Chicagoans. The charities that offered health tips to the masses, in the years before the city eventually appropriated the task, were popular causes. Wealthy women and men donated portions of their vast fortunes and large chunks of their time to these organizations.[2] The germ theory of disease aroused the upper class's keen interest in public health efforts, awakening them to the fact that illness was not caused by inferior ancestry or individual moral, physical, and intellectual weakness, but by bacteria that could—and would and did—attack anyone.[3] Thus medical charities, vehicles for self-protection as well as benevolent gestures, became a popular cause of the rich. Tens of thousands of urban poor were recipients of this largesse each year.

The city's medical community hailed the efforts. The editors of the *Chicago Medical Recorder* deemed philanthropy so important to public welfare that they argued in 1891 that preventive medicine was beyond the ken of mere doctors. Better, they argued, that the moralist, publicist, philosopher and, "most of all," the philanthropist define the parameters of preventive medicine.[4] Wealthy industrialists and their wives were not the city's only medical philanthropists, however; many of Chicago's doctors also donated their services to medical charities. Free medical dispensaries,[5] the Chicago Visiting Nurse Association (VNA), and the Chicago Infant Welfare Society (IWS) burgeoned under this aid and encouragement.

The charitable institutions in Chicago that provided for the health needs of the poor were numerous, easily accessed, and heavily used. By 1921 the public health nurses working for the Chicago VNA were making 247,914 visits to 32,827 patients annually. Mothers with newborns made up nearly one-third of these patients.[6] The IWS provided well-baby care at dozens of infant welfare stations; in 1923 IWS doctors examined 11,005 babies monthly.[7] Settlement house workers provided additional neighborhood health services: hygiene classes for mothers, mobile hospitals that treated sick babies during the summer, and pasteurized milk for infants whose mothers did not breastfeed.

In Chicago, the services of medical charities became models for the city's health department to emulate. Eventually, the health department operated its own infant welfare stations, in addition to those run by the IWS, and employed public health nurses whose work mimicked the VNA's. In 1925, when roughly 58,000 babies were born in Chicago, the twenty-six IWS stations and the twenty-five health department stations cared for almost 57 percent of them.[8]

There was a measure of rivalry among the free medical services, particularly between medical charities and the health department. It was commonly believed—as Edna Foley, the VNA superintendent from 1912 to 1937, argued—that the personal service offered by volunteers was less expensive and more attentive than the services offered by publicly funded medical agencies.[9] That sentiment was so widespread that from their beginnings in the mid-nineteenth century through the first quarter of the twentieth century, the public health efforts of medical charities in Chicago were at least as visible, and certainly more numerous, than the health department's. Their messages—delivered via free health care services, milk stations, newspaper columns, pamphlets, and posters—reached virtually every woman in Chicago.

A favorite theme of all public health organizations, charitable and municipal alike, was infant feeding. These groups deemed lactation failure not just a problem of individual women and their babies but a grave public health crisis. In Chicago, as elsewhere, philanthropic organizations and municipalities responded to high infant mortality with campaigns urging mothers to breastfeed and to avoid artificial food. In keeping with the nature of the emergency, the propaganda was dramatic. A Civic Federation of Chicago poster explaining that "Mother's Milk is Best of All" was headlined "Don't Kill Your Baby."[10] A 1911 Department of Health broadside pleaded, "You can't improve on God's plan. For Your Baby's Sake—Nurse It!"[11] Women learned from one newsletter that before birth a baby needs mothers' blood, "after birth it needs her milk."[12] The Health Department's booklet *Our Babies* called human milk "The Child's Life Insurance" and admonished women that "no mother who has only a spark of mother love in her heart would deprive a child of its natural nourishment either on purpose or selfishly."[13]

Some historians argue that these histrionic pleas to breastfeed were, in large part, a ploy to shame women back into their traditional roles.[14] The breastfeeding campaign rhetoric in Chicago, however, which admittedly emphasized mothers' duty, was an attempt to elicit womens' aid in alleviating a serious public health problem caused by too little breastfeeding and too much artificial feeding. Helpless in the face of sick, artificially fed babies, physicians believed and public health workers strongly suggested that if more mothers breastfed their babies for longer periods, infant health would improve and the number of infant deaths would decline. The medical community viewed the slogan "To Lessen Baby Deaths Let Us Have More Mother-Fed Babies" as a dramatic but simple truth.[15]

An equally dramatic truth was "clean milk makes healthy children; dirty milk makes nice, clean grave stones."[16] Although public health activists favored human milk and damned artificial food, like private physicians they could not in good conscience simply push breastfeeding and ignore bottle use. One doctor urged Chicago Medical Society members in 1891 to teach women how to use artificial food safely. Only then would "a sour nursing-bottle in the house of the rich or the poor . . . be considered as much of a disgrace as personal uncleanliness, and far more dangerous to the life of the child."[17] While their rhetoric on the importance of breastfeeding never wavered, within ten years of this doctor's plea public health workers not only explained to mothers how to prepare artificial food but also *provided* palatable artificial food to babies, even as they continued to beg women to breastfeed. Public health advocates, like individual physicians, found themselves in the contradictory position of declaring that "the proper food for babies is mother's milk, no sensible mother needs advice on this point," while giving away certified cows' milk at street-corner milk stations.[18]

The contradictory activities took their toll on public health workers, much as they had with private physicians. By the 1930s the medical charities that provided health care to women and their babies were taking a nonjudgmental stance toward bottle-feeding. Artificial food no longer killed large numbers of babies, and apparently, medical personnel had decided there was little they could do to stem the tide of artificially fed babies anyway. Although stressing the importance of breastfeeding to mothers remained a primary purpose of its infant welfare stations, even the Chicago Department of Health ceased to make the distinction between breastfeeding and mixed feeding when conducting field surveys of mothers with newborns. Now breastfeeding almost always meant mixed feeding. This was an important, albeit unacknowledged, sign that the health department had given up prodding mothers to breastfeed exclusively, and avoid artificial food, for the sake of their babies' health.[19]

Despite this latter-day capitulation, from their origins in the nineteenth century until, roughly, the 1930s, medical charities and the Chicago Department of Health advised all mothers to breastfeed their babies and chastised them if they did not. This staunch, remarkably uniform stance on breastfeeding was a cornerstone of the city's public health policy for forty years.

The Chicago Visiting Nurse Association: "Breast Feeding Is a Mother's Duty"

Visiting nurses, among the original public health workers in Chicago, cared for the sick poor in their homes gratis. The Chicago Ethical Society sponsored Chicago's first group of young, dedicated visiting nurses in 1883. The Society abandoned the charity in 1887, and Mary Shumway, a wealthy young woman who had observed the enormous benefits of visiting-nurse work during her European travels, promptly offered to fund the orphaned group. She dubbed the organization the Augusta Memorial Visiting Nurses in memory of her mother, Augusta Huntington. After Shumway married and moved to Boston, a number of physicians whose patients had been cared for by Augusta Memorial nurses prevailed on Shumway's wealthy friends to keep the organization alive. Through the collective efforts of these doctors and wealthy Chicagoans, the Chicago Visiting Nurse Association was born in late 1889.[20] The service was a popular one. In 1908 VNA nurses made 85,318 visits to 13,804 patients.[21] In 1920 they made 226,615 calls to 32,845 patients, including 8,167 mothers and their newborns.[22]

VNA nurses served the sick poor in their homes, almost always without charge. The VNA asked only a "very small minority" of patients who could afford it to pay ten cents for the service. Charitable contributions, raised by the wealthy women who served on the VNA board of directors, paid for the bulk of nurses' salaries and other VNA services. One popular gesture among the charity's patrons was to donate enough money to pay the annual salary of a nurse in memory of a relative. In return, donors received detailed monthly accounts of their nurse's activities, although some renditions were a little too vivid for some benefactors. VNA superintendent Edna Foley had to apologize to at least one woman: "I am sorry that we seem to be sending you particularly harrowing . . . [reports]. Instead of letting them distress you, will you not feel that your support is of tremendous assistance to them, for without it we could not do a great many of the pleasant things that we are able to give them."[23]

The VNA easily attracted donors because visiting nurses served "the people whose mode of living contributes to the poverty, uncleanness, and unsanitary conditions of any community," and so benefactors viewed the VNA as a particularly effective bulwark against transmission of disease to the community at large.[24] The women on the VNA board of directors were neither romantic about nor sympathetic toward the population that they served. Quite the contrary, they perceived VNA patients as threatening and burdensome. According to the fashion of the day, VNA board members embraced eugenics as a means of eradicating any future need for the VNA or similar efforts. "We want the science of eugenics to be studied and mastered and put into effect," explained VNA president Mary Aldis in 1911, "so that we shall not have the degenerate and foredoomed sufferers to care for that we have now."[25]

So that their sermons did not fall on deaf ears, visiting nurses learned "to . . . secure such a firm footing in each home . . . [that] the inmates follow[ed] and acknowledge[d] the nurse's advice and authority without question." Assorted public health leaders considered district nurses' advice a primary vehicle for the permanent moral and physical uplift of impoverished mothers and their children. "When the Visiting Nurse . . . goes into the squalor of the tenement house . . . [and] bathes and dresses the untended infant and neglected children," wrote the Chicago Commissioner of Health in 1895, "[she] gives an object lesson in cleanliness . . . she is walking in the footsteps of the Master. . . . She lifts up and civilizes, humanizes and Christianizes those whom she serves."[26] The VNA was so successful in this regard that doctors and other philanthropic workers often asked for their help when attempting to tame recalcitrant patients.

Nurses served patients from all ethnic and racial groups and almost always spoke the language(s) that predominated in the neighborhood they were assigned to. African American nurses, however, served only African

American patients; white nurses only white patients. Edna Foley explained to one benefactor that the district her family had supported in her father's memory for many years "is now almost entirely given over to colored people and we have very little work in it for our white nurse. . . . Do you mind if we transfer the support of District 3 to District 5. . . . There are comparatively few colored people there, a good many Italians, and a great many poor people."[27]

VNA nurses were incredibly hardworking women. Each nurse made her way to eight to ten homes daily, homes that were sometimes a mile or more from the nearest streetcar. Wearing ankle-length skirts and carrying medical equipment, baby clothes, and linens, visiting nurses often crossed muddy prairies "unbroken by paved streets but decorated here and there with small shacks not unlike one-story chicken-coops." A visit to a single home often entailed numerous other journeys as well: to summon an ambulance or a doctor, to purchase medicine from a drugstore, or to find a caretaker for a patient's children.[28]

Although visiting nurses did not attend births—"she has not the time," explained one VNA officer—they did give periodic prenatal examinations and postpartum care to women who requested the service.[29] At prenatal visits, nurses gave pregnant women written instructions on how to prepare for home birth. Mothers learned from nurses how to clean their houses, bathe, and prepare their breasts for breastfeeding.[30] After a birth, a nurse visited a woman daily for ten days and then every other day until she deemed the new mother strong enough to care for her baby without assistance.[31]

The VNA considered pregnant women and new mothers prime candidates for lessons in health and hygiene. Consequently, their indoctrination by the VNA was incessant—subtle as well as overt. For example, postpartum women were the only patients asked to pay for nursing service, whether or not they could afford it. Request for payment had little to do with funding the VNA and everything to do with the instruction that visiting nurses constantly imparted to poverty-stricken mothers. Demand for payment taught mothers—who had seven or eight months to plan for their postpartum care—to save money in anticipation of items that their children would need in the future.[32] The schooling often stuck. Harriet Fulmer, the VNA's second superintendent, reported in 1909 that "in revisiting many of the babies cared for during July and August, we found more than two-thirds of the mothers not only grateful but carrying out what the nurses had taught them . . . with a steady pressure of advice and instruction throughout the year, we would be an immense factor in reducing infant mortality."[33]

One of the district nurses' most important public health mandates was

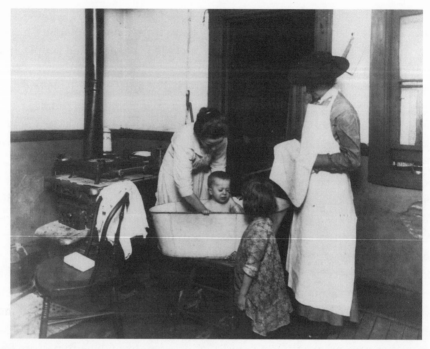

Figure 9 A Chicago Infant Welfare Society visiting nurse teaches a mother how to bathe her baby. 1911. *Source:* Chicago Historical Society.

advising new mothers on infant feeding. The Chicago VNA *Visiting Nurse Manual*—dubbed "the Bible of the public health nurse" nationwide—instructed all public health nurses to "insist upon breast feeding."[34] Visiting nurses learned to encourage mothers to breastfeed for the first year of their babies' lives and never to help a patient dry up her milk unless ordered to do so by a physician. Nurses told pregnant patients that "breast feeding is a mother's duty" and encouraged fathers to "make it possible for the mother to give this care to her child." Nurses also anticipated and prevented problems that mothers occasionally encountered while breastfeeding. If a mother's milk came in so rapidly that it caused discomfort, nurses applied a "comfortable" breast-binder for a few days. Fearing that a mother's nipples might transmit germs to her baby—like an unwashed nipple on a bottle—nurses taught mothers to cleanse their breasts daily with boric solution.[35] This practice, which the VNA was not alone in championing, may have made some mothers feel that their breasts posed some of the same threats to babies as bottles.

It is unlikely, however, that this type of advice from VNA nurses was instrumental in discouraging breastfeeding. Rather, like upper- and middle-class mothers, working-class mothers seem to have taken the lead in choosing bottles. Despite the VNA's mandate to nurses to "insist upon breast feeding" and the breastfeeding instruction given by nurses to patients, a significant number of the VNA's patients did not breastfeed their babies. Because VNA nurses customarily referred to all sick babies as "feeding cases,"[36] nurses apparently had plenty of firsthand experience with the health problems engendered by the "feeding question." Thus it is little wonder that the Chicago *Visiting Nurse Manual,* despite its breastfeeding decree, also described the intricacies of artificial feeding at length.[37]

It is not clear, however, if the VNA patients who fed their babies artificially were among the women who also received the copious prenatal care and instruction for which the VNA was known. Rather, it seems that most of the mothers who bottle-fed had started to do so before contact with the VNA. In one 1906 case, a visiting nurse discovered an Irish mother of eight children, whose husband worked in the stockyards for $1.50 a day, feeding her twin babies oatmeal water. The babies "were practically starving to death." The nurse immediately purchased malted milk for the babies and taught their mother how to prepare it. On subsequent visits the nurse brought a change of clothes for the twins and showed their mother how to bathe them. The nurse reported that the altered food regimen, clean clothing, and regular baths set the babies on the road to recovery.[38]

In another case, when the visiting nurse arrived, an exasperated doctor was attempting to persuade a bewildered, non-English-speaking woman whose baby was born prematurely to breastfeed. The nurse immediately intervened and, acting as the mother's interpreter, explained to the angry doctor that a neighbor, who was also in attendance and shouting louder than the doctor, had just brought the new mother something to feed the baby. The neighbor insisted her brew was ideal for premature babies. "Of course," reported the nurse, "the doctor thought we were in league against him to send that baby to Paradise sooner than was necessary and we had a difficult time placating him, getting rid of our volunteer and quieting the mother and fixing the baby." With help from the nurse, the mother recuperated and the baby thrived.[39] It is not clear how the mother ended up feeding the baby, but it is likely that the nurse backed up the doctor and persuaded her to breastfeed.

The VNA's familiarity with artificially fed babies is evident in other ways as well. Through the joint effort of the VNA (which provided the personnel), the Northwestern University Settlement House (which provided the space), and the Chicago Relief and Aid Society (which provided the equipment), baby tents, portable hospitals for sick infants, were brought to congested neighborhoods each summer between 1905 and 1917.[40] Only babies from poverty-stricken families received care in the tents; nurses referred families able to pay for medical service to a private physician. Thus, the heavily used baby tents, largely for infants suffering from digestive ailments, were one indication of widespread "feeding problems" among the VNA's clientele.[41]

The VNA, Northwestern Settlement House, and Chicago Relief and Aid Society maintained the tents each year from at least July 1 to September 15; longer if the summer's heat remained oppressive. The canvas hospitals reflected the long-held notion that "fresh air" cured. Just a few hours of "complete rest" in a tent's open air, doctors contended, would leave children "in a far better condition." Doctors argued that, minimally, baby tents were "preferable to the homes of many poor people." Each tent contained cribs, a hammock, electric lights, and a telephone. Two electric fans and frequent sprinkling with water of a tent's canvas roof kept interiors cool.[42]

The mothers of breastfed babies returned to the tents at regular intervals to nurse their infants. No records exist indicating how many of the babies cared for in the tents were exclusively breastfed, fed by both breast and bottle, or artificially fed, but it is likely that mothers actually fed "breastfed" babies additional foods at home. Hence, doctors permitted breastfed infants no other sustenance as long as they resided in a baby tent. Nurses supplied artificially fed babies with the certified-pasteurized-modified milk produced by the Chicago Milk Commission (CMC), another medical charity. Until the CMC closed its milk stations in 1910, the organization maintained a certified milk depot for general neighborhood use outside every baby tent.[43]

Chicago's first baby tents opened on the city's northwest side, where, visiting nurses observed, "while the Polish mothers love their little ones as much as we do, they are still clannish, ignorant, and superstitious" and reluctant to allow their sick babies to be cared for in distant hospitals.[44] The Department of Health likewise noted, "The foreign mother is timid and afraid to leave home, and more afraid to let the baby go."[45] Neighborhood baby tents soothed women's anxiety. Since the tents were located only blocks from a baby's tenement, nervous mothers could reassure themselves periodically "by peeking through uncurtained, screened windows, that the attendants were as kind as they looked and that the babies were being tenderly cared for." Mothers brought their sick infants to the tents each morning to be tended by nurses and doctors and picked them up each evening. Only when a doctor judged an infant critically ill did a baby remain in a tent all night.[46] Organizations in New York City, Cincinnati, Cleveland, Minneapolis, Nashville, and Hartford soon imitated Chicago, setting up similar tents in their poorest neighborhoods.[47]

Thousands of mothers brought their babies to these tents each summer. During the summer of 1910 alone, the personnel at baby tents cared for more than four thousand babies in ten tents scattered throughout the city.[48] In 1916, the year the Chicago Commissioner of Health issued an emergency executive order instructing that all the city's milk be pasteurized, the VNA reported remarkable improvement in the condition of babies brought to the tents. They were not nearly so ill as in previous years. Although the babies' healthier status likely was due to pasteurized milk, when very few mothers brought babies to the tents in 1917 the VNA crowed, "we feel that at last our long years of teaching are bearing fruit and that the preventive work . . . is showing good results in our second generation families." At the end of that summer the tents closed permanently.[49]

In the 1920s and 1930s, VNA nurses continued to teach mothers about infant feeding, pushing breastfeeding as well as advising and assisting women who fed their babies artificially. However, they seemed to have softened their earlier stance on artificial food and now looked upon it much less harshly. In the 1927 VNA *Annual Report* there are two photographs under the heading "Nursing Care to the New-Born and Instruction to Mothers Are Important Parts of Our Work." Baby bottles are visible in both pictures. Moreover, in one of the photographs artificial food preparation is clearly the purpose of the instruction: a nurse pours milk through a siphon into a bottle as a mother, her infant in arms, watches attentively.[50] The VNA's 1937 boast that "our babies, at the end of their fifth week, are breast-fed babies, sleeping alone and cared for by well-taught mothers" was likely apocryphal.[51] As one nurse reported in 1938, she had spent part of her day calming a chaotic household. Eventually she left the "mother . . . more comfortable than she had been all night" and her newborn "twins . . . bathed, fed and sleeping, and their bottle feedings for the day prepared and in the ice box." Although the VNA still preferred that their tiny patients be breastfed, an encounter with an artificially fed baby was no longer an automatic emergency. Visits with bottle-fed infants were now standard and uneventful, so routine that the VNA described this particular nurse's visit as "typical."[52]

The Chicago Infant Welfare Society: "Keep Babies Well by . . . Encouraging Breast Feeding"

While pregnant and postpartum mothers were the VNA's largest group of clients, VNA nurses cared for everyone—old and young, men and women, infants and children. In contrast, the Chicago Infant Welfare Society (IWS),

formed several decades after the inception of the VNA at the height of concern over the high mortality among Chicago's babies, concentrated solely on
the care and well-being of infants.[53]

The "feeding question" was directly responsible for the birth of the IWS.
The wealthy benefactors of the Children's Hospital Society formed the
Chicago Milk Commission (CMC) in 1903 to disseminate clean milk to babies
and children via neighborhood milk stations. When doctors protested in
1910 that milk stations by their very existence discouraged breastfeeding,
the CMC closed its milk stations and metamorphosed into the IWS, one of
whose principal purposes was to promote breastfeeding. (I describe the birth
and demise of the CMC in chapter 6.)

The IWS opened its first infant welfare stations in neighborhoods where
infant mortality was greatest, with one glaring exception. Because infant
welfare activists attributed the high infant death rate to the ignorance of
immigrant mothers, they ignored the high death rate among native-born
African American babies. Consequently, infant welfare stations were situated
overwhelmingly in white, immigrant neighborhoods. The IWS focus on
immigrants was so strong that the IWS only assigned nurses to stations if
they could speak whatever languages predominated in the neighborhood.[54]
IWS literature was likewise available in myriad languages.[55] Not until 1914
did the IWS board of directors give some thought to opening a station "in a
neighborhood inhabited by colored people."[56] During its first year, the IWS
operated ten stations located in park field houses, settlement houses, and day
nurseries. Between 1911 and 1912 the number of stations increased from ten
to thirteen, but the number of babies cared for almost doubled. By 1916 the
IWS operated twenty-two stations.[57]

IWS doctors and nurses provided free well-baby care via the neighborhood stations. Mothers took advantage of the service in droves. During the
summer, doctors examined babies at stations three days each week. When the
weather cooled, they offered only biweekly hours. The IWS held these
"Mothers Conferences" at well-publicized times. After a baby's initial examination, an IWS nurse followed up by going to the baby's home to observe
conditions there, to watch the mother care for her baby, and to instruct the
baby's mother in proper infant feeding. At all visits, station and home alike,
nurses emphasized the importance of breastfeeding.[58]

The stations aimed "to keep babies well by advice, by supervision, by
encouraging breast feeding, by instruction of the mothers in the rules of
hygiene and by furnishing certified milk below cost." Although the IWS
board was "very desirous" of caring for breastfed babies—to keep them

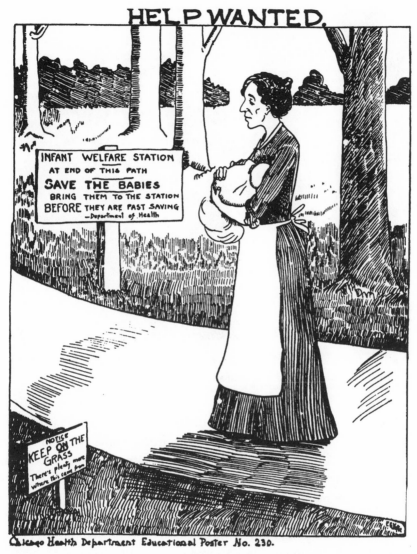

Figure 10   The Chicago Department of Health hung this poster in congested neighborhoods in 1914 to steer mothers with babies to the local infant welfare station. *Source: Bulletin Chicago School of Sanitary Instruction,* 11 July 1914.

exclusively breastfed—IWS employees, like private physicians, could not ignore artificial food; too many mothers fed it to their babies. Consequently, the IWS also taught bottle-using mothers how to modify milk in their homes. If "home conditions" made a mother's modification of milk inherently unsafe, the Borden Dairy, at the request of an infant station doctor, delivered one of three certified milk formulas to a patient's home for ten cents a quart.[59]

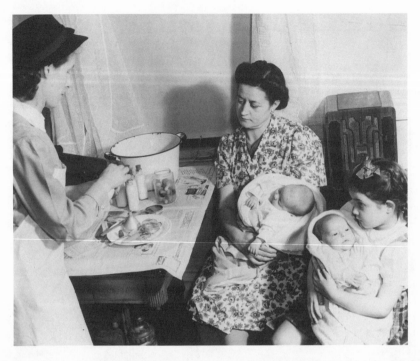

Figure 11 A Chicago Infant Welfare Society nurse explains to a mother of twins how to prepare infant formula. Undated. *Source:* Chicago Historical Society.

IWS doctors did not recommend artificial food lightly. They made it clear that milk distribution was not the primary purpose of the IWS and deliberately made certified milk formulas difficult to obtain. This was in stark contrast to the IWS's predecessor, the CMC, whose personnel distributed certified milk to the mothers of babies for the asking. In order to obtain milk through the IWS, mothers had to produce a milk card signed by an IWS physician. And unlike the CMC, whose workers advertised their wares via posters, placards, pamphlets, and newspapers, the IWS declined to publicize the availability of formulas. They even refused to provide non-IWS physicians with a list of standard formulas.[60]

To attract clients, the IWS relied on both word of mouth and their nurses, who traversed neighborhoods in an effort to get acquainted with mothers. Nurses reported that the question "How much does your baby weigh?" never failed to arouse a mother's curiosity. "Bring her over Tuesday and let the Doctor weigh her," nurses urged. Nurses, particularly those able to speak to mothers in their native language, found that mothers readily confided in them, "coming to us full of confidence and faith in our judgment."[61] Peer pressure also induced women to bring their babies in for examinations. When one stubborn woman told her neighbor that she had no intention of taking her newborn to the local station, the neighbor admonished her, "If you do not, you will be sure to get fits from the Nurse, so you had better go."[62] By the end of 1911 at least one nurse was able to say, "Oh, I don't have to urge them anymore, they just come." Some mothers brought their babies to their local station as often as every other week.[63]

Assorted medical organizations also helped persuade mothers to take their babies to the local infant welfare station. Presbyterian Hospital employees had long watched babies, discharged in fine condition after birth, return sick as many as fifteen times: "victims of ignorance and neglect, until finally their frail lives went out in this unequal struggle." With the advent of the IWS, a Presbyterian Hospital nurse began accompanying postpartum mothers home to introduce them to the nearest infant welfare station and to encourage them to use its services regularly.[64] By 1913 Chicago Department of Health visiting nurses likewise referred all their mothers to IWS stations.[65]

Infant welfare stations attracted mothers not only because they assured healthier babies but also because they promised women some fun. Each station held monthly mothers' meetings where nurses spent fifteen to twenty minutes teaching mothers about infant care. They devoted the rest of the meeting to socializing. Mothers talked, played games, listened to music, and ate. "I hate to go home, I have . . . such a good time," said one woman. The meetings encouraged friendly relations between mothers and IWS personnel and mutual aid among neighborhood women. For example, one mother who was breastfeeding her baby gladly provided breast milk each day to a neighbor's premature baby when an IWS doctor told her that the baby would not survive without human milk.[66]

The medical attention provided by the IWS, and the concomitant conscientiousness stirred in mothers, had dramatic results. In 1911, 112 babies died in Chicago for every 1,000 born. But the death rate among IWS babies was considerably less than half that: 42 per 1,000 babies cared for.[67] The numbers continued to improve. In 1915 doctors cared for 9,313 babies at IWS stations. Only 320 of the babies died. If they could locate the baby's parents, IWS workers investigated the cause of every death. Of the 300 infant deaths that they were able to track in 1915, 49 of the dead had been breastfed and 251 had been artificially fed. Fifty-four babies were born of American parents, 127 of Polish parents, and 45 of Italian parents; the rest were lumped together as "miscellaneous." "Our worst hygienic conditions are found in districts inhabited largely by Poles," one doctor concluded.[68] Ninety of the families had no regular income, ninety-seven had an income of ten dollars a week or less, and eighty-six earned between ten and fifteen dollars a week. Only twenty-seven families had weekly incomes over fifteen dollars. "Low wages," lamented doctors, "are unquestionably an important factor in the high death rate of the slums."[69]

While lobbying for a living wage was not within IWS purview, bettering breastfeeding rates certainly was. To ensure that the babies they cared for would be breastfed, the IWS encouraged their doctors and nurses to promote breastfeeding at every opportunity. When examining infants, IWS doctors and nurses discussed breastfeeding with the baby's mother. The IWS required doctors and nurses to note on each baby's medical record the baby's weight, the hygienic condition of the home, how that home was ventilated, whether the baby's mother worked outside the home,[70] and whether the baby was breastfed. If a child was not breastfed, doctors recorded the reason. If a child consumed artificial food, doctors noted whether conditions in the home permitted its safe preparation.[71]

The myriad IWS services required funding. Unlike the VNA, which relied mainly on the largesse of the wealthy, fund-raising for the IWS took place in several arenas and prompted the participation of women of all classes. One direct appeal chided Chicagoans, "Today when so much is being said regarding efficiency, we cannot consider a community efficient when it is willing to spend forty-five dollars to bury an infant while fifteen dollars would save it." Another entreaty begged the middle class, "Think of your own clean, comfortable babies and your own white porcelain tubs—and then give all you can to aid the Infant Welfare Society in its efforts to make and keep *all* Chicago babies well and happy."[72]

IWS superintendent Minnie Ahrens solicited the help of the wealthy as well. In 1913 Ahrens organized discussion groups for well-to-do women interested in infant welfare. Talk of the tragedy of infant morbidity and mortality was followed by a plea for funds. Pediatricians Isaac Abt, Clifford Grulee, Frank Churchill, and Henry Helmholz often joined Ahrens to give "splendid talks" to rich women; their wives hosted meetings in their homes. Grulee's mother-in-law, Mrs. L. H. Freer, was particularly instrumental in fund-raising. After an engaging speech before thirty-five women in suburban Hinsdale in March 1913, Freer offered to take interested women into the city to see an infant welfare station. The women who joined her were so enthralled by their visit, and offered so much money to the society as a result, that similar trips became integral to IWS fund-raising.[73]

In May 1913, Freer organized the IWS Woman's Auxiliary to solicit volunteers to register and weigh babies at infant welfare stations. Volunteers consequently freed station nurses so they could spend the bulk of their time talking with mothers about infant care. The Woman's Auxiliary also took charge of all fund-raising activities, overseeing the activity of many small, local fund-raising groups.[74]

One group of girls, living in Chicago's wealthy south side Kenwood neighborhood, began raising money for infant welfare stations as members of the Kenwood Social Service Club. The founder of the club reminisced in 1960 that members visited the station that they funded in the Back-of-the-Yards neighborhood adjacent to the Union Stockyards twice each week in groups of two, driven there by a chauffeur because their parents would not permit them to go into that neighborhood alone. These girls devoted many hours each week to the IWS, not only raising money but sewing hundreds of flannelette blankets for IWS babies, often working through the night to finish them in time for a birth.[75]

The Woman's Auxiliary created an intricate bureaucracy to handle the burgeoning money-raising and volunteer activities. For each twenty-five donors in an area, the Woman's Auxiliary formed a fund-raising center. Each center established a sewing circle to keep stations supplied with infant layettes and children's clothes. Centers elected their own officers and center officers made up the Woman's Auxiliary Board of Directors. Fund-raising centers quickly formed in suburbs on all sides of Chicago including Winnetka, Glencoe, Kenilworth, La Grange, Woodlawn, Riverside, and Oak Park.[76] Women all over Chicago—young and old, rich and middle-class—heard and responded to the baby-saving pleas.

In January 1914, flush with success, members of the Woman's Auxiliary planned a citywide Baby Week campaign both to raise the money needed to increase the number of infant welfare stations from thirteen to fifty and to disseminate an "intelligent knowledge of infant needs" to the public.[77] What constituted appropriate infant food—first and foremost human milk—was a major theme of the week's events. Nude, robust, smiling babies decorated one poster designed to advertise Baby Week. The infants implored, "Deliver us from our friends who know not our need. Give us mothers who are mothers in deed. Take not away from us that food which God in His wisdom provides. Except of extreme necessity, force not upon us an unnatural food."[78]

Many organizations—public, private, and philanthropic—agreed to participate in and publicize the weeklong campaign. Churches and synagogues repeatedly announced the Baby Week schedule to their congregations. The city hung 780 billboards announcing events. Newspapers

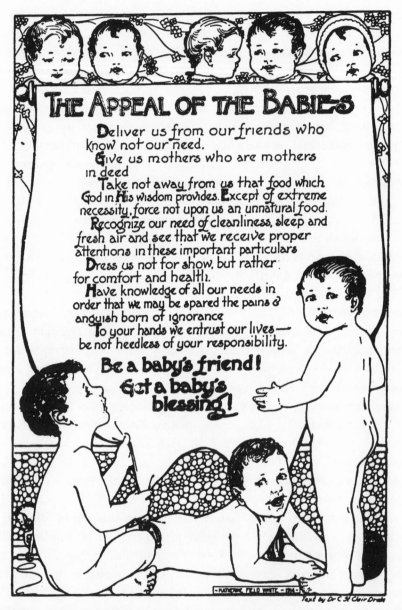

Figure 12 The Chicago Infant Welfare Society commissioned this poster in conjunction with their first Baby Week campaign in 1914. *Source: Bulletin Chicago School of Sanitary Instruction,* 18 April 1914, 70.

promised pages of free advertising for all Baby Week activities. An electric sign heralding the week swung over State Street, downtown Chicago's main thoroughfare. The sculptor Lorado Taft designed *Mother and Child,* a statue to symbolize the event, and the IWS placed copies of the statue around the city. On their milk routes, five local dairies distributed 200,000 booklets describing the effort.[79] Two years before Chicago required that all milk sold in the city be pasteurized, and before the infant death rate from diarrhea began to plummet, dairies were already taking advantage of all the concern over infant welfare and helping the public link infant health with cows' milk.

Unfortunately, the IWS had to shelve their elaborate plans when President Woodrow Wilson sent U.S. troops into Mexico and the city's and country's attention turned to events there. Only one of the planned events took place: a mass meeting in Chicago's Loop at which U.S. Children's Bureau representatives Julia Lathrop and Josephine Baker spoke. Grulee's mother-in-law wrote of the disappointment in her diary: "The pages of the newspapers were filled with War instead of Charity, and where there had been dreams of hundreds of thousands of dollars, only $53,000 was secured. But that was worthwhile and the women started with fresh energy to fortify all the territory taken."[80]

The vision of the IWS Woman's Auxiliary came to fruition the following year when Chicago mayor William Hale Thompson declared July 17 to 24, 1915, "Baby Week." The IWS packed the week with educational and fundraising events. On Saturday, July 17, rabbis discussed infant care in their synagogues. On Sunday priests and pastors spoke to their congregations. Physicians delivered daily lectures in parks throughout the city.[81] New York, Pittsburgh, Toledo, and Grand Rapids all followed Chicago's example within a year, and the instructional celebration soon became a national event. Inspired by the shocking results of the physical exams given to American draftees during World War I—almost 30 percent of men were declared unfit for military service owing to permanent defects caused by early childhood diseases or inadequate care as infants—the U.S. Children's Bureau declared 1918 "Children's Year."[82] Josephine Baker called the war "a backhanded break for children" because it prompted the nation "to see that new lives, which grow up to replace brutally extinguished lives, were extremely valuable national assets."[83] As part of the yearlong campaign, the Children's Bureau asked parents to record their children's weight and height at regular intervals, and the bureau furnished interested parents with growth charts. Each chart listed "normal" heights and weights for children at given ages. The Children's Bureau emphasized in particular the relationship between height, weight, and the proper feeding of children.[84]

The overwhelmingly positive response throughout the country to the mere notion of infant welfare ensured an expansion of local activities. The initial efforts of the IWS, concentrated only in the most poverty-stricken neighborhoods, were soon duplicated citywide thanks to the IWS Woman's

Auxiliary and the Philanthropy Department of the Chicago Woman's Club, which joined forces in 1917 to sponsor nurses to visit the home of every newborn in the city. The single visit guaranteed that every mother giving birth in Chicago heard a breastfeeding lecture. Nurses also urged mothers to take their babies to the nearest infant welfare station for regular examinations.[85]

In another outreach effort, some stations sponsored Little Mothers' Club classes to train the girls who cared for younger siblings. Usually, noted one IWS worker, these eight to ten year olds knew more about their infant siblings than their harried mothers did. One girl, whose mother worked long hours in what IWS workers described as a "sweat shop," was devoted to a baby brother who suffered from rickets. She brought her brother to an IWS station for examination, attended Little Mothers' Club classes, and applied her newly acquired knowledge meticulously to her brother's care. IWS superintendent Minnie Ahrens was so impressed by this "little mother's" conscientiousness that she marveled, "One can hardly realize he is the same baby."[86]

In 1912 the Chicago Department of Health relocated the IWS Little Mothers' Clubs to public and parochial schools and sponsored and promoted them as after-school programs. Two afternoons each week, health department nurses taught "practical instruction in the care of infants" to hundreds of girls. By 1918 almost nine thousand girls had completed Little Mothers' training.[87] In 1921 the Chicago Board of Education voted to add Little Mothers' Club classes to the regular curriculum for seventh- and eighth-grade girls. Two nurses taught the classes full time, four part time.[88] The in-school classes were similar to the original IWS Little Mothers' Clubs in that each class focused on a different lesson. In one class girls learned the importance of hygiene in the home. In another they learned how to make a baby's bed, what kind of bed covers to use, and where to position a baby's bed in a room. Other lessons included how to bathe a baby, how to dress a baby, how to care for a baby during the summer, and how to recognize when a baby was sick.[89]

There were also two lessons on infant feeding that likely left an indelible mark on students. Because public health nurses trained these girls not as future mothers but as present-day big sisters who cared for infant siblings in their mother's absence, the lessons emphasized artificial food and only perfunctorily mentioned breastfeeding. During the first infant-feeding lesson, nurses taught girls the advantages of "natural feeding," the importance of scheduled feeding, and the dangers of overfeeding. They described the artificial foods available to babies not fed "naturally." At the second lesson girls learned how to modify, sterilize, and pasteurize cows' milk and why these processes were important.[90] It is likely that these Little Mothers passed on what they learned about infant feeding to their own mothers. Moreover, these classes probably had a lifelong influence on students. Having been "Little Mothers" in their youth, these girls were practiced in artificial feeding when they became actual mothers. The method already familiar to them would logically have been their feeding mode of choice.

By 1924 the reach of the twenty-seven IWS stations was incontrovertible.[91] The IWS served babies who normally would not have received medical care; two-thirds of children cared for in 1924 came from families earning less than eight dollars a week per capita, the sum that United Charities determined put a family below the poverty level.[92] Despite their ubiquitous presence, large clientele, and incessant messages, however, the IWS did not have a profound influence on breastfeeding rates.

Although breastfeeding remained an emphasis of the IWS, it appears that, despite its efforts, the organization did not better *exclusive* breastfeeding rates among its clientele. Grulee claimed in 1934, for example, that of 20,000 babies cared for by the IWS between 1925 and 1929 inclusive, more than 91 percent were breastfed "either partially or wholly." His terminology demonstrates the Infant Welfare Society's new breastfeeding stance.[93] Chicago doctors had previously been careful to distinguish between exclusive breastfeeding and "mixed feeding," that is, feeding a baby human milk as well as artificial food. In this earlier era physicians did not refer to mixed feeding as "breastfeeding"; all infant mortality, infant morbidity, and infant feeding studies placed the two feeding practices in separate categories.[94] Infants' lives had depended on these distinctions. By the 1920s, however, that difference was apparently moot because the medical community now deemed cows' milk safe. To breastfeed "either partially or wholly" was now a single acceptable category when in years past such sloppy practice might have ended in a baby's death. Big decreases in infant deaths from diarrhea in Chicago ultimately coincided with the universal pasteurization of milk in 1916 and the refrigeration of milk during shipping in 1920. Exclusive or prolonged breastfeeding, which was not increasing but drastically decreasing, had little, if anything, to do with it.[95]

The Chicago Department of Health: "Let Us Have More Mother-Fed Babies"

By 1907 the city was following medical charities into the infant welfare arena in earnest. Department of Health efforts to quiz and educate mothers about infant-care practices signaled the start of the transformation in public health in Chicago from being wholly charity-driven to wholly government-driven.

Before 1907 city officials paid little attention to infant welfare other than to offer women occasional tips on proper infant care via one of their publications. In 1895 F. W. Reilly, Chicago's assistant commissioner of health, wrote, "THE PROPER FOOD FOR BABIES IS MOTHER'S MILK.—No sensible mother needs advice on this point."[96] In 1899 Health Commissioner Arthur R. Reynolds sent physician volunteers into "thickly populated" city neighborhoods to teach mothers how to feed and care for their babies. But before the summer of 1907 the Department of Health made no prolonged effort to work with mothers to control the biggest killer of babies, infant diarrhea.[97] In fact, health department officials admitted in 1911 that they had long dismissed the rash of deaths among infants each summer as unavoidable.[98]

Once the Department of Health inaugurated its infant welfare work, however, the city's assorted campaigns to prevent diarrhea were ubiquitous. Posters and weekly bulletins taught women to keep food away from flies, to pasteurize milk, to use ice to keep milk cold, to keep homes clean, to get prenatal care, to immunize children, and to breastfeed. The health department pinpointed the location of every infant death from diarrhea to determine the neighborhoods at greatest risk. They found the highest infant mortality in the west side river wards, in the district southwest of the Union Stockyards, and in the South Chicago rolling mills district near the mouth of the Calumet River.[99]

In the summer of 1907 the Department of Health employed seventy-five medical inspectors to go door-to-door in these three areas to teach mothers how to care for their babies during hot weather. That summer alone medical inspectors visited 43,784 families with infants. "[I]n decided contrast with the infant feeding conditions in the better residence portions of the city where the proportion breastfed is much lower," 76.2 percent of the babies examined were breastfed. Nevertheless, these medical inspectors attributed the high rate of infant diarrhea in these neighborhoods to the additional "feeding of improper foods."[100]

Department of Health field surveys, like this 1907 effort, proved an efficient way to uncover and rectify infants' health problems, and the city continued to conduct them, in various forms, for decades. In a Department of Health field survey conducted in the summer of 1909, fourteen doctors and twenty nurses knocked on doors looking for households with babies. When they found one, the doctor or nurse offered to examine the baby. If they encountered a sick baby, they immediately reported the case to the VNA. The

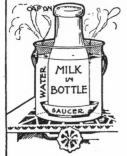

MAKE BABY'S MILK SAFE
PASTEURIZE IT AT HOME
THIS KILLS DISEASE-PRODUCING GERMS in MILK

Directions for Pasteurizing

Use a pail a little shorter than the milk bottle.
Place saucer in bottom of pail and stand the.
bottle of milk on this saucer. Leave cap on bottle.
Pour hot water into pail until water level is
about four inches below top of bottle.
Place on stove and bring water to boiling
point.
When water begins to boil immediately
remove bottle of milk from pail.
Cool the milk in bottle as rapidly as you
can and place it in ice-box as soon as possible.

MILK MUST BE KEPT COLD & TIGHTLY COVERED IN CLEAN BOTTLES TO PREVENT DEVELOPMENT of GERMS IN IT.

Chicago Department of Health, Educational Poster № 55   *Designed by. Dr C. St. Clair Drake*

Figure 13   Before 1916, when the health commissioner ordered that all milk sold in Chicago be pasteurized, the Chicago Department of Health encouraged mothers to pasteurize milk at home. *Source: Bulletin Chicago School of Sanitary Instruction,* 31 May 1913, 88.

number of desperately ill infants quickly overwhelmed the VNA, and health department officials hired their own visiting nurses to supplement the VNA's work.[101] Those nurses became permanent fixtures on the urban landscape. The myriad activities stemming from the field surveys had dramatic effect. One doctor noted that only 25 percent of the babies he saw at his clinic during the summer of 1909 suffered from digestive disorders, a sharp decline from previous summers.[102]

Given this tangible success, the Department of Health sought to further its entrance into the infant welfare arena and began to work with assorted medical charities specializing in infant welfare. Public health officials now referred to what had been multiple, isolated efforts to keep babies well as "united agencies working under an organized plan."[103] During the summer of 1910, under the auspices of the newly formed Infant Welfare Committee—whose primary agencies were the Department of Health, United Charities, and the VNA—an army of five hundred nurses visited 23,984 newborns. Nurses visited homes in the city's most congested wards housing mainly

ADDRESS					Flat House Floor	Rear Middle Front	WARD	SANITARY SCORE		
NAME						Age	Registered	CLEANLINESS 15		VENTILATION 10
NATIVITY OF MOTHER	OCCUPATION	FOOD	MILK	STOOLS	SICKNESS	REFERRED		Floor 3		Rt. Angles 2
	Housework	Breast Only	Raw	Color	Acute Enteritis	Dispensary		Walls 2		1 Opening 10
Lithuanian	Other	Breast and	Boiled	Blood	Chronic Enteritis	Hospital		Ceiling 2		Opposite Openings 3
Polish	Father's Occupation	Cond. Milk or	Past.	Curds	Marasmus	Tent		Lodgers 2		Windows that do not open 6
Bohemian	CHILDREN	Cow's Milk or	Prep. Mod.	Mucous	Rickets	V. N. A.		Windows 2		Open on same side 5
Russian	5 or more	Pat. Food or	Certified	No. in 24 hrs.	Bronchitis	I. W. S.		Poor H'kpg. 4		CROWDING 10
Other Slavic	Fewer than 5	Other Food	On Ice or In Water	Constipation	Pneumonia	Physician		LIGHTING 10		400 cu. ft. per adult No. Rooms
Italian	No. sleeping in Baby's room	Artificial Only	Covered	Diarrhoea	Skin Disease	Co. Dr.		Deduct for Each Dark Room		Men in Family
Other Latin	CHILD'S COND.	FEEDING	BATHING	SLEEP	Sore Eyes	Co. Agt.		PLUMBING 10		Women in Family
Austrian	Healthy—Sick	Irregular	Sponge	Alone	Other	Red Cross		Leaking 4		Children in Family
Dutch	CARE OF BABY	Day—Night	Tub		OUTING	Other		Clogged 4		No. Roomers
German	Kept Where	Water	Ice Tickets					Odor 2		ACCUMULATION 10
Other Germanic	Rel. Temp.	MOTHER'S DIET						S. Trap 3		Garbage 10
Danish	Rel. Humid.	DEMONSTRATION						Enclosed 3		Rubbish 4
Swedish	Ventilation	INSTRUCTIONS						Hopper Closet 5		Manure 10
Norwegian	Covered with Netting							Privy Vaults 10		FLIES 15
Hungarian	CLOTHING	REMARKS						Yard Closet 7		Many 15 Few 5
United Kingdom	Too much							Basement flooded or damp 9		SCREENS 10
other Foreign	Too little							YARD 10		On Doors 5
U. S. A.	Airing	DISTRICT			DATE OF VISIT			Small 5 None 10		On Windows 5
	Date	Result	Date	Result	Date	Result	Date	Result	Date	Result	Date	Result	Date	Result	TOTAL		
Revisits								Dropped	Date	Transferred Date

NOTE.—Except when direct statement is required, indicate your answer by a neat V on the line after the word.

H. D.—M. 541 d 35M—5-18.   **NURSE'S CASE HISTORY**

Weighed and Measured   Yes / No

Nurse

Figure 14   During the summer of 1910, under the auspices of the newly formed Infant Welfare Committee, 500 public health nurses visited the homes of 23,984 newborns to gather the information on this form. *Source: Report and Handbook of the Department of Health of the City of Chicago for the Years 1911 to 1918 Inclusive, 583.*

Polish, Italian, Bohemian, and German immigrants.[104] They chose the homes to visit from a "Baby Register" compiled from myriad sources, including the Department of Health's erratic birth records, visiting nurses' reports on pre-natal visits, records kept by day nurseries, baby tent reports, CMC records, and assorted data kept by churches and hospitals.[105] With Department of Health survey forms in hand, these "hot weather nurses" quizzed mothers about infant care. What did they feed their babies? How often did they feed them? If their babies consumed any cows' milk, how did mothers prepare it? What did their babies' stools look like? Nurses also observed and recorded the condition of each home they visited: its sanitary condition, method of ventilation, lighting, crowding, and presence or absence of flies. Education was an equally important part of the interview. Nurses talked to mothers about proper infant care, "watch[ed] over the milk and warn[ed] against flies."[106]

Surveys and interviews were not the health department's only infant welfare activities. In 1911 the department produced the film *Summer Babies,* a documentary for mothers explaining how to care for infants during the summer. The film, which ran in local theaters, urged mothers to feed their babies pure milk and not to give their babies beer.[107] Also that summer, the Department of Health wrote and distributed infant-care literature in nine languages. Health department physicians spoke on infant care at churches and settlement houses, likewise in an array of foreign languages.[108] The Civic Federation of Chicago aided the effort by printing ten thousand four-color placards headlined "Don't Kill Your Baby"—in English, Polish, Yiddish, Bohemian, German, Lithuanian, and Italian—and posted them on walls, fences, and billboards throughout the city. The placard depicted two infants, one glowing with health, the other looking like an emaciated old man. The healthy infant drank only mother's milk, dubbed "Best of All"; cool, sterilized water; and properly prepared clean milk. The shriveled baby drank tea, coffee, and beer and ate meat, bread, and sweets.[109]

The Department of Health soon institutionalized its field work. Dividing the city into forty-acre districts and selecting the most congested according to the U.S. census, health officials assigned one of their nurses to each district. Nurses started with thirty-five cases from the baby register and visited an average of fifteen homes daily. Gradually, the health department increased nurses' caseloads until each had one hundred active cases. Nurses triaged

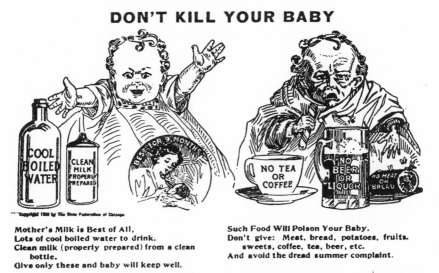

Figure 15 The Civic Federation of Chicago, in conjunction with the Chicago Department of Health, printed this as a four-color placard in seven languages: English, Polish, Yiddish, Bohemian, German, Lithuanian, and Italian. The health department commonly translated its public health messages into multiple languages to reach assorted immigrant communities. *Source: Bulletin Chicago School of Sanitary Instruction,* 8 January 1910.

their cases, giving priority to babies living in poor housing, babies getting poor care, babies delivered by midwives, and, especially, bottle-fed babies.[110]

Nurses kept detailed records of their visits. They rated infants' homes on scorecards, deducting points for dirty floors, inadequate ventilation, poor lighting and plumbing, excessive flies, and lack of screens. They also noted an infant's health and feeding history and the mother's ethnicity.[111] Nurses conducted their investigations "sympathetically, tactfully, and as far as possible without giving offense," using "the simplest language possible." If a mother breastfed her baby, the nurse confirmed that breastfeeding was going well. Nurses taught the mothers of artificially fed babies how to modify and pasteurize milk. They left a copy of the Department of Health pamphlet on infant care with every mother they visited. Given the personal attention they received from the city's nurses, new mothers had special incentive to read the pamphlet.[112]

Meanwhile, the health department's breastfeeding propaganda did not ebb. The city continued to take every opportunity to glorify human milk and warn of the dangers of cows' milk at a time when the milk wars were in full swing and few battles were yet won. One 1911 poster depicted a long tube with one end attached to a cows' udder and the other end in a dying baby's mouth. Between the cow donor and human recipient, the tube snaked through a filthy barn, a railroad station, a steam engine, and a bottling plant. Eventually the tube wrapped itself around a horse-drawn milk wagon pulled slowly through city streets. Its last stop before baby's mouth was a fly-covered, open milk bottle sitting on the hapless infant's porch. "And yet some people wonder why so many babies die!" the broadside scolded. The necessary preventive measure was obvious, the poster explained: "To Lessen Baby Deaths Let Us Have More Mother-Fed Babies."[113]

In 1913 the Chicago City Council funded four Department of Health infant welfare stations to augment the thirteen stations already operated by the IWS.[114] By 1918 the Department of Health still operated only four stations, while the IWS had expanded to twenty-three facilities. The health department encouraged mothers to bring their babies to stations right after birth and to keep bringing them in regularly for free checkups.[115]

Like the IWS, doctors and nurses at the health department stations examined babies under the age of two, offered infant-care advice to mothers, and referred sick babies—"unless the sickness is due to mistakes in feeding"—to the appropriate agency. Station physicians emphasized the importance of breastfeeding and taught mothers how to manually express milk from their

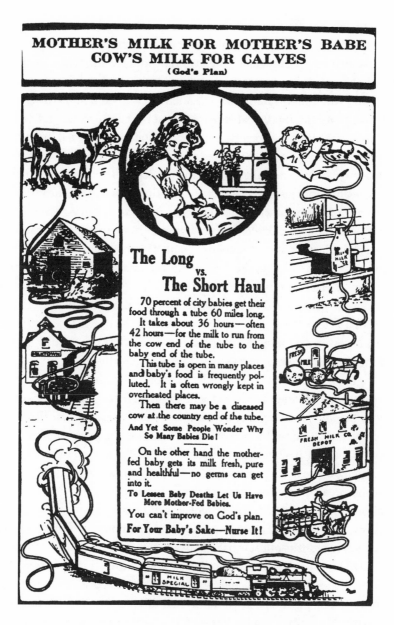

Figure 16 Many cities used this illustration as part of their campaign to increase breast-feeding rates. The wording on the poster, however, changed from city to city. This is Chicago's version. *Source: Bulletin Chicago School of Sanitary Instruction,* 3 June 1911.

breasts "so that the flow of milk may be stimulated and the baby continued on breastfeeding as long as possible." Doctors documented a baby's medical history, as well as a mother's age, health, reproductive history, "personality . . . [and] general ability to comprehend and follow instructions."[116]

In 1921, while infant mortality was 89.33 per 1,000 live births citywide, the mortality rate among the babies cared for at the twenty-four stations operated by the Infant Welfare Society and the four stations operated by the health department was 15.7 per 1,000 babies registered.[117] Given the stations' obvious impact on infant mortality, Herman Bundesen, Chicago's new commissioner of health, increased the number of stations run by the health department from four at the start of his tenure in 1922 to twenty-five in 1923.[118] Public schools and park field houses housed the new stations, saving the department its largest station expense, rent. In 1925, when roughly 58,000 babies were born in Chicago, the twenty-six IWS stations and the twenty-five Department of Health stations cared for more than 33,000 of them.[119]

Bundesen, who served as commissioner of health from 1922 to 1927 and again from 1931 to 1960 and was remarkably well-known to Chicago's citizens, made lowering infant mortality a top priority throughout his tenure. Beginning in 1923 every mother in Chicago, shortly after giving birth, received a health department pamphlet explaining the importance of breastfeeding. In 1925 Bundesen revised and expanded the health department's pamphlet *Our Babies* to seventy-two pages. A Department of Health visiting nurse delivered the booklet personally to each new mother's home. Bundesen took to reading his favorite paragraph in *Our Babies* "aloud with the fervor of a person preaching salvation." The paragraph began, "To nurse her baby at the breast is the first duty of every healthy mother."[120]

Chicago's infant-care advice for mothers did not end with the delivery of *Our Babies*. Mothers continued to receive one pamphlet a month by mail for the first twelve months of their babies' lives: *How to Care for Your One Month Old, How to Care for Your Two Month Old,* and so on. During extremely hot and cold weather—"summer complaint time and . . . cold catching time"— mothers received postcards with additional advice. The health department provided mothers with a binder labeled "The Baby and You" in which to store all the information for handy reference.[121]

In 1925 the American Medical Association recommended that all municipalities hire public health nurses to visit the home of each new mother to ensure, specifically, that breastfeeding was going well. Nassau County, New York, implemented such a plan in 1924 with great success. Infant mortality dropped from an average seventy-two deaths per 1,000 live births during the three years preceding the universal visit to forty-nine deaths per 1,000 live births in 1924.[122] Beginning in August 1925, Chicago Department of Health field nurses followed the example of Nassau County nurses and visited all the city's babies regularly with an eye on maintaining breastfeeding. They visited each infant who received regular medical attention from a private or public physician every ninety days. They examined babies who never saw a doctor every thirty days. Nurses recorded a baby's name, address, and birth date, whether the baby was breastfed, when and why breastfeeding was discontinued, and whether the baby was under the care of a private physician or an infant welfare station.[123]

Increasing the breastfeeding rate of Chicago's mothers continued to be a priority of the city's infant welfare work. Bundesen held Department of Health infant welfare station doctors "strictly responsible" for assuring that the mothers who brought their babies to the city's infant welfare stations breastfed. If an artificially fed infant welfare station baby died, Henry Niblack, chief of the Bureau of Child Welfare, told colleagues in 1936, "we want to know why; if that baby had been taken off the breast, we want to know the indication." Station doctors and nurses kept infants' medical records on colored charts—yellow for breastfed babies and blue for artificially fed babies. "If there are too many blues," said Niblack, "we expect an explanation." Infant welfare station records indicated that in 1936 more than 90 percent of African American babies were breastfed.[124] "These mothers still take breast feeding for granted," Niblack explained. "It seems," he mused, "that the higher class a neighborhood, the fewer the breast-fed babies."[125]

No matter how expansive or seemingly successful the effort to increase breastfeeding rates, however, Chicago's medical community continued to fear that a significant number of women would feed their babies artificially. Thus, even as public health nurses visited mothers to encourage them to breastfeed, the health department outfitted their infant welfare stations with equipment to teach mothers how to modify cows' milk. The Chicago Department of Health touted the two seemingly contradictory efforts as part of the same baby-saving crusade: "the campaign for breast-feeding of babies whenever possible, [and spreading] knowledge of the proper use of cows' milk in artificial feeding."[126]

The Department of Health further diluted its pleas to breastfeed by changing radically its definition of breastfeeding, much as the IWS had done. In its earliest infant welfare field surveys, the health department defined breastfeeding as giving only human milk to a newborn, as opposed to mixed feeding. Giving any amount of artificial food to a newborn, even if the baby received substantially more breast milk than cows' milk, was not considered breastfeeding. Now that women rarely breastfed exclusively, however, health officials helped their cause by changing the meaning of breastfeeding to the vague "give your baby at least a little human milk for a while." The July 1925 issue of the health department's monthly publication *Chicago's Health,* which implored mothers to "Give the Baby a Fair Chance," illustrates this. Health officials told mothers, "Breast fed children are the strongest and healthiest. Therefore, breast milk, *no matter how little,* [emphasis mine] should always be given when available as it is the perfect baby food and almost always agrees with the child."[127]

Bundesen claimed that at the start of his tenure as health commissioner in 1922 only 20 percent of Chicago's babies under the age of one were breastfed. Consequently, he ordered health department workers to make increasing breastfeeding rates a priority. In 1927 he bragged that, thanks largely to health department efforts, 90 percent of Chicago's babies now consumed breast milk.[128] If Bundesen's claim is true—and extant surveys contradict his figures for both 1922 and 1927 (see appendix C)—it is likely that most of Chicago's "breastfed" babies were fed a mixed diet of both human and cows' milk, as was by then long the custom. The commissioner's claim that breastfeeding rates had increased drastically under his watch was most likely typical Bundesen bravado. The surveys of 1925 do indicate that breastfeeding rates in Chicago soared that year (again, see appendix C), but 1925 is an anomaly. I cannot say definitively why, except that 1925 was the first year Department of Health visiting nurses called on all new mothers. Perhaps their messages did affect mothers in the week or two after their babies were born, the same weeks nurses gathered breastfeeding data. Or maybe mothers were simply telling nurses what they wanted to hear. Or possibly, the health department exaggerated breastfeeding statistics to reflect positively on their high-profile breastfeeding campaign.

The city's doctors, in fact, continued to complain that even breastfed babies were commonly weaned before their digestive systems were mature enough to tolerate solid food. No doctors complained of this more vociferously than the doctors working at the health department's infant welfare stations. In 1924 station physicians were dismayed to learn that 63.5 percent of the infants they examined regularly were weaned at or before their third month of life. Bundesen's triumphant claim notwithstanding, doctors' warning that "there is no substitute for mother's milk" apparently did not have the desired effect.[129]

◆

Medical charities were widespread, heavily used, and extraordinarily influential in Chicago at the end of the nineteenth and well into the twentieth centuries. Virtually all of them, as well as the Chicago Department of Health, which entered the infant-welfare fray in 1907, made the care of pregnant women and babies and insistence on breastfeeding a top priority. Refusing to be coy in their pronouncements, they did not speak of infant-feeding options as an array of equal choices. Rather, they told mothers unequivocally that human milk was good for babies and other foods were bad.

They also recognized, however, that the consumers in this situation were not mothers, but babies who ate what their mothers gave them to eat. And if mothers, for whatever reason, fed their babies artificial food, then the medical community, and particularly the public health community, had an obligation to provide safe sustenance. Thus, virtually all of Chicago's public health agencies, charitable and otherwise, took what seemed to be a contradictory approach to infant feeding. They lauded breastfeeding as the only way to feed babies while simultaneously, and at great expense, providing alternatives to breastfeeding. As more women turned to bottles, doctors, in their attempt to provide what they touted as "safe" (or at least "safer") artificial food, rationalized that they were providing a product to mothers who *already* bottle-fed. But the certified, pasteurized, and modified milk provided by medical charities paved the way for even more mothers to bottle-feed.

This stance of the public health community eventually created a new infant-feeding mentality for both physicians and mothers. Importance-of-breastfeeding messages became so diluted that the longtime distinction between exclusive breastfeeding, mixed feeding, and artificial feeding no longer applied. Getting a mother to breastfeed at all, for any amount of time, became the new goal of public health services. Eventually mothers, doctors, and public health bodies discarded even that weakened missive.

5

"Mercenary Hirelings" or "A Great Blessing"?: Wet Nurses as Private and Institutional Employees

Two incompatible realities in the late nineteenth century—the dangers of artificial food and its growing use—ensured that wet nurses were a presence in some families' lives from the 1880s through the 1920s. Faced with the consequences of mothers' move to bottles, the medical community consistently recommended hiring a wet nurse rather than employing artificial food if a baby was not "mother-fed." As one irate physician said after listening to several papers on infant feeding at a 1908 American Medical Association meeting, "There would be just as much sense in feeding a man on hay as in feeding a baby on cows' milk. . . . Only one circumstance justifies a man in eating hay, and that is that he can not get any other food. . . . As long as we can find breast milk there is nothing to justify our giving the baby cows' milk."[1] The vast majority of doctors demonstrated their agreement with this sentiment by going to unusual lengths to procure wet nurses, not only for the sick babies of the wealthy but for infants housed in hospitals and foundling homes as well.

When a physician recommended that a family hire a wet nurse, however, parents usually reacted with dismay. According to the families who employed them, wet nurses were immoral, unruly, ignorant, and coarse, much more often a curse than a blessing. This animosity was due largely to class tensions. Families who could hire wet nurses were exceptionally well-off, while wet nurses tended to be poor women in unusually desperate circumstances. This dichotomy was a recipe for disaster. Chicago pediatrician Isaac Abt echoed the complaints of most mothers when he wrote of wet nurses, "Their price was above rubies and they made the family pay it in submission to their whims, accession to their demands, and forbearance with their bad habits."[2]

Wet nursing has a long, varied history in the United States. Women brought the custom with them from England to colonial America. In New England the habit of "placing out" babies to live in wet nurses' homes burgeoned among the wealthy, and advertisements for wet nurses were common.[3] Even in the colonial era, however, ministers and medical literature praised the nursing mother and disparaged the women who placed out their babies, charging that mothers performed only part of their duty by giving birth and that breast-feeding truly fulfilled their motherly obligation.[4] Given this increasingly articulated view, the use of wet nurses waned over time in the United States. As their use diminished, wet nurses came to live in the infant's home, not vice versa, and employers forced wet nurses to "place out" their own babies, usually to foundling homes where caretakers fed them artificially.[5]

By the late nineteenth and early twentieth centuries, some families routinely hired a wet nurse in anticipation of a baby's birth if the expectant mother was unable or unwilling to breastfeed. Most often, however, parents hired wet nurses only after the health of their artificially fed baby deteriorated. In these cases, emergencies all, it was usually the family physician who traversed the city hunting for a wet nurse. By the 1910s doctors in some cities—weary of these frantic, eleventh-hour searches—instituted more efficient, and less traditional, ways of finding human milk. They organized employment agencies for wet nurses. They urged the hospitals that housed sick infants to keep wet nurses on staff. Eventually they distributed pasteurized human milk in bottles via breast milk stations.

Use of the conventional wet nurse waned in proportion to the growing safety of artificial food. This occurred in several stages; the advent of clean water supplies started the decline, followed by assorted efforts to halt the adulteration of cows' milk, the legal requirement that all milk sold be bottled, sealed, and pasteurized, and, finally, consumers' increased access to refrigeration.[6] By the 1930s the traditional wet nurse—both the one who worked in private homes and the one who lived and worked in hospitals—had vanished. In her stead, medical personnel in many American cities collected milk daily from lactating women, paying them by the ounce for their milk. For the few babies in precarious health who continued to require breast milk, human milk stations became the latter-day equivalent of the wet nurse. From 1938 until the early 1960s, the Chicago Board of Health operated a Mothers' Breast Milk Station where public health nurses collected milk from healthy mothers and distributed it free of charge in bottles to sick and premature infants.

Along with this change in human milk distribution came a shift in attitude toward human milk providers. The personnel who gathered, pasteurized, and bottled human milk for the eventual use of sick or premature babies deemed their donor-mothers respectable, thrifty women who wanted only to supplement their family's income, utterly unlike their slovenly, "mercenary-hireling" predecessors. These latter-day wet nurses provided their milk in a discreet manner, immediately and appropriately detaching themselves from their product. By the end of the 1960s human milk stations like the one run by the Chicago Board of Health were out of business, and the meaning of giving human milk to an infant not one's own metamorphosed once again. Breast milk, like blood, became a priceless gift donated by selfless individuals and available through milk banks.[7] The giving of human milk became as far removed from a mercenary act as it could possibly be.[8]

The employment of wet nurses through the first quarter of the twentieth century and the conflict that their use engendered are telling phenomena. Doctors' lactation-failure theories, which had discouraged many women from breastfeeding for a host of often contradictory and illogical reasons (see chapter 3), became even more elaborate when physicians discussed wet nurses' milk. Physicians warned, for example, that some wet nurses came from ethnic groups known for being inherently poor milk producers. Mothers who hired wet nurses repeated and embellished these complaints. The angriest protest was that wet nurses' indulgent diets ruined their milk and sickened babies. Lactation-failure theories were now clearly part of the larger culture and not simply confined to the medical community. That a woman's genetic makeup, character, or lack of conscientiousness could make her milk "bad" was becoming part of well-to-do mothers' consciousness.

The harsh relations between wet nurses and their employers shed light on upper- and middle-class attitudes toward, not just the working class, but also the act of breastfeeding. While the employers of wet nurses might grudgingly laud nurses' beneficial product, they deemed wet nurses themselves troublesome. Many linked breastfeeding with these allegedly inferior and immoral employees. Among the well-to-do, breastfeeding was becoming less an activity of biological necessity and motherly love and more an activity associated with the uncontrollable, unworthy, and vulgar lower class.

◆

Much of the history of wet nursing in the United States is obscure because little evidence remains of wet nurses' lives and work. Since private families in the late nineteenth and early twentieth centuries employed wet nurses far more frequently than did record-keeping institutions, it is not even possible to ascertain the precise extent of their use. Doctors' anecdotes and mothers' letters to women's magazines confirm that they were hired well into the twentieth century.[9] In addition, help-wanted and situation-wanted ads for wet nurses appeared occasionally in the *Chicago Tribune*. There were not many ads, however—an average of three or four on most Sundays in the last quarter of the nineteenth century—because wet nurses were most often procured, not via a newspaper advertisement or even an employment agency, but privately and discreetly through the family physician.

Women who did hire private wet nurses to suckle their babies were usually vague about their reasons for not breastfeeding. One Massachusetts mother began a letter to *Babyhood* magazine quite casually: "When it became evident after my daughter's birth that a wet-nurse or artificial feeding were the only alternatives . . ."[10] Her letter implied, as did many others, that an inability to lactate was so commonplace that explanations were unnecessary.

Physicians complained, however, that when a mother hired a wet nurse it was often a selfish decision. One New York City doctor claimed that some mothers who were capable of breastfeeding hired wet nurses because many wealthy families assumed that lactation impaired women's health by sapping their strength. He also contended that some well-to-do mothers employed wet nurses so they would be free to socialize. Joseph DeLee, one of the first obstetricians in Chicago, agreed with the latter charge. He complained in 1898 that "women of fashionable society" chose to pursue "a busy round of pleasures, late parties, dinners, theater, champagne" rather than breastfeed their infants. He accused wealthy mothers of recklessly abandoning their babies to life-threatening diseases precipitated by the bottle or "the cold comfort of a mercenary hireling wetnurse."[11]

Exactly what types of families used wet nurses is as nebulous as how many families used them and why, although only upper-class families could easily afford them. Isaac Abt seemed to have this in mind in 1917 when he explained that he deliberately kept the salaries of the wet nurses who worked at Sarah Morris Children's Hospital in Chicago at a low eight dollars a week. "It is the middle and lower class people, of no great means, who need them most," he explained, and he wanted to keep their milk affordable. Another Chicago doctor agreed with Abt's reasoning, but pointed out that even at eight dollars a week the cost of human milk far exceeded what most families could pay. A Detroit doctor suggested that if wealthier families paid considerably more for human milk, effectively subsidizing those who could not afford it, breast milk would be available to all babies.[12]

Alleviating "Disastrous Results"

The proposal was a radical one but this physician was by no means alone in believing that almost any means of getting human milk to a sick baby was worth the effort. Since doctors advised mothers that human milk was necessary for the normal, healthy development of an infant, if forced to choose between a wet nurse and a bottle most doctors thought there was no contest. They favored mothers' milk, *any* mother's milk.

They based their preference on bitter experience. At the New York Infant Asylum, opened in 1865, employees fed babies artificial food with such "disastrous results" that although the asylum had cribs for 150, no more than twenty-five or thirty beds were ever occupied because the death rate was so high. Not until the asylum's directors added a large maternity ward to the building, in order to supply babies with a steady stream of wet nurses, did the institution become "one of the best-conducted, and most successful of the charitable institutions in New York."[13]

Opened in 1871, the Chicago Foundlings' Home likewise employed wet nurses. The Home housed poverty-stricken mothers and their babies, as well as abandoned infants and babies brought in by distraught fathers whose wives had died. From the start, the babies living at the Home unaccompanied by their mothers suffered by far the highest death rates. Cognizant of this, the Home's directors were "always glad to take all the wet-nurses" they could get and required the mothers living there to breastfeed one other baby in addition to their own.[14] In 1874 the Home housed, over the course of twelve months, one hundred women who wet-nursed infants.[15] But even with that extraordinary number, the Home almost never had enough human milk to keep all the babies well. So distressing was this lack of breast milk that workers noted an unprecedented event in September 1879: there were briefly more wet nurses available than babies who needed them.[16]

The Home's directors found that few babies survived artificial feeding, hence they never permitted more than ten artificially fed infants at a time to live there and lamented in 1882, "[O]ur experience has shown us that [even that] . . . is too many." When the two rooms in the Home set aside for bottle-fed babies were full, employees turned over infants left on the doorstep to other charities for care. Even when Chicago's hospitals made special pleas to the Home to take in a baby whose mother had died in childbirth, employees did so only when they had sufficient wet nurses.[17]

Given the high diarrheal death rate among artificially fed infants, the medical community preferred wet nurses to bottles well into the twentieth century. In 1886, editors of the popular infant-care magazine *Babyhood* encouraged mothers who did not breastfeed to hire a wet nurse. Editors assured women, "A wet-nurse *is* a nuisance, but no one who has tried one will ever take any other way of bringing up a baby that she cannot suckle herself." In 1910 the Chicago Board of Health urged mothers to hire a wet nurse rather than bottle-feed, "for there are certain elements in mother's milk that we cannot supply in any artificial food." As late as 1927 the U.S. Children's Bureau recommended in their extremely popular pamphlet *Infant Care* that mothers who did not breastfeed hire a wet nurse.[18]

"One-Quarter Cow and Three-Quarters Devil"

If a mother agreed to hire a wet nurse, it was almost always the responsibility of the family doctor to locate one immediately. Doctors searched and negotiated for wet nurses without complaint; they considered the task part of their job. One doctor, curious about how many physicians customarily found wet nurses for families, queried doctors around the country in 1913. Of the eighty who responded, only eight claimed never to have found a wet nurse for a patient. Most said they hired six or more a year.[19]

Isaac Abt was typical. He often found artificially fed infants near death on first examination. They were usually in such dire straits that he found their "recovery extremely doubtful, unless something could be done at once." His advice to these infants' mothers was always the same. "First of all," he told them, "we must get a wet nurse." On one of his many sojourns to find a wet nurse, Abt bargained frantically with the matron of a maternity home, eventually trading new lace curtains for a wet nurse's services. Boston physician Fritz Talbot likewise spent hours each week hunting for wet nurses. During one particularly trying search in 1908, he scoured the city on electric car lines for the better part of three days.[20]

Although most doctors agreed that wet nurses were the best choice, they warned that wet nurses heralded serious problems for employers. Doctors typically sympathized with the mothers who employed wet nurses; rarely did they pity the wet nurse. Arthur Meigs, who toiled for many years to create an artificial food that carbon-copied human milk, warned, "The class of society from which wet-nurses are drawn is a very low one . . . and therefore the chance of their being diseased is very great; and, besides, they are generally of such a low order as to be difficult to manage." Another doctor claimed that a wet nurse could pose an even greater risk to a baby's health than a bottle if she did not have "the proper mental . . . qualifications, such as temperance, equanimity, [and] sense of duty." Frank Spooner Churchill, a prominent Chicago pediatrician, had similar qualms. Although he told colleagues at a meeting of the Chicago Medical Society that "a good wet nurse" would provide a better substitute for mother's milk than any artificial food, he simultaneously cautioned, "A wet nurse is one-quarter cow and three-quarters devil."[21]

These complaints, directed at the immigrants and the working poor who toiled as wet nurses, were not particularly unusual during the Gilded Age and Progressive Era. Class rancor and nativism were rife and, accordingly, the families who hired wet nurses often complained that "suitable" wet nurses were impossible to procure. Wet nurses were usually poor women forced to sell their milk either because they were unwed mothers abandoned by their families—in which case they were also subjected to their employers' moral judgment—or because their husbands had died or deserted them. The wet nurses at the Chicago Foundlings' Home were typical. Their only choice, if they wanted to keep their babies, was between moving into the Home and suckling another infant in addition to their own or living in the county poorhouse.[22]

Chicago pediatrician Julius Hess tried to blur what so many employers saw as a clear dichotomy—they were well-bred and superior, the wet nurses they hired were crude and inferior—by explaining that there were actually two types of wet nurses. One was "well-born" but had fallen on hard times. An advertisement in the Chicago Medical Society's weekly publication, *The Chicago Medical Recorder,* hinted at just such a situation in 1899: "A Widowed Lady, age nineteen, educated, refined, would accept situation as wet-nurse. A good home in a refined family is desired for her." The other type of wet nurse, Hess explained, was born of poverty and likely to gain an exaggerated sense of self-importance if showered with too many unaccustomed luxuries. He suggested, to avoid problems, that the wet nurse "be treated neither as a guest nor as a menial, but so far as possible should be graded according to her previous station in life." *Babyhood* magazine likewise differentiated between types of wet nurses, that is, types of *unmarried* wet nurses. Because women born in the United States should know proper from improper behavior, *Babyhood* deemed them of immoral character and deserving of scorn if they had a baby while unmarried. But if a woman was raised in a country where marriage among the poor was illegal, or where marriage essentially began with an engagement, *Babyhood* argued that single motherhood did not necessarily indicate an immoral character. "In these people," *Babyhood* explained, "unchastity does not presuppose the same laxity of principle as among us, and the chances of vicious character are correspondingly less."[23]

Chicago pediatrician Clifford Grulee sympathized with the plight of wet nurse and employer alike. "The natural independence of the lower classes and their failure to appreciate superiority of any sort," he wrote, "combined with the frequent haughtiness of their employers as a result of newly acquired prosperity, raises almost insuperable barriers to domestic peace." A less sympathetic doctor observed, "The wet-nurse—who often comes from a life of hardship and toil to one of luxury and idleness—naturally eats anything and everything. . . . As a result, she grows ill, her milk fails, and a change has to be made." He suggested, "notwithstanding the moral objections," that unmarried wet nurses made the best employees as they could "be more easily controlled."[24]

While employers usually attributed a wet nurse's undesirable personality to her class background, most doctors' judgments of wet nurses' lactation ability were colored by racial and ethnic stereotypes. "One class [of wet nurses] consists of those who have plenty of milk," wrote one doctor, "e.g. Italians and colored mothers." Hess thought precisely the opposite. "The phlegmatic temperaments as seen in women of Northern and Central Europe and of Teutonic and Slavic descent, offer the ideal material," he advised, while "Italians and Southern negroes when removed from their home environment . . . secrete a milk poor in quality." But he also demonstrated the measure of most parents' desperation when he added, "However, even the latter in an emergency should not be neglected." Another doctor argued that American-born females made poor wet nurses compared with Irish and German immigrants because the former had "flat and narrow chests."[25]

While most physicians believed that ethnicity dictated body type and that body type dictated lactation ability, others rejected these sentiments. One such physician found, after a lengthy search, an African American woman willing to breastfeed a very sick white baby. The baby's shocked mother objected strenuously to the doctor's choice of a wet nurse. The angry doctor promptly offered to find a cow in lieu of the unsuitable wet nurse. What kind of a cow would you prefer, he sarcastically asked the infant's mother, "a black, a white or a red one?"[26]

Given the low opinion of wet nurses, there were doctors who wholly objected to their use, although these physicians were a minority. One declared that a woman was driven to wet nurse for only two reasons—poverty or to make money—and that both motives made her inherently unsuitable. A poverty-stricken woman, he argued, was too weak "to undergo the hardships of double nursing." A woman belonging to the "mercenary class," on the other hand, was "endowed with so little moral obligation as to require constant watching to protect the child." How could any physician assume responsibility, he mused, for the actions of a potentially "corrupt or vicious woman" who may "carry out the vilest schemes or indulge in the most demoralizing practices"? Another physician, lecturing before the Practitioners' Society of New York in 1884, contended, "The physical defects of the bottle we understand pretty well, and can, to a great extent, guard against them. Its moral qualifications, compared with those of the wet-nurse, are simply sublime."[27]

W. S. Christopher, a Chicago pediatrician, was similarly concerned that when the advantages of breast milk were weighed against a wet nurse's personality, "the balance is not always on the side of the wet nurse." Christopher argued in 1892 that the "modern methods" of artificial feeding had advanced sufficiently so "that in the hands of intelligent and conscientious parents, they prove more efficient than wet nursing."[28] Physician Leonard Keene Hirshberg warned, "Wet-nurses, at their best, are unsatisfactory, and at their worst they are exceedingly dangerous. . . . Taken as a class, they are ignorant, careless and unclean. Setting aside the occasional gem among them, they seldom provide their charges with nourishment as wholesome as that to be had from the milk laboratory."[29] Joseph Edcil Winters, a New York physician, preferred bottles when a mother did not breastfeed because the mortality rate among wet-nursed infants was higher than among mother-nursed infants. "When a mother cannot nurse her child," he asked angrily, "shall we recommend it to the perilous care of that most remarkable and incomprehensible of creatures, the wet-nurse?" Winters theorized that the death rate among wet-nursed babies was so high because those infants consumed "the milk of a hired nurse, whose passions, emotions, nervous organization, and whole constitution are totally different from those of the mother."[30]

Adamant opponents of wet nursing in the medical community remained the exceptions, however. Most doctors believed that a "satisfactory" wet nurse was possible to find if "sufficient trouble" was taken.[31] Even the most reluctant advocates acknowledged that the practice saved lives. Emelyn Lincoln Coolidge, a physician and popular *Ladies' Home Journal* columnist, contended that wet nurses were unduly expensive and "very uncertain as to temper, sometimes making a great deal of trouble in a house," but she consistently recommended them as a last resort for sick infants.[32] And although the editors of *Babyhood* magazine acknowledged that "wet-nurses are not selected from the highly-intelligent classes," they nevertheless defended wet nursing as better for a baby than bottle-feeding. Mothers learned in *Baby-hood* that a wet nurse is chosen for one quality and one quality only—"a good breast of milk." Wet nurses "are neither better nor worse than other women in their rank in life," contended *Babyhood* editors, "and come with an honest intent to do their duty."[33]

"The End of All Peace in the Household"

The reassurances comforted employers little. "The natural repugnance of the mother" for wet nurses was often, in the words of one doctor, "an insurmountable obstacle."[34] Most mothers who did not breastfeed, "having a deeply-rooted prejudice against the whole race of substitute mothers," usually tried bottle-feeding first.[35] Only after that led to disaster did a woman bring a wet nurse into her home, replacing one distressing experience with another. Mothers felt simultaneously superior to and jealous of their wet nurses and hid that jealousy behind an impenetrable wall of moral judgment.[36] *Babyhood* magazine defended mothers' behavior: "Nothing can be more repugnant to one's instincts than to trust the dear child, whose natural nourishment has failed, to the care of a woman whose very fitness for the task is evidence of her unchastity."[37]

A letter from one Massachusetts mother, Fanny B. Workman,[38] to *Baby-hood* magazine in 1886 describes a host of trials suffered by her as an employer of wet nurses. The letter also vividly illustrates, although it clearly was not Workman's intent to do so, the terrible predicament of wet nurses who worked in private households. Workman's letter is unusual only in its detail; many shorter letters to women's magazines voice similar complaints and describe similar situations.

According to Workman, her bottle-fed daughter sickened soon after birth. In dismay, Workman summoned two doctors who immediately suggested hiring a wet nurse. "With a sigh of despair," Workman immediately anticipated "the end of all peace in the household."[39] Reluctantly, she employed "a simple, unintelligent-looking Irish girl" who, at Workman's insistence, "placed out" her own baby before starting the job. Workman then devoted a week "to the renovation of the person of the Irish Mary, whom it was necessary to clothe anew from head to foot." Eventually satisfied with her servant's appearance and basking in the compliments of neighbors who admired the wet nurse's new look, Workman lamented, "If only the look of intelligence were not wanting!"

A litany of complaints followed. The nurse was slow in getting out of the way of oncoming carriages when she took the baby for a walk. When the wet nurse carried the infant, "the child's head hung over her arm and vibrated like a pendulum." An extremely annoyed Workman followed the wet nurse around for weeks adjusting her daughter's head. The sneaky wet nurse consumed all the foods that Workman forbade her (tea, ice water, and pickles) lest they spoil her milk, slyly persuading the cook to give them to her. The cook, "that weak-minded individual," had to be fired. When the wet nurse learned that her own baby had taken ill, she wanted to go to the baby at once. In order to dissuade the wet nurse from leaving, Workman arranged to have the wet nurse's sick baby cared for—at Workman's expense—by a woman at a nearby farmhouse. After two weeks the farmer's wife declared that caring for the wet nurse's baby was too much work "and when the nurse was told her baby must be changed again she became greatly agitated, and consequently her milk had a decidedly bad effect upon her charge." The distraught wet nurse demanded to care for her baby herself in Workman's home, alongside Workman's child. Appalled, Workman fired her and began the hunt for another wet nurse.

She quickly found another candidate, who was "decidedly unattractive, with a face of most heavy, unintelligent mould." When the woman arrived for her job interview with her infant in arms Workman asked, "Did you not understand that you were to leave your baby?" The woman quickly agreed to "place out" her baby and accepted the job. Two weeks later the new wet nurse received a telegram informing her of her baby's death. Frantic with grief, she prepared to attend the funeral. An irate Workman complained, "I decided that would never do. . . . After an hour or two spent in argument I prevailed upon her not to go to the funeral. How I made her see that it could in no way benefit her to go, and might kill my child, I do not know, but finally she did see it all."

After the death of her child, however, the wet nurse was not as easily ordered about. She "became very unruly and obstinate" and ate foods that did not agree with the baby. Workman fired her. Rather than hire a third wet nurse, Workman offered her baby Mellin's Food "with perfect success." Her baby consumed the Mellin's Food "with an appetite she had never known for the nurse's milk." Workman concluded that "the milk of the gentle cow has the advantage over that of the wet-nurse—it is not affected by indulgence in peanuts, cucumbers, and ice-cream."

Mothers wrote to *Babyhood* to commiserate with Workman. Even a mother who defended wet nurses against Workman's assault—because her second child had been rescued from the ill effects of artificial food by the milk of a wet nurse—agreed that "it would seem superfluous to look for even average mental or moral qualification in persons of the class that furnish wet nurses." Another mother who "thoroughly believed" in wet nurses, because her son had become so robust at their breasts, hired seven wet nurses in twenty months. "Many and manifold have been my trials and tribulations," she grumbled.[40] Mothers who defended wet nurses praised their product; rarely, if ever, did they commend the producer.

Mothers fretted most over a wet nurse's character. As one women asked, "How can any mother dare . . . risk . . . the effect upon her child of a wet-nurse in whose family some terrible disease may be hereditary, or, what is worse than disease or death, who is an immoral woman?" A steady stream of anecdotes reinforced the fear that wet-nursed babies absorbed their nurse's unsavory character as easily as they digested their milk. One mother reported that a friend's child became a replica of her wet nurse, with identical facial expressions and mannerisms. "There could be no doubt that the milk which she drank, being nothing less than the veritable blood of the wet-nurse, undoubtedly changed the character."[41]

Babyhood magazine editors tried to disabuse women of the conviction that the disposition of the wet nurse could be transmitted through her milk, declaring the notion an absurdity "raised . . . by mothers whose characters were far less deserving of admiration than that of the despised nurse." Food, explained *Babyhood* editors, does not affect personality. Abt advised his patients' mothers to hire wet nurses "of phlegmatic temperament and good morals," but likewise reminded them not to dwell too much on this issue as "moral qualities are not transmitted through the milk."[42]

"Wanted—A Wet-Nurse WITHOUT A Baby"

Despite employers' incessant, vociferous complaints, the dilemmas inherent in wet nursing—as illustrated by Fanny Workman's two hapless employees— were far greater for the wet nurse. Like Workman, private employers almost always refused to allow a wet nurse's baby to live in their home. As one *Chicago Tribune* ad unabashedly put it, "Wanted—A Wet-Nurse, WITHOUT A Baby."[43] Thus wet nurses commonly placed their own babies in foundling homes where caretakers gave them artificial food. The death rate of these infants was enormous.[44]

Physicians readily acknowledged that hiring a private wet nurse usually meant a poor baby died in order to save a rich one. Doctors constantly discussed solutions to the problem. One New York physician, noting that wet nurses worked "even in families in which the mothers are fully competent to suckle their own infants," suggested that doctors refuse to find wet nurses for women capable of breastfeeding because of the "gross injustice . . . done to the infants of the wet-nurses." Hess counseled employers to permit a wet nurse to keep her baby with her. That largesse, he advised, would benefit the employer as well as the wet nurse. He explained, "The presence of the wet-nurse's baby predisposes to her peace of mind," and, consequently, the household would benefit from her tranquillity. The U.S. Children's Bureau concurred, recommending that a wet nurse be allowed to keep her baby and nurse it alongside her employer's infant because "her peace of mind will insure better breast milk." Grulee told doctors who placed wet nurses with families to feel "morally bound" to assure that the wet nurse's infant "receives the most careful attention." A New York doctor who had treated many "a wet-nurse's starved baby" proposed legislation in 1886 making it illegal for any woman to leave her baby in an institution so she could work as a private wet nurse. But the only state to do anything about the situation was Maryland, whose legislature passed a law in 1916 forbidding the separation of a mother and baby during the first six months of the baby's life. Between 1915 and 1921, Maryland reduced the death rate of babies born to unwed mothers from one out of three to one out of eight. The U.S. Children's Bureau attributed the decrease in deaths to the fact that the six-months law made it more likely that single mothers would stay with their babies and, consequently, breastfeed them.[45]

The wet nurses forced to trade their babies for employment could expect no job security in return, as Fanny Workman's letter demonstrates. One physician noted that the mother of one patient fired thirteen wet nurses in fourteen days. He did not consider this particularly unusual. Disturbed by the trend, Grulee suggested that no wet nurse be judged by her first days on the job. "The complete change of surroundings and diet are frequently the cause of disturbances in the flow of milk," he explained, "and until the woman becomes accustomed to these one should not judge of her fitness as a nurse."[46]

Wet nurses faced hazards in addition to job insecurity and losing their babies, syphilis infection among them.[47] Grulee advised, "[U]nder no circumstances allow a syphilitic baby or the offspring of syphilitic parents, whether that child shows signs of syphilis or not, to suckle a healthy woman."[48] The city of Baltimore, whose Board of Supervisors of City Charities was responsible for the care of foundlings, ignored this warning when they hired wet nurses. This practice had dire consequences: a mechanic's wife paid by the city to take in a baby to breastfeed (her own infant twins had died) contracted congenital syphilis from the infant, whose mother was a prostitute. The illness remained undiagnosed until the mechanic's wife developed a chancre on her breast from nursing the baby. The angry doctor who treated the woman charged that the Baltimore Board of Supervisors of City Charities treated the health of its wet nurses far too casually. "If a man knowingly put my wife . . . in danger of syphilis," he wrote, "and gave no warning and . . . [she] acquired it, I would consider a bullet too good for him."[49]

As this physician observed, the damage a baby could do a wet nurse's health was usually ignored. Customarily, mothers and doctors who hired wet nurses usually worried about the opposite possibility—that a wet nurse might egregiously affect her nursling's health. Thus, wet nurses hired through physicians always received rigorous physical examinations. Physicians who hired wet nurses to work in hospitals considered physical examinations even more vital. Doctors wanted to prevent a wet nurse from passing an infectious disease, first to a weak and susceptible infant, and then to the entire hospital.[50] When examining potential wet nurses, doctors administered Wasserman reaction tests for syphilis and examined wet nurses' vaginal secretions for signs of gonorrhea. They inspected wet nurses' teeth because they deemed a nurse's ability to chew a wide variety of foods essential to good milk. Physicians also checked nurses for symptoms of tuberculosis.[51] Although it was common knowledge by the end of the nineteenth century that bacteria rather than habits, character, or class caused tuberculosis, the poverty-stricken still shouldered disproportionate blame for the disease. Weakened by constant exposure to substandard housing, unhealthy working conditions, and poor diets, they were, after all, the most susceptible to TB.[52] Dread of infectious disease made the myriad imagined threats posed by wet nurses all the more frightening.

To ascertain her ability to produce milk, physicians also examined the wet nurse's baby. If her baby was healthy, that was the surest sign she was capable of producing ample quality milk. Some doctors also put stock in determining the chemical composition of a wet nurse's milk.[53] Hess looked for specific physical attributes in a wet nurse. She had to be eighteen to thirty-five years old and in good health, and to have "good quality" mammary glands and "sufficiently developed" nipples. Having more than one living child was an additional asset, he argued, because her children's good health demonstrated a woman's long-term ability to successfully breastfeed.

Hess also advised that multiparas were less likely to be perturbed by the unfamiliar surroundings they faced in private homes.[54]

Systematizing the Search for Wet Nurses

Because fewer women in the early twentieth century were willing to wet-nurse for meager, insecure livings, the hunt for wet nurses became more taxing. Physicians, municipalities, and medical charities consequently proposed ways to make the search easier. In 1906 one doctor suggested that the American Pediatric Society spearhead a campaign in every sizable community to organize the registration of wet nurses. Without a systematic way to locate a wet nurse, he protested, "there is an abundance of mother's milk going to waste all over the country." Another physician complained in 1908 of "something twisted in our arrangement of preventive medicine," because every large American city housed a milk commission to disseminate clean cows' milk to babies, but not a single organization existed to address "the many perplexing problems of the human milk supply." He suggested creating a national human milk commission both to maintain a corps of wet nurses and to establish human milk stations for the sale of bottled breast milk. Yet another doctor proposed that each community appoint one local organization to maintain a list of mothers with a "superabundance" of milk. There was "plenty of human milk to be had," he contended, if only the country's pediatric societies would "facilitate its being obtained."[55]

Women began to cooperate voluntarily with such endeavors. One mother wrote an article for *American Motherhood* magazine urging prolific women to share their excess milk ("a veritable elixir of life") with mothers unable to nurse because of illness or "failure of milk." The author herself supplied fifteen to twenty-six ounces of milk each day to a sick baby. Aided by instructions from her family physician, she learned to pump milk from one breast while her baby nursed on the other. Twice each day the sick baby's father picked up the milk that the woman stored on ice in sterile bottles until his arrival.[56]

The call to share this precious commodity in lieu of the traditional wet nurse continued.[57] One Detroit physician suggested that if mothers with abundant milk would make their milk available to less-fortunate mothers, "it would be a great factor in reducing infant mortality as well as preventing a great economic waste."[58] The sharing of human milk came naturally in some locales. In Chicago, mothers who brought their breastfed babies to Infant Welfare Society stations for regular well-baby examinations occasionally breastfed babies whose mothers did not nurse. Station doctors facilitated this aid by telling lactating mothers about particular infants in desperate need of human milk.[59] In Jewish and Italian neighborhoods in New York City women commonly nursed each other's babies, particularly if one mother found her milk supply waning.[60] In these environments, the need for the traditional wet nurse was virtually nonexistent.

This largesse was not ubiquitous, however, and medical personnel continued to devise unconventional methods to locate wet nurses. In Chicago, the Mother and Baby Welfare Association opened a Wet Nurse Bureau of Information in 1905. The bureau "carefully investigated" all their wet nurses and issued them certificates of health. The bureau charged employers five dollars to find and certify a wet nurse. If any wet nurse proved "unsatisfactory," the bureau provided another at no additional charge.[61] The Chicago Visiting Nurse Association (VNA)—whose public health nurses had perpetual access to potential wet nurses because of their large postpartum-care service for the poor—routinely told their patients that if they had more milk than they needed to sustain their own baby, and if they wanted to work as wet nurses, they should "report to any large obstetrical service . . . and ask if a wet-nurse is needed."[62] In Boston, one doctor obtained breast milk from mothers residing at the local Salvation Army Home.[63] New York City pursued a more macabre route. Employees of the city's infant welfare program perused incoming death certificates looking for stillbirths. When they learned of one, a worker immediately visited the dead baby's mother to ask if she would be willing to wet nurse an infant.[64]

Medical societies in some cities throughout the United States struggled to provide wet nurses through an institution designed solely for that purpose. Members of the Chicago Pediatric Society recommended in 1907 that a bureau to register wet nurses be established in the Chicago VNA central office. Society members suggested that the bureau advertise its services in the *Bulletin of the Chicago Medical Society* and that data on potential wet nurses—their personality, age, health status, and general history—be made available to interested physicians. VNA superintendent Harriet Fulmer agreed to the proposition. The wealthy women who ran the Children's Hospital Society, however, thwarted the Pediatric Society's efforts when they established their own bureau for wet nurses first. Pediatric Society members then decided that their own work on such a project was "unnecessary."[65]

Boston pediatricians established a Wet Nurse Directory in 1910.[66] Initial efforts in 1900 to simply list the wet nurses in Boston and make the list available to doctors and mothers failed because women forced to wet-nurse for a living could not afford to wait on a list to be hired. Wet nurses were invariably single mothers who needed immediate and steady work. So, to guarantee these women full-time employment and the medical community instant access to them, the Massachusetts Babies' Hospital obtained a house and hired eight women to live there with their babies. Residents earned room and board and eight dollars a week whether or not they were working. By 1915 the Boston Wet Nurse Directory paid their wet nurses fifteen dollars a week and enlarged the house to accommodate fourteen residents. Physicians in Massachusetts and in every large New England town learned of the directory via eight thousand postal cards.[67]

The wet nurses who moved from the directory to work in private homes brought their own babies with them "in every instance."[68] Directory doctors formulated the rule primarily to benefit the employer's baby, however. The sick babies breastfed by wet nurses were usually very weak and did not, at first, require much milk. If the wet nurse's own baby was not with her to nurse often and vigorously, directory doctors feared that her milk supply would quickly dwindle to the detriment of the employer's infant. Once the employer's baby regained strength and health, the doctors instructed wet nurses to nurse their own infants only if they had enough milk for both babies. If they did not, they were to feed their own babies artificially.[69]

The directory's physicians had the same ambivalent attitude toward their wet nurses as doctors in general did. Although they bragged of having healthy nurses with milk of fine quality, they also warned potential employers that "no guarantees as to their characters, habits and dispositions" could be made.[70] Hence, one mission of the Directory was the rehabilitation of their wet nurses. One reason Directory physicians required wet nurses' babies to accompany their mothers at all times—aside from the fact that it kept employers' babies in better health—was that doctors worried that if they forced a wet nurse to board her baby, her entire salary would go to that expense. If a wet nurse had no money accumulated at the end of her tenure, she would find herself in the same dire situation after as before her relatively short-term employment. Doctors also quizzed employers about the women's appearance and attitude. Directory doctors informed wet nurses of their employers' assessments and expected them to alter undesirable behaviors.[71]

The Boston Wet Nurse Directory obtained their residents through queries sent to private physicians and maternity hospitals. Maternity hospitals of that era delivered only the babies of poor or single women (married women of means summoned doctors to their homes[72]) and so hospitals welcomed the chance to place "friendless mothers who had to go penniless out into the world."[73]

Like so many of the institutions that either hired wet nurses for their own use or supplied them to families, by the end of the 1910s the Wet Nurse Directory of Boston began looking for additional means of gathering and supplying human milk. Eventually they hired a public health nurse to gather milk from healthy mothers in their homes. The nurse brought the milk to a central office where it was sterilized, bottled, and then delivered to the homes of sick, artificially fed infants. The endeavor was so successful that by 1927 the Directory hired a supervisor and second nurse and closed the home that housed wet nurses.[74]

Wet Nurses as Hospital Employees

By the 1910s, the ongoing shortage of wet nurses prompted doctors to urge hospitals to follow the example of foundling homes and hire wet nurses as live-in employees. Churchill told colleagues at a meeting of the American Pediatric Society, "I am sure that breast feeding is a most valuable factor in the reduction of our mortality and think wet-nurses should be a part of the regular equipment of a hospital." Grulee insisted that "every well-organized children's department must have a wet nurse." Abt contended, "An infants' hospital, which necessarily must receive the babies who have been most neglected and who require the most expert treatment, should consequently have at hand an ample supply of breast milk."[75]

In Chicago, wet nurses worked in hospitals to a greater extent than in other cities because members of the Chicago medical community pioneered both obstetric techniques and the care of premature infants. In doing so they deemed human milk essential to infants' survival, especially infants born prematurely. Joseph DeLee, the Chicago physician dubbed the "father of modern obstetrics," observed after years of medical practice that "without mother's milk, it is almost impossible to raise a premature infant—certainly to be a healthy one." DeLee explained that he had "given up all attempts with artificial feeding [of premature babies], and get mothers' milk at any trouble and expense."[76] Chicago was also home to Julius Hess, the "father of neonatal medicine,"[77] who opened the largest premature infant station in the country at Sarah Morris Children's Hospital in 1922. It was there that Hess and Evelyn Lundeen, the station's longtime supervising nurse, determined the three goals of premature infant care: maintenance of body temperature, prevention of infection, and provision of adequate nutrition. Hess and Lundeen defined this adequate nutrition quite simply—human milk. Breast milk, they argued, was "of paramount importance in the feeding of premature infants."

Thus, if a mother did not supply her premature baby with breast milk, one of Sarah Morris's resident wet nurses did.[78]

At Abt's behest, wet nurses lived in a wing of Sarah Morris—the pediatric department of Chicago's Michael Reese Hospital—from its inception in 1913.[79] Abt observed that at Sarah Morris, "babies are brought in to us marantic, with cold extremities, on the very edge of the hereafter, and we give them a few teaspoonfuls of breast milk, and keep on giving it, and the babies revive. We do this day after day." With human milk, he contended, most sick babies could be saved, without it, "we would lose nearly every one."[80]

Like other doctors who hired wet nurses to work in hospitals, Abt insisted that wet nurses live with and breastfeed their own babies. The practice not only kept the babies healthy, he explained, but the "natural stimulation to . . . [their mothers'] breasts" ensured an ample milk supply for the hospitalized infants who received their human milk in bottles. Wet nurses at Sarah Morris produced, on average, thirty-seven ounces of milk per day, in addition to the milk they supplied their own babies. They nursed their own babies at 7 A.M., 11 A.M., 3 P.M., and 9 P.M. and slept a hefty ten hours—from 9 P.M. to 7 A.M.—because hospital nurses woke them up every four hours to express the milk to be given in bottles to sick and premature babies.[81]

Sarah Morris's wet nurses earned eight dollars a week plus room and board. In addition to providing milk, they did light cleaning around the hospital. Initially, they learned to express their milk manually. Abt disliked breast pumps, charging that they were inefficient and occasionally injured the breast.[82] In 1922, after Abt invented an electric breast pump, wet nurses at Sarah Morris learned to use it. His pump proved remarkably efficient, sucking the breast forty-five times a minute and providing more stimulation, consequently causing more milk to be produced, than a hungry infant. Women adjusted suction pressure to minimize injuries. The pump worked so well that it procured milk even after women swore that their milk had been depleted by hand expression.[83]

Beginning in 1909, Chicago's Children's Memorial Hospital found women willing to wet-nurse through the local Salvation Army headquarters. Wet nurses fed their own babies on one breast and a sick infant on the other.[84] Churchill noted that it was "astonishing" how much milk these wet nurses supplied the hospital after a few week's employ, owing to frequent nipple stimulation. One woman, he claimed proudly, produced five quarts in a single day.[85]

When employees at Chicago's Presbyterian Hospital discovered in 1914 that of the ten hospitalized babies in their nursery only two were nursed by their own mothers, they too hired a wet nurse.[86] The lone wet nurse was rarely able to supply ample milk for all the hospitalized babies who needed it, so her milk was given only to the sickest ones.[87] Like at Sarah Morris, Presbyterian's wet nurse earned eight dollars a week plus room and board. Her baby lived in the children's ward. In the first four months of her employment, doctors credited her with saving the lives of twenty-five babies. Between July 1916 and September 1916, inclusive, doctors and nurses cared for 136 infants at Presbyterian. Thirty-eight of them received milk from the wet nurse. In 1917, seventy babies drank the wet nurse's milk. One, fed artificially from birth, came to Presbyterian "quite lifeless," and nurses had to give him human milk through a feeding tube because he was too weak to suck. Presbyterian doctors attributed his survival to breast milk.[88]

In order to prevent infection from being passed from wet nurse to baby and vice versa, wet nurses at Presbyterian put only their own babies to their breast. They withdrew the milk fed to hospitalized babies with the Caldwell breast pump, a suction device, after sterilizing their breasts with boracic acid. Hospital personnel kept human milk on ice for two to twenty-four hours, as demand dictated. In 1928 Presbyterian ceased having a wet nurse in its permanent employ and hired one only "as needed."[89]

Although doctors who worked with wet nurses in hospitals held them in higher esteem than did private families, physicians nevertheless spoke of them in similarly derisive, wary tones. Hess helped design a uniform "to overcome the slovenly appearance of the wet nurse as she is usually seen wandering about the wards of an infants' hospital." Grulee cautioned that "careful supervsion [sic] of the wet nurse is very necessary." Abt acknowledged that babies "usually flourished on their milk, which fortunately, could not transmit moral qualities along with its health-giving properties."[90]

Abt's distrust of wet nurses was so profound that he took special "precautions . . . to guard against . . . [their] vagaries" at Sarah Morris Children's Hospital, placing them under constant surveillance.[91] "It has happened more than once," Abt explained, "that a woman desiring to engage herself as wet-nurse has presented some other woman's baby borrowed temporarily for the purpose" of getting hired. Consequently, Abt ordered the monitoring of each wet nurse's milk output and fired women at the first sign of diminished production. In this manner, he claimed to have caught some unscrupulous wet nurses diluting their milk with cows' milk and others wholly substituting cows' milk for their own.[92]

The precarious nature of their jobs—and not wanton disregard for babies' health—probably forced some Sarah Morris wet nurses into this dangerous mischief, for the involuntary turnover rate of wet nurses living in hospitals was as high as in private homes. Some hospitals automatically fired a wet nurse when her menstrual cycle resumed, although this did not occur at Sarah Morris, where doctors found that, contrary to popular belief, menstruation had little, if any, effect on milk quantity and quality. Like at other hospitals, however, Sarah Morris's wet nurses did lose their jobs when their babies reached a certain age because many physicians believed that human milk had little nutritive value after nine months. Abt was characteristic in this regard. Even though he knew that a mother's breasts would continue to produce milk as long as nursing babies stimulated them, he feared that milk quality hopelessly deteriorated by the end of the first year. Thus he was uncomfortable keeping any wet nurse for more than nine to ten months.[93]

The quick turnover of wet nurses at Presbyterian Hospital demonstrates the insecurity of wet nurses' lives. Six months after hiring their first wet nurse in 1914, Presbyterian replaced her. Though the second nurse's milk output was not as great as the first's, Presbyterian dubbed her "a great blessing." Their satisfaction with her was fleeting, however. She lost her job one month later to be replaced by a third wet nurse, an Italian woman who spoke no English. This woman stayed eight and one-half months and was fired in May 1915. The new wet nurse lost her job two months later. The subsequent wet nurse was fired in September. Her successor likewise lasted only two months. The wet nurse hired in November left on April 15, 1916, when another wet nurse took up residence. She was replaced on June 16. On November 1, that wet nurse was fired.[94]

The anxiety of wet nurses working in hospitals was likely exacerbated by the desperate circumstances that drove them to the job in the first place. The nurse hired by Presbyterian Hospital in November 1915 was a Canadian whose husband had been killed the previous February. She was left with three children to care for and pregnant with a fourth. Another Presbyterian wet nurse, hired in June 1916, was a Hungarian woman deserted by her husband. She kept her infant with her at the hospital and used her salary to board her eighteen month old. After a stint as a wet nurse, a woman's life usually reverted to its bleak origins. In June 1917 the wet nurse fired by Presbyterian Hospital—"as her infant was eight months old"—was the first in three years of rapid hirings and firings who "had a real home to go to" when she left the hospital. She went to live with her parents.[95]

Human Milk Stations: "Eliminating Difficult Problems"

In the 1920s wet nursing took on yet another form. By 1929 at least twenty American cities provided bottled breast milk to sick and premature infants through human milk stations.[96] Doctors heralded the stations as an improvement in labor relations. As one physician noted, "The feeding of breast milk through the intermediary of a wet nurse is . . . an age long procedure, but here is a new venture, of passing the milk of the wetnurse through a bottle to the baby, thus eliminating . . . any difficult problems."[97] Physicians deemed breast milk depots cost-effective as well. One Detroit doctor estimated that human milk stations, as opposed to conventional wet nurses, cut the cost of providing an ounce of human milk to a sick baby from twenty-one cents an ounce in 1916 to fifteen cents an ounce in 1923.[98]

Stations continued to rely on historically proven methods to find donors. One doctor declared that as long as a city had a maternity hospital, an ample supply of breast milk was guaranteed.[99] Nurses and doctors routinely asked—"in the most natural way"—any hospitalized postpartum woman with abundant breast milk to share milk "with a less fortunate infant whose mother had died in childbirth or who for some good reason could not supply her infant from her own breast." Most mothers agreed to do so with no thought of payment. Physicians soon discovered, however, that when these mothers' maternity bills came due and additional expenses for their babies piled up, money was a reliable incentive to continue milk donation.[100]

In Chicago, the Board of Health began paying women for their milk when public health officials opened the Chicago Board of Health Mothers' Breast Milk Station in 1938.[101] The milk station's bottled and pasteurized human milk effectively replaced Chicago's resident hospital wet nurses. The Board of Health's Revised Code of 1931 likely made the milk station imperative—the Code required that every hospitalized premature infant be fed breast milk and that the Board furnish the milk to a hospital immediately upon request. If the baby's mother did not provide breast milk, hospitals now turned to the Breast Milk Station, which supplied the milk at no charge. In 1938 the station furnished 624 babies with 99,210 ounces of milk purchased from 302 mothers. In 1940, 920 babies consumed 101,561½ ounces from 246 mothers.[102]

The Board's public health nurses, who visited all new mothers and babies in their homes, located most of the station's human milk donors. On a nurse's first visit to a home, she asked any woman with a lot of milk if she would be interested in selling excess milk to the milk station. If a mother was interested, the nurse brought her in for a thorough physical and dental examination. After a mother was accepted as a donor, as long as she continued to come in each morning to express her milk, she received free medical examinations. Nurses cultured her throat each week for bacteria and drew her blood each month to check for sexually transmitted diseases. They examined her baby weekly as well and were especially careful to chart her baby's weight gains. If a donor's baby was not gaining weight, the station's nurses stopped accepting milk from the mother and urged her to give all her milk to her baby.[103]

Gertrude Plotzke, the public health nurse who opened the Breast Milk Station at the behest of Chicago Commissioner of Health Herman Bundesen and who remained its superintendent until the station closed in 1961, described its early days as part social event and part sanitary training experience. Each morning thirty-five to forty-five donors lined up at the station's three sinks to take turns washing their hands and breasts in a carefully devised hygienic ritual. Mothers took the daily washing routine so seriously that when public health nurses occasionally came to the station to observe, mothers protested that the nurses were not washing their hands properly. "They would watch the nurses and then they would complain the nurses didn't know how to scrub," explained an amused Plotzke years later. "I said, 'Well, they'll learn.'"[104]

After washing, mothers sat at a table wearing sterile masks over their mouths. Placing disinfected towels under their breasts, they hand-expressed their milk into sterile tin cups for about an hour. After donors left, Plotzke and her assistant, gowned and masked as if to perform surgery, measured the milk, poured it into bottles, and placed the bottles on ice in buckets. Then they pasteurized the milk in a fifteen-gallon pasteurizer and sterilized equipment for use the following day. Later they filled the orders that came in daily from both hospitals and families. Plotzke froze excess milk in the station's Deepfreeze, a rare piece of equipment for any enterprise in those days. Customers picked up their own milk—the station had no delivery service until much later in its history.[105]

The Board of Health paid milk donors five cents an ounce for their milk in 1938 (selling milk was a particularly convenient way for a mother with a baby to earn money during the Great Depression), nine cents by 1944, and thirteen cents an ounce by the time the station closed in the early 1960s. In addition, mothers earned streetcar tokens for their trek to and from the station and a quart of cows' milk to supplement their diets. Nurses working at the station insisted that mothers drink half the milk before leaving for the day. If mothers failed to down the milk, recalled Josephine Sobolewski, who became the station's supervisor in 1948 under Plotzke's auspices, "we knew what they would do. They would take it home and give it to the kids." According to Sobolewski, mothers ordinarily provided their milk for eight to nine months after the birth of their own babies, but she remembered at least one mother who donated for two to two-and-a-half years with each of her several babies.[106]

The occupation of wet nursing, which continued to be a necessary service for at least two decades into the twentieth century, ended with a public largely unaware that many cities housed human milk stations to replace the vanished wet nurse. Breast milk was delivered quietly to hospitals and homes, where mothers and nurses fed it to premature and dangerously ill infants until they revived. Janet Golden has called this the "commodification" of human milk. Breast milk, via human milk stations, became a commodity with its own inherent value, untainted by the unsavory characteristics of its supplier. Most recently, Golden points out, breast milk is not sold at all but donated in a "moral transaction."[107]

Despite her demise, memory of the unsavory wet nurse long remained. The employees at human milk bureaus took great pains to differentiate their respectable donor-mothers from wet nurses. As one doctor wrote, "This service in no way interferes with the duties of housewife and mother, and exposes her in no way to the public view. The only person with whom she need come in contact is the supervising nurse."[108] Bottled breast milk was said to be a "better foster-mother" than the "perennial wetnurse, that necessary but often slatternly female."[109] Human milk stations now provided milk from disembodied women—not troublesome, omnipresent employees who fed infants directly from their breasts.

Some mothers whose babies received this milk nevertheless had the same objection to using human milk from milk stations as women in previous decades had to using wet nurses; they doubted the "suitability" of the donor. In Detroit, for example, some white women refused to patronize the local milk bureau, fearing that the milk was from a "colored mother." Objections were so numerous that the bureau "virtually ceased" accepting milk from African American women. Milk from African American donors that was accepted in Detroit went only to hospitals to be pooled with the milk of white mothers "and furnished to those who have no objections."[110] Thus, milk stations began where wet nursing ended—amid class rancor, nativism, racism, ethnocentrism, and distrust of human milk.[111]

♦

Wet nursing was not an insignificant practice in the late nineteenth- and early twentieth-century United States. Conflicted attitudes toward wet nurses and their milk were so commonplace and influential that they helped some women justify their own aversion to maternal breastfeeding. In

Chicago, between 1871, when the Chicago Foundlings Home opened its door to orphaned babies and the women willing to wet-nurse them, and 1961, when the Board of Health closed the Mothers' Breast Milk Station, which had supplied bottled human milk at no cost to premature and sick infants for more than twenty years, mothers and doctors alike remained conflicted about wet nurses, their product, and their function. The precipitous decline in maternal breastfeeding rates beginning in the late nineteenth century reflects this ambivalence.

Physicians' take on human milk was equally contradictory. On the one hand, doctors believed human milk to be so essential to babies' health that they went to extraordinary lengths to hire wet nurses for the use of private families and to employ, outfit, house, and supervise them in medical and charitable institutions. They publicly derided the "selfish" mothers who did not breastfeed. They believed that human milk was so superior to artificial food that it was worth almost any trouble and expense to obtain. On the other hand, they feared that a wet nurse's milk supply might so utterly lack essential nutritive elements by the time a wet nurse's baby was eight or nine months old that the milk might harm any baby who consumed it. Similarly, mothers and doctors worried that any change in a wet nurse's unreliable personality or diet could taint her milk and poison her tiny charge. Many physicians also believed that certain women—depending on their racial or ethnic backgrounds—were inherently incapable of working as wet nurses because their bodies could not possibly produce milk either quantitatively or qualitatively acceptable to any baby. This sentiment—that breast milk is very good but that any one of a number of variables in women's lives, personality, history, and physical makeup could make it very bad—explains, in part, the move from breast to bottle.

So does class conflict. Fanny Workman's letter to *Babyhood* magazine is evidence that doctors did not exaggerate the difficulties inherent in wet nursing. In times of unabashed class antagonism, women who hired wet nurses exhibited animosity toward their employees without compunction. The harsh relationship between wet nurses and the mothers who employed them sheds light, not only on upper- and middle-class attitudes toward the poor, immigrant women who worked as their servants, but on upper- and middle-class perceptions of breastfeeding. While wet nurses' employers occasionally lauded their employees' beneficial product, they invariably deemed wet nurses themselves impossibly troublesome, linking breastfeeding with immoral, unworthy women.

Never for a moment did Workman acknowledge that she owed her daughter's life to the efforts of wet nurses. Rather, she expressed outrage that she had been forced to permit these irresponsible, ignorant, and uncouth women to handle her baby at all. Workman exhibited no compassion for or understanding of her wet nurses' plight. Instead, she forced them to abandon their own babies to strangers who fed them artificial food. Workman remained angry and unsympathetic even after her second wet nurse's baby died—a baby who was essentially sacrificed so Workman's daughter could live. Almost all the mothers who employed wet nurses were similarly hostile toward them. The interests of women who worked as wet nurses and the women who employed them could not have been more diametrically opposed. The women who hired wet nurses steadfastly refused to acknowledge even what little they did share with their employees—motherhood.

Women who hired wet nurses linked the product so closely with the producer that any benefit the product provided was overshadowed by what employers perceived as the producers' utter lack of attractiveness and morality. It is not a far cry from thinking a person is beneath one's station to thinking a person's function is beneath one's station. Wet nursing was an occupation limited to only the most desperate women. For the women able to hire private wet nurses, human milk may have been what their babies needed, but they could not uncouple the milk from the act of breastfeeding, an activity that they associated with poverty, vulgarity, ignorance, even sin (in the case of unwed wet nurses).

Upper- and middle-class women who decided not to nurse their own babies did not choose their own comfort and convenience over their baby's health. Rather, they chose between an activity that was appropriate for their class and an activity that was increasingly inappropriate. Contempt for wet nurses does not just illuminate a microscopic chapter in American labor and class relations. The attitudes and convictions of these doctors and well-to-do mothers helped orchestrate the move from breast to bottle.

6

"Give It the Nearest Thing to Mother's Milk": Human Milk Substitutes

When human milk was unavailable from any source, physicians reluctantly turned to what they derisively called "artificial food." Doctors did not dub human milk substitutes "artificial foods" lightly. The phrase was a pointed one, meant to signify an "unnatural" substance and, as such, an inherently undesirable one. It was no coincidence that a poster designed to promote Chicago's first Baby Week campaign in 1914 featured babies begging, "Take not away from us that food which God in His wisdom provides. Except of extreme necessity, force not upon us an unnatural food."[1]

In the realm of artificial food, physicians and mothers had three basic options: canned cows' milk, proprietary infant foods to be mixed with cows' milk or water, and "fresh" cows' milk. Mothers who bottle-fed their babies usually chose fresh cows' milk in any one of several forms: raw, certified, pasteurized, sterilized, modified, or some combination of the latter four. Since some of these choices were clearly safer for babies than others, the Chicago Department of Health and the city's assorted medical charities targeted mothers almost exclusively when they designed the city's clean-milk campaigns.

Raw milk, mothers learned, came straight from the cow, although this was true only in theory. In reality, raw milk was often three days old before it reached a consumer and by that time likely had been adulterated by dirt, dyes, and worse. Thus, public health authorities advised mothers to avoid this option. Certified milk—if it was not pasteurized, sterilized, or modified—was also raw, but because a conscientious organization gathered, bottled, shipped, and distributed it according to strict hygienic standards, medical authorities deemed it significantly safer, and certainly purer, than raw milk. Pasteurized milk was heated to a certain temperature for a specified amount of time—but never boiled—to kill dangerous bacteria. Sterile milk was heated to boiling to kill all bacteria. Modified milk, usually made from certified milk that was also pasteurized, had the percentages of protein, fat, and sugar altered to resemble more closely the percentages in human milk.

Long before doctors considered certifying, pasteurizing, sterilizing, and modifying milk, families concocted their own human milk substitutes. During the colonial era, if human milk was unavailable, caretakers fed babies pap and panada—mixtures of meat or rice broth, cows' milk, sugar, and water— via sucking rags or nursing bottles.[2] Feeding infants this type of ad hoc food was probably not uncommon. The initial inventors of mass-produced breast milk substitutes uniformly reported that the haunting image of sick babies deprived of mother's milk inspired their product. Among these products were canned condensed milk, which made its debut in the United States in 1856, and canned evaporated milk, sold widely in the United States by the 1880s. Mothers could also choose from an array of proprietary infant foods. Drugstores sold these commercially manufactured powders—to be mixed with cows' milk or water or both—by the 1870s.

Whatever the artificial food, its developer had one aim: to mimic "average" breast milk in order to give babies "so unfortunate as to be deprived of their natural source of nourishment . . . a food as nearly like that natural supply as possible."[3] Human milk substitutes, however, consistently fell far short of this ideal and doctors remained wary of them. Charles Warrington Earle, a Chicago physician, claimed that he had tried every conceivable artificial food on countless babies. When one infant occasionally took to a particular food, Earle had frequently been tricked into thinking that, finally, he had discovered the perfect human milk substitute. By 1891, however, he was not so easily fooled. Earle urged his colleagues to explain to mothers that no artificial food was equally effective for all babies—a food that agreed with one baby might not agree with other infants. And if a baby did do well for a time on one food, the food would not necessarily continue to agree with that infant. All artificial foods, he now argued, were potential health threats to all babies at all times.[4] Yet the "scientific" development of infant food continued, fueled both by mothers' abandonment of prolonged breastfeeding and physicians' alternating high and dashed hopes for artificial food as described by Earle.

Condensed and Evaporated Milks: "The Milk of Contented Cows"

Obtaining fresh, pure milk had long been a problem for both urban dwellers and travelers, so canned milk proved a boon. Canned milk is preserved in one of two ways, condensing or evaporating.[5] Condensed milk, developed in 1856, is whole milk reduced in volume by evaporation and preserved with sugar. Evaporated milk, invented in 1885, is also reduced in volume by evaporation but is preserved by boiling and quick canning and contains no extraneous sugar.[6] Both are to be diluted with water before serving. Evaporated and condensed milks, which do not spoil and are easy to carry and store, attracted droves of mothers.

Gail Borden opened the first canned milk factory in the United States in 1856.[7] The specter of sick infants with no access to human milk initially inspired Borden, as it would in later years the many physicians involved in artificial infant food formulation. Although his canned milk did not find an appreciative audience immediately, during the Civil War the Union Army opted to give the milk to its soldiers. When the war ended, returning soldiers spoke enthusiastically about the canned miracle that provided sustenance to the ill and wounded.[8] Mothers took note.

While Borden manufactured condensed milk in the United States, Swiss chemist Henri Nestlé, similarly moved by the suffering of European babies who were not breastfed, invented a powdered infant food. His milk food, primarily composed of cows' milk, was to be mixed with water. By 1868 his product was being sold in Switzerland, Germany, France, and England. Five years later, Nestlé's milk food was available throughout Europe, the Americas, and Australia. Unable to keep up with the demand, Nestlé sold the company in 1875. In 1878, when Nestlé's arch rival, the Anglo-Swiss Condensed Milk Company, started manufacturing its own powdered milk food, the Nestlé Company retaliated by producing its own condensed milk. In 1905 Nestlé and the Anglo-Swiss Condensed Milk Company merged.[9]

Borden's most successful imitators—Nestlé in Europe and eventually Pet Milk and Carnation Milk in the United States—shared one intriguing connection, John Meyenberg, described by all who knew him as a temperamental inventor. Meyenberg invented evaporated milk while he was employed by the Anglo-Swiss Condensed Milk Company, but when the owners of the company scorned his innovation—probably because given their great success with condensed milk they saw no need for a change in manufacture—the disgruntled inventor moved to the United States. In 1885 Meyenberg opened the Helvetia Milk Condensing Company in Highland, Illinois, a small town near St. Louis, where he marketed his unsweetened evaporated milk under the name Highland Brand Condensed Milk. Meyenberg, ever the disgruntled drifter, soon left the company to others. The Helvetia Company eventually changed its name to Pet and advertised its product as "far closer to the ideal" infant food than other condensed milks because it was unsweetened. In 1899 Meyenberg resurfaced in the state of Washington where he aided the start-up of another company that eventually became Carnation Milk.[10]

E. A. Stuart, Carnation's founder, learned of evaporated milk when, as the owner of a small grocery store, he purchased one hundred cases of Highland Brand Condensed Milk from a Helvetia salesman. When Stuart's son was born two years later, Stuart fretted over the baby's slow weight gain. Remembering the dozens of Highland cans still on his shelves, he fed them to the baby. The milk fattened up his son nicely, and Stuart ordered one hundred more cases. In 1899 Stuart became a partner in the Pacific Coast Condensed Milk Company in Washington State. For technical expertise Stuart and his partner relied wholly on John Meyenberg. In 1901, Stuart bought out his partner's share of the floundering company and paid Meyenberg $25,000 for his assorted secrets. Meyenberg disappeared again, and in 1916 Pacific Coast became the Carnation Milk Products Company.[11]

In its advertising, Pacific Coast exploited the fears generated by years of milk campaigns. The cows that produced Pacific Coast milk were not diseased. Pacific Coast milk was not dirty and adulterated. Pacific Coast milk would never spoil. While talking to an advertising copywriter in 1907, Stuart spoke eloquently. The cows that provided his company with milk roamed lush, sheltered valleys, grazed lazily on tender grass, and drank cool, clear, spring water. "Ah," the copywriter reportedly said dreamily, "the milk of contented cows." And so a slogan was born. Generations of American mothers proceeded to feed their babies Carnation milk—from "contented cows"— not the milk produced by the emaciated, filthy, and TB-infested creatures that milk reformers railed about. Carnation recommended its milk for infants and assured mothers that their product solved "the problem of getting safe milk in hot weather."[12]

The Pacific Coast Company encountered a minor setback in September 1913 when Dr. Harvey W. Wiley revealed in *Good Housekeeping* magazine that, rather than being "contented," Carnation's cows were actually a rather sorry lot. Wiley charged that the animals providing milk to Pacific Coast were housed "in dark, ill-smelling rooms . . . and milked without sanitary precautions." Some of the cows, he complained, "were so plastered with manure that I could hardly tell their color." Wiley explained to an editor of the *Journal of the American Medical Association* that Pacific Coast did not own a single cow and never had. Like all condensed milk companies, Pacific Coast purchased milk from assorted dairies, some quite disreputable, and in this they were no better or worse than any other milk manufacturer—just decep-tive in their advertising.[13]

Bad publicity, however, was a fleeting setback. The high cost of fresh milk in cities assured the popularity of canned milks. Boston municipal health workers noted in 1907 that as the price of whole milk rose so did the sale of condensed milk. This aroused considerable consternation among doc-tors because the cheapest condensed milk was more expensive than the best whole milk, at least when it was properly diluted. Boston milk inspectors feared that the vague instructions on cans of evaporated and condensed milks encouraged mothers to add too much water.[14] Since condensed milk was supposed to be served diluted anyway, adding too much water likely seemed to mothers to be less sinful than sanctified.

Chicago doctors validated the concern of Boston's health officials, charg-ing that mothers commonly added far too much water to canned milks. Earle warned in 1891 that one teaspoon of condensed milk made twelve ounces of water look hearty, when in reality it was a "starvation diet." James Warren Van Derslice agreed. "How many of these cases have each of us seen," he asked physicians at a meeting of the Illinois Medical Society in 1910, "where the child is brought in on the end of a long tube-bottle and find the child is being given one or two teaspoons of condensed milk, diluted with 6 or 8 ounces of water?" Clifford Grulee asked, "How many see the poor, puny, marantic infant brought up on condensed milk or malted milk, as the result of the efforts of the mother to give it a food which contains none of the death-dealing . . . bacteria?" Joseph Brennemann confessed in 1928 to "a fondness for condensed milk" but only, he emphasized, "in weakly, poorly nursing, and premature babies, in the absence of mothers' milk . . . *in this very limited period only.*" Otherwise he called condensed milk a "dangerous, not to say damnable, food" and hesitated to contribute to its "harmful employment by furnishing fuel to the peculiarly pernicious practices and propaganda on the part of certain condensed milk producers."[15]

Proprietary Infant Foods: "Worse Than Useless"

Proprietary (also called commercial) infant foods became available in the United States not long after the Civil War, just as Borden's condensed milk was becoming popular. Private companies manufactured the foods—pow-ders composed largely of starches and malt sugars to be mixed with either cows' milk or water or both—and sold them in drugstores. Physicians detested them, deeming them unscientific and too readily available to untrained mothers. Chicago pediatrician Frank Spooner Churchill called proprietary foods "utterly worthless as foods for infants, nay worse than useless, inasmuch as mothers do their babies much harm by giving them these 'foods.'"[16]

The sheer number of commercial infant foods and the array of ingredients they contained were staggering. Mellin's Food, invented by London chemist Gustav Mellin in 1866, was a "soluble, dry extract of wheat, malted barley and bicarbonate of potassium . . . converted into soluble carbohydrates, maltose and dextrins, and by evaporation reduced to a dry powder consisting of maltose, dextrins, proteins and salts."[17] Other foods included Eskay's Albumenized Food (eggs, barley, oats, wheat, and milk sugar, to be mixed with cows' milk), Peptogenic Milk Powder (said to convert the casein of cows' milk into the "softer albuminoids" in mothers' milk after being mixed with equal parts milk and water and a "stated amount" of cream), Just's Food (partly digested cereal to be mixed with milk and water), Horlick's Malted Milk (milk, malted barley, and wheat, to be mixed with water); Lactopreparata (dried modified cows' milk, sugar, and starches, to be mixed with water), Lactated Food (wheat, partially predigested barley malt, phosphate of lime, and milk sugar, to be mixed with cows' milk and water), and Nestlé's Food (condensed cows' milk, "wheaten bread, so treated that the insoluble starch has been transformed into soluble dextrin," and cane sugar, to be mixed with water).[18]

Advertisements for proprietary infant foods often appeared in women's and infant-care magazines, but none claimed superiority over human milk. "Nurse your baby if you can," recommended one 1914 Nestlé's Food ad. "If you can't, give it the nearest thing to mother's milk—Nestlé's Food." Most ads, in fact, carried dire warnings about the dangers of artificial food, not unlike those issued by doctors. Their only claim was that their product was considerably less likely to lead to disaster than others were. Thus, babies might be "Brought Past the Danger Time" by Lactated Food. Nestlé's Food, to be mixed with water and not adulterated, bacteria-laden, easily soured milk, alerted mothers to the dangers of cows' milk. Nestlé's fumed, "If mothers only knew that the Government inspectors found throughout the land only eight clean dairies in a hundred!"[19]

Mellin's Food ads—via testimonials from once-distraught but now-pleased parents—were particularly adept at warning mothers away from deadly competitors.[20] Mrs. Fred C. Eaton of Warren, Pennsylvania, informed *Ladies' Home Journal* readers in 1902 that her artificially fed son, Hamlen

How Long Does Your Baby Sleep?

Twenty hours each day is right for the first month, then gradually less till at six months sixteen hours a day is just right.

Your baby must have that sleep to get fat and rosy. And it will have that sleep if you feed it regularly and evenly on its mother's milk or the nearest substitute—

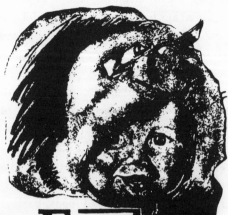

Nestlé's Food

If mothers would only realize the every-day danger of carrying consumption and other dread diseases to babies in cows' milk! If mothers only knew that in one State, where the laws are strict, there are 200,000 infected cows—one for nearly every baby in the State.

If mothers only knew that the Government inspectors found throughout the land only eight clean dairies in a hundred!

Nurse your baby if you can. If you can't, give it the nearest thing to mother's milk—Nestlé's Food.

Safe because you add only water to prepare it. *Safe* because it is made under the strictest scientific condi-

tions. *Safe* because no reach it in its airtight can.

Nestlé's is made from the milk of healthy cows kept in sanitary dairies. All the heavy parts of milk are modified, so that the curd is soft and fleecy as in mother's milk. All that your baby needs and the calf doesn't is added. And—there you have Nestlé's on which three generations have grown healthy and strong.

Send the Coupon. It will bring you a box of Nestlé's Food—enough for twelve feedings—and a book by specialists, filled with things you should know.

NESTLÉ'S FOOD COMPANY, 239 Broadway, New York

Please send me, FREE, your book and trial package.

Name ....

Address ....

Figure 17   This advertisement for Nestlé's Food, from an April 1914 issue of *American Motherhood,* contends that Nestlé's Food is safe because mothers mix it with water, not invariably dirty, spoiled, and adulterated cows' milk.

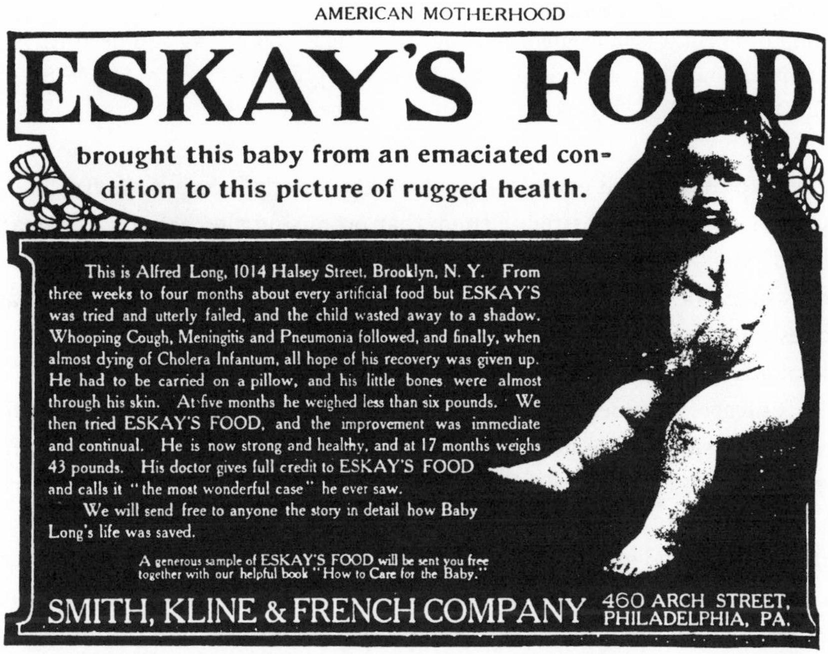

AMERICAN MOTHERHOOD

ESKAY'S FOOD

brought this baby from an emaciated condition to this picture of rugged health.

This is Alfred Long, 1014 Halsey Street, Brooklyn, N. Y. From
three weeks to four months about every artificial food but ESKAY'S
was tried and utterly failed, and the child wasted away to a shadow.
Whooping Cough, Meningitis and Pneumonia followed, and finally, when
almost dying of Cholera Infantum, all hope of his recovery was given up.
He had to be carried on a pillow, and his little bones were almost
through his skin. At five months he weighed less than six pounds. We
then tried ESKAY'S FOOD, and the improvement was immediate
and continual. He is now strong and healthy, and at 17 months weighs
43 pounds. His doctor gives full credit to ESKAY'S FOOD
and calls it "the most wonderful case" he ever saw.

We will send free to anyone the story in detail how Baby
Long's life was saved.

A generous sample of ESKAY'S FOOD will be sent you free
together with our helpful book "How to Care for the Baby."

SMITH, KLINE & FRENCH COMPANY 460 ARCH STREET,
PHILADELPHIA, PA.

Figure 18   This advertisement for Eskay's Food, from a December 1905 issue of *American Motherhood,* is typical of early twentieth-century pitches for proprietary infant foods, which never failed to warn mothers about the deadly effects of artificial feeding. All the messages in these advertisements were strikingly similar: only the advertiser's product did not kill.

Cowley Eaton, weighed nine pounds at birth but only six and three-quarters pounds at four weeks. "We feared and all our friends were certain we would lose him," Mrs. Eaton explained, "but we began the use of Mellin's Food, and now every one says 'a typical Mellin's Food baby.' We are confident Mellin's Food saved his life."[21]

Eskay's Albumenized Food also used testimonials in its ads, and the company received many unsolicited pictures of happy, healthy babies reared on Eskay's.[22] One typically horrifying story accompanied by a picture of a rotund baby appeared in *American Motherhood* in 1905:

This is Alfred Long, 1015 Halsey Street, Brooklyn, N.Y. From three weeks to four months about every artificial food but ESKAY'S was tried and utterly failed, and the child wasted away to a shadow. Whooping Cough, Meningitis and Pneumonia followed, and finally, when almost dying of Cholera Infantum, all hope of his recovery was given up. He had to be carried on a pillow, and his little bones were almost through his skin. At five months he weighed less than six pounds. We then tried ESKAY'S FOOD, and the improvement was immediate and continual. He is now strong and healthy, and at 17 months weighs 43 pounds. His doctor gives full credit to ESKAY'S FOOD and calls it "the most wonderful case" he ever saw.[23]

Despite the implicit caveats, the ads likely softened some women's determination to breastfeed, assuring them that promising alternatives to human milk did exist. As one mother complained in 1889, "Our New England grandparents knew of no other way than to nurse their own children. There was no question of anything else. . . . The 'only true substitute for mother's milk' was not advertised in every paper and placarded in public places."[24]

In Chicago, commercial infant foods were peddled less through traditional advertising and more by door-to-door salesmen. When Herman Bundesen became Chicago's Health Commissioner in 1922 he was shocked to learn that every new mother in Chicago received dozens of visits from assorted proprietary infant food salesmen. Bundesen, who was soon to appear on his own twice-weekly radio program sponsored by the Milk Foundation, apparently differentiated between commercial infant foods and cows' milk, proprietary food manufacturers and dairies. In order "to stop the traffic in baby decoctions and devices with its consequences of deceived mothers and ailing babies," he immediately ordered the Department of Health to stop publishing the daily birth register from which salesmen obtained mothers' names and addresses. The distressed representatives of one infant food company pleaded with the Department of Health to reverse the new policy and went so far as to offer the department fifty cents for each new mother's name and address. Health officials refused. The new policy became a cornerstone of Bundesen's subsequent breastfeeding campaigns, described in chapter 4.[25]

Modified Milk: "Absolutely No Mathematical Work"

Rather than permit mothers to rely on the wares peddled by commercial companies, doctors began to offer their own solutions to the infant-feeding problem. Beginning in the early 1890s, inspired by the theory and work of Harvard pediatrician Thomas Rotch, doctors began to recommend modified milk—cows' milk with the percentage of fat, protein, sugar, and ash altered to more closely resemble the percentages in human milk. When milk was modified, it was done either in the home, by a mother following a complicated set of instructions, or in a milk laboratory, by chemists following a doctor's prescription.

Different milk modification methods abounded. One Chicago doctor preferred L. Emmett Holt's recipes, described in Holt's popular *Diseases of Infancy and Childhood*. Holt recommended combining varying proportions of cream, skimmed milk, and sugar of milk—depending on a baby's age and physical condition—dissolving the mix in boiling water, adding one part lime-water for every twenty parts milk to minimize the acidity, and reducing the water used in the milk-sugar solution in relation to the amount of lime-water.[26] Although this solution was troublesome to mix, it was relatively simple compared with recipes to come.

Mellin's Food Company touted a method to modify milk using its product as the key ingredient. Mellin's Food, the company claimed, was not simply nourishment but a "true modifier of milk," capable of altering the casein in cows' milk so profoundly that it eliminated the "tough, indigestible curds in the stomach so trying to the infant digestion." Mellin's Food published a book-length tome for physicians—*The Mellin's Food Method of Percentage Feeding,* based on Rotch's theories—that contained recipes for 474 formulas guaranteed to quell doctors' objections to artificial food.[27]

The Mellin's percentage feeding system was complex. Each formula listed assorted "creams," "top milks," "bottom milks," and "skimmed milks" essential to the mix. A lengthy "Percentage Table Index" at the start of the book listed every known "safe" percentage combination of protein, fat, and carbohydrate for babies, what page to find the formula's recipe on, and the formula's number. So, for example, a physician requiring a food containing 1.25 percent proteids, 4 percent fat, and 5 percent carbohydrates for a particular baby could find the formula's recipe—numbered 183 on the Percentage Table Index—on page 47. Formulas close to each other in number differed only in minute gradations, so that formula 184 had 1.25 percent proteids, 4 percent fats, and 5.5 percent carbohydrates, and so on. To concoct each formula, chefs needed a kaleidoscopic array of ingredients. Formula 306, for example— composed of 2 percent proteids, 1.5 percent fat, and 5 percent carbohydrates—contained two level teaspoons of Mellin's Food, three ounces of fresh milk, four and one-half ounces of bottom milk with 3 percent fat, and eight and one-half ounces of water. There were additional tables containing recipes for the top, bottom, and skimmed milks and creams, each with different percentages of fat, to be used in the hundreds of formulas.[28] Mellin's did not explain how the sizeable variation in fat among milks in this era of no dairy regulation would affect their exacting recipes.[29]

The Mellin's Food Method of Percentage Feeding even contained descriptions of babies' typical digestive ailments so doctors, if necessary, could make a diagnosis and alter a particular formula accordingly. "We will say that the baby is being fed with a mixture which, perhaps, contains too much Proteid, indicated by the undigested curds found in the stools. . . . We turn to the Percentage Table Index, find the percentage formula which shows Proteids ½ of 1% less than the one now being used, but in which the other constituents are the same." The Mellin's Food Company heralded their lengthy book as the first attempt ever "to furnish a simple, automatic, practical table, which calls for absolutely no mathematical work on the part of the physician." They urged physicians to write to them with their comments and suggestions.[30]

Milk Laboratories: "Out of the Hands of Ignorant, Money-Making Manufacturers"

The aid provided by Mellin's Food notwithstanding, modifying milk at home was extremely difficult. When mothers did feed their babies modified milk, usually either they obtained a standard, ready-made formula from a milk station or filled a doctor's prescription at a milk laboratory where a chemist prepared a unique formula based on the prescription. Thomas Rotch's percentage feeding method, described in chapter 3 and heralded as "the most distinctively American principle of pediatric practice," used "by almost all careful practitioners who have any skill in the feeding of infants," inspired this new urban industry.[31] Frank Churchill lauded milk laboratories because "the feeding of the infant is thus taken out of the hands of ignorant, money-making manufacturers and placed as its importance demands in the hands of the educated physician."[32]

Milk laboratories ostensibly furnished babies with a flexible but precise product capable of mimicking the "variety of good breast-milks" which, Rotch argued, nature provided for "the individual idiosyncrasy of the especial infant." Theoretically, chemists at milk laboratories did not just turn cows' milk into generic human milk, they transformed cows' milk into the unique version of human milk suited to a particular baby. Chicago physician Junius Hoag agreed with Rotch that "what is meant for one infant seems to be poison for another" and blessed the milk laboratories that provided "food so arranged as to meet the necessities of each child."[33]

For a time virtually every large city in the United States had at least one milk laboratory. The best known—originating in Boston and quickly setting up subsidiaries across the country—was the Walker-Gordon Laboratory. George Walker, a wealthy businessman and lithographer, and G. E. Gordon, a dairy farmer, were intimates of Rotch. Rotch credited Gordon with enhancing his knowledge of cows' milk.[34] As a farmer, Gordon invented a device that separated protein curds from cows' milk to make it easier for calves to digest. (Gordon never explained why calves needed human intervention to digest cows' milk, but since Rotch and others were theorizing at the time that human milk could mean trouble for human babies his invention likely seemed of use to dairy farmers.) Gordon, who had never considered altering cows' milk for human consumption, discovered Rotch's work when he came across an article on reducing the protein in human milk by diluting it. Gordon was so impressed that, after meeting Rotch, he decided to devote his knowledge of the dairy industry to a cows' milk laboratory for human babies. Rotch contacted Walker, who agreed to finance the venture, and the first Walker-Gordon Laboratory was born in Boston in 1891. By 1907 there were twenty Walker-Gordon Laboratories in the United States, Canada, and London.[35]

Walker-Gordon Laboratories used only certified milk, with company employees acting as the certifying body.[36] Because the birth of milk laboratories coincided with the invention of certified milk in New Jersey, the milk produced by a Walker-Gordon dairy farm was often the only clean milk to be had in some cities. The Chicago Medical Society credited Walker-Gordon with "holding . . . the highest position of rank among certified milk producers and distributors in America."[37] Even Earle, who continued to stand "upon the ground where I have always stood," believing that mother's milk is best for babies, praised the enterprise. "If it were possible for us to place in the hands of every mother who is obliged to bring up her child on an artificial food, such milk as is prepared there," he wrote rhapsodically in 1892, "this entire [feeding] question would be nearly solved."[38]

The first Walker-Gordon Laboratory in Chicago appeared in 1895. Ninety percent of the 111 physicians who used the laboratory that first year reported a wholly favorable experience.[39] Mothers were pleased as well. When Josephine Laflin gave birth to her second child in Chicago in 1898, she fed him a Walker-Gordon formula which "seemed to agree perfectly" with him. Access to the formula soon dictated Laflin family life. Making plans to spend the summer in the East, Laflin was attracted to the homes for rent near Buffalo because Buffalo housed a Walker-Gordon Laboratory "for Baby's milk." When the Laflin household—with father, older son, and dog in one carriage and cook, nurse, baby, and mother in another—left for Buffalo that June, servants carefully loaded "a square box with Walker-Gordon Modified milk packed with ice" onto the baby's carriage.[40]

Walker-Gordon and other milk laboratories customarily operated from one of two bases. They had stand-alone facilities, like in Boston and Chicago, or they were affiliated with a reputable dairy, like in St. Louis.[41] In Chicago, Walker-Gordon was located for many years at 2112 Michigan Avenue. In mid-1908 the lab moved to new facilities at 2450-52-54 Calumet Avenue, which the Chicago Medical Society dubbed "the finest and most thoroughly equipped milk laboratory in the world."[42]

Chicago housed at least one other for-profit milk laboratory. The Soesman Laboratory Co. provided physicians with preprinted forms, allowing them to designate the percentage of fat, milk sugar, albuminoids, mineral matter, total solids, and water in a formula, the number of feedings to be prepared daily, and the number of ounces in each feeding. The Soesman Laboratory advertised their ability to provide physicians with "a new instrument of precision for carrying out their ideas."[43]

The popularity of milk laboratories was short-lived, however. In 1902 A. H. Wentworth, a Boston physician, analyzed some laboratory-produced formulas and found that none matched their prescriptions. In most cases the fat percentage was lower and the protein percentage higher than the prescribed formula. The percentage of sugar commonly erred in both directions. Wentworth found every error "appreciable." Since Rotch based percentage feeding on the theory that the minutest change in a baby's formula had the potential to seriously affect a baby's health, Wentworth's findings created serious doubt that milk laboratories were a potent infant feeding tool. "Within certain limits," Wentworth argued, "accurate percentage modifications of milk are not essential to the well-being of a majority of the babies that are fed on modified milk." The only advantage milk laboratories offered consumers, Wentworth concluded, was convenience. Disadvantages included their inaccuracy, "stale" milk, and the extraordinary expense.[44]

The cost of modified milk did indeed concern most doctors. Chicago physicians Isaac Abt and Frank Spooner Churchill lamented in 1897 that at forty-five to fifty cents daily for eight feedings, only an elite minority of families could afford laboratory-produced modified milk. Even after modified milk was made available in bulk at twenty cents a quart, it remained costly.[45] Accordingly, during its first year in Chicago, Walker-Gordon served only 281 babies.[46]

Standardized formulas eventually overcame the cost hurdle. Although percentage feeding by prescription was largely discredited by the early 1910s, generic modified milk formulas based on a baby's age and physical condition remained available through philanthropic milk stations in Chicago and elsewhere well into the 1920s, even the 1930s. Hull House was the first charity in Chicago to sell (and in many cases to give away) standardized-pasteurized milk formulas at its neighborhood milk station beginning in 1901. From early July until mid-October, Hull House workers provided formulas to neighborhood families with infants sickened by digestive ailments. Neighborhood physicians actively supported the enterprise, steering families to the service. In August and September of 1902 Hull House sold an average of two hundred bottles of milk each day.[47] In July 1903, when the Chicago Milk Commission (CMC) made standardized-modified milk available at dozens of milk stations throughout the city, the Hull House milk station became an official CMC station.

Chicago had several other philanthropic milk laboratories scattered throughout the city, most affiliated with medical institutions. Alarmed at the number of women reporting an inability to breastfeed and fearing that it would become a permanent trend, doctors at the Northwestern University Medical School established a diet kitchen in 1902 to provide babies with certified-modified cows' milk in standard concentrations. Dr. F. X. Walls, the diet kitchen's founder, argued there was no "philanthropy of greater value to the race" than diet kitchens, especially in poor neighborhoods. Mothers paid the Northwestern University Medical School Diet Kitchen five to fifteen cents a day for modified milk if they could afford it and nothing at all if they could not.[48] Because Northwestern University doctors recognized the importance of human milk backup for babies, the kitchen also sold bottled breast milk provided by a staff of wet nurses.[49]

Sarah Morris Children's Hospital, the pediatric department of Chicago's Michael Reese Hospital, also housed a milk laboratory complete with sterilizer and pasteurizer. One Michael Reese annual report boasted, "The old days of working in the dark with children's foods are gone, we hope, forever, and in their stead has come a time when the microscope in the laboratory of the chemist has made the feeding of children almost an exact science." Abt was especially pleased with the Sarah Morris setup after working for years in hospitals where, he charged, workers made little effort to distinguish between the food served infants and the food served adults.[50] Like the Northwestern University Medical School Diet Kitchen, however, the Sarah Morris Hospital milk laboratory did not confine itself to supplying artificial food to infants. It too provided bottled human milk furnished by Sarah Morris's resident wet nurses.[51]

Although enthusiasm for percentage feeding waned relatively quickly, hospital milk laboratories continued to keep the concept alive for quite some time. In 1936 Chicago's Presbyterian Hospital heralded the opening of their new milk laboratory, which manufactured "at least 25 different formulas, sometimes more, in order to serve the individual needs of each small patient."[52] Like their forerunners, however, the lab's nurses also processed and distributed human milk for babies unable to digest any of the laboratory's twenty-five "individual needs" formulas.[53]

Certified Milk: "Fancy Milk"

Every artificial food—canned, raw, pasteurized, sterilized, and modified milk, and proprietary infant food—relied on one basic ingredient, cows' milk. In most urban areas before the 1920s, however, palatable cows' milk was hard to come by. Certified milk, invented in 1892 by Henry L. Coit, a New Jersey physician, was touted for decades as the only clean and unadulterated milk many cities had to offer.[54] Produced under the stringent hygienic rules and vigilance of a milk commission—usually a group of doctors working for a municipality or medical charity—certified milk was sold or given away at milk depots.[55]

A personal crisis precipitated Coit's interest in certifying milk. In 1887, "maternal failure" (presumably his wife's inability to breastfeed) prompted him to begin what became a two-year search for decent cows' milk for his infant son. "The vicissitudes through which I passed on the question of pure materials with which to nourish this child, will never be told," he remarked at the first gathering of the American Association of Medical Milk Commissions. "Driven from one source of impoverished and contaminated milk to another," Coit eventually found a suburban dairyman with four clean, healthy cows. His peace of mind was short-lived, however. Arriving at the tidy farm one day to pick up milk for his baby, he discovered three members of the dairy farmer's immediate family stricken with diphtheria. The farmer, who displayed no symptoms of the disease, was frantically busy, milking cows by day and nursing sick family members by night. Coit recalled that this "honest and industrious man, but without a knowledg [sic] of hygiene . . . became unwittingly a dangerous element in my family life."[56]

When John Summerfield Coit died, his angry and distraught father proposed that members of the New Jersey State Medical Society form a commission—composed of two doctors from every New Jersey county—to investigate the relationship between infant mortality and the urban milk supply.[57] The resulting Milk Committee of the Medical Society of New Jersey drafted regulations to govern the production of milk. Both the New Jersey State

Board of Health and the New Jersey State Dairy Commissioner rejected the rules, calling them radical and utopian.[58]

Exasperated, Coit formed the Essex County Medical Milk Commission, an organization with no legal authority, to oversee the production of milk in his own county. In the contract signed by the Essex Commission and their first dairyman, the dairy farmer agreed to pay all costs incurred for milk certification, including the frequent laboratory examination of his milk and the bimonthly veterinary checks of his cows. The Milk Commission, in turn, enforced the contract and periodically published the analyses of the dairyman's certified milk.[59] An ecstatic Coit declared that certified milk leveled the playing field for infants everywhere. "The poorest baby in Coomes Alley," he exulted, "will now fare equally well with Thomas Edison's baby in Lewellen Park."[60]

Doctors in Buffalo and Newark soon followed the example of Essex County doctors and set up their own "Committee of Physicians" to supervise dairies in those cities.[61] By 1907 twenty-two cities in the United States, including Chicago, had medical milk commissions operating an estimated 159 milk depots. Hospitals and settlement houses also operated additional certified milk stations in their neighborhoods as one of many health-related services.[62] Milk stations burgeoned in spots frequented by women and children like settlement houses, public schools, parks, nurseries, and medical dispensaries. Some stations carried certified milk, most offered certified milk that was also pasteurized, long before pasteurization was required by law.[63]

The certified milk commissions springing up around the country orchestrated not just mammoth logistical efforts—negotiating contracts, inspecting farms, testing milk, examining dairy cattle, and pasteurizing, bottling, shipping, and distributing milk—but educational ones as well. Milk commissions sought to enlighten two groups: dairy farmers and the general public. Dairy farmers were first on the agenda. Before coming under the scrutiny of the milk commissions, dairy workers seldom washed their hands before milking. Farmers rarely, if ever, bathed their cows. Dirt and bacteria dropped from cows' filthy bellies and udders into milk pails.[64] During the early years of medical milk commissions, convincing even one dairy farmer in a community to adhere to certified standards was a formidable task. Bitterly resenting interference in their industry, dairymen scorned certified milk as "fancy milk" and eschewed new production methods.[65]

When a milk commission did convince a dairyman of the benefits of certification, the commission defined all standards and work procedures for his farm. Dairy workers learned to employ surgeons' hygienic practices: they scrubbed their hands; ventilated, drained, and scoured barns; groomed cows; sterilized milking utensils; and fed cows abundant and appropriate food. Dairy farmers' contracts with certified milk commissions also required that all dairy cows be healthy; described the precise steps to be used when collecting milk; and explained how to cool milk, prepare it for shipment, and transport it.[66] Coit reasoned that the time put into educating dairy farmers was well worth it. He argued, "Soap, water, scrubbing-brush, sunshine, and disinfectants are of no avail without the thought which effectively employs them."[67]

Certified medical milk commissions educated the public with equal vigor and precision. Volunteers at certified milk stations instructed women to breastfeed their babies and to give babies cows' milk only if human milk was unavailable. They warned women never to save money by buying cheap milk. They taught mothers how to detect impurities in milk and how to care for it after purchase.[68]

This daily bombardment, not only from workers at certified milk stations but from women's magazines and municipal health departments, created an appreciation for precise infant care that became part of mothers' daily routines. In some circles, and certainly among the upper- and middle-class mothers who read women's magazines, the care of infants' food became a particular obsession. Mothers exchanged complex tips on how to care for babies' milk when traveling, quizzed doctors about appropriate formula preparations, and studied and experimented with assorted milk recipes.[69]

Despite all this attention to milk preparation, certified milk never became the answer to the "feeding question." As the public came to recognize the benefits of clean cows' milk, charlatans sought to cash in on the certified milk business. Although Coit registered the term "certified" with the United States Patent Office in 1904 to prevent its use by unscrupulous milk dealers, his effort was in vain.[70] Some dairies, to circumvent the patent, formed their own sham certifying commissions. The high cost of producing certified milk also dashed the lofty hopes of most milk commissions. The original medical milk commission in New Jersey charged twelve cents a quart for its milk in 1894, twice the cost of raw, uncertified milk.[71] Few could afford to purchase it.

The mere existence of certified milk depots generated the biggest problem of all. Despite the admonition of one doctor that "it must always be recalled that the responsibility of the depot is not to sell milk but to avoid selling it by fostering the maternal milk supply," clean cows' milk became an enemy of maternal nursing.[72] Certified milk commissions advertised their milk widely, imbuing the public with the notion that safe and wholesome cows' milk was something all children needed. Even as milk station workers told women that human milk was better for their babies than certified milk, mothers learned of the "special training, skill, and hard work of a high character" that went into certified milk production.[73]

On its face, certified milk and the educational efforts of certified milk stations were to be celebrated. The messages pouring forth from these stations permeated homes, where mothers began putting extra effort into the care of cows' milk, and dairy farms, where the practices of just one sanitary farm in a community often spread to adjacent farms.[74] At some point, however, women internalized the news that, with care, cows' milk could be as safe and effective a food for babies as human milk. In 1904 French doctors angrily accused milk stations in France of encouraging artificial feeding by their very existence.[75] In 1910 physicians hurled this accusation at the Chicago Milk Commission as well.

The Chicago Milk Commission: "Apt to Encourage Artificial Feeding"

There were only sixty-four hospital beds for children with contagious diseases in the entire city of Chicago in 1902. In February 1903 the Chicago Woman's Club formed the Children's Hospital Society, whose board proceeded to lobby every Chicago-area hospital to devote a portion of its facility to the care of sick children.[76]

The focus of the Children's Hospital Society quickly expanded. Among other activities, the society's board attempted to persuade hospital personnel to give only the highest-grade milk to hospitalized children, to little avail.[77] Because of this initial involvement in "the milk question," however, when Chicago's milkmen announced in May 1903 that they were going to cut their customary two deliveries per day during the summer to only one, the Hospital Society acted immediately to prevent a citywide crisis. Once-a-day milk delivery meant that milk would be at least forty-eight to sixty-five hours old by the time it reached consumers, who often had no ice. Equally distressing, the once-a-day delivery routes began at 8 A.M., several hours after the summer sun rose, rather than at 3 A.M., their traditional starting time. The specter of Chicago's oppressive summer heat spoiling the milk sitting on delivery wagons and porches haunted Chicago's citizenry. The Chicago Medical Society called on every citizen to "raise a mighty clamor" in protest.[78]

The Children's Hospital Society formed an offshoot—the Chicago Milk

Commission (CMC)—to provide the city's babies with certified milk during the crisis. Aided by Nathan Straus, a wealthy New York merchant who for many years operated philanthropic milk stations in New York City, the CMC moved quickly.[79] Straus donated pasteurizing and bottling equipment to the organization and sent one of his aides, a young New York physician, to install the pasteurizer.[80] The Chicago School Board offered the CMC a basement in a public school at Cass and Illinois Streets to use as its office and laboratory. CMC members scurried to ready the building according to Straus's specifications. Seven weeks after milkmen announced their decision to cut back deliveries, the CMC was selling certified-pasteurized and certified-pasteurized-modified milk from stations located in the city's most congested neighborhoods.[81]

Although Chicago's citizens feared that the milkmen's move would increase the city's infant death rate markedly, infant mortality did not rise that summer. Chicago Health Commissioner Arthur Reynolds credited the CMC with thwarting disaster. The milk commission's success was due in part to its ability to deliver milk in a remarkably timely manner. The CMC's certified dairies milked at 5:30 P.M., and the milk reached Chicago no later than 10:00 P.M., when it was immediately pasteurized, modified, bottled, and readied for delivery by 7:00 A.M.[82]

The CMC was not the first medical charity in Chicago to run a certified milk station, but it was the first to do so on a citywide scale. The few charities that had been making isolated attempts to provide clean milk to families in their neighborhoods—the Northwestern University Settlement House and Hull House, for example—quickly joined the CMC endeavor.[83] That first summer and fall volunteers distributed 222,000 bottles of pasteurized-certified and pasteurized-certified-modified milk. CMC milk distribution steadily increased: in 1908 workers dispensed 735,079 bottles of milk.[84]

The first CMC executive committee, formed in 1903, included eleven physicians—Isaac Abt (the commission's first chairman), F. X. Walls, John Cook (the first president of the Chicago Pediatric Society), and Frank Spooner Churchill among them. Also on the executive committee were prominent Chicagoans like Jane Addams, Stanley McCormick, son of industrialist Cyrus McCormick, and Julia Lathrop, who was to become the first head of the U.S. Children's Bureau. These reform-minded citizens followed in Coit's and Straus's footsteps as they investigated the conditions under which milk was produced and made clean milk available to children of the poor at a reasonable price. "The infant cannot draw from the udder direct," Mary Plummer, the CMC's first secretary, explained, "and it is between the udder and the child that most of the contamination occurs." If a child is bottle-fed, asked

Plummer, should not the cow, as the baby's "foster mother," be healthy and clean?[85]

Executive committee members had no difficulty agreeing that only mothers already artificially feeding their babies would be permitted to obtain the CMC's modified milk. Realizing that their widely advertised clean milk might persuade some lactating mothers to try bottle-feeding, CMC members refused to provide their milk simply for the asking. The CMC required customers to provide a voucher from a physician, visiting nurse, or priest to ensure "that they are people the Commission desire [*sic*] to reach."[86]

But the extensive advertising of CMC services ended up undermining the no-voucher, no-milk policy. Few, if any, of the city's mothers could have missed notification of the service. The *Chicago Tribune* printed and posted five hundred placards describing the whole milk, barley water, and modified milk formulas available at CMC milk stations. The CMC solicited weekly articles on infant health matters and published them in the Domestic Science column of the *Tribune*. The commission mailed the cost and content of its modified milk formulas to all Chicago physicians.[87] Editors for the *Chicago Medical Recorder* lauded the CMC in their weekly bulletin: "This activity has merit. It breathes the spirit of the age of preventive medicine."[88] The CMC marked each milk station with large posters, one in English and the others in whatever languages predominated in the neighborhood:[89]

40% of CHILDREN
under five years die principally from improper feeding.
SAVE THE BABIES
**Pure, Pasteurized and Properly prepared milk for Babies of all ages and
conditions.**
SOLD HERE AT COST.

It soon became difficult to turn insistent customers away.

The CMC did not ignore breastfeeding education, however. CMC physicians instructed station workers to encourage mothers to breastfeed, and in order to discourage the use of modified milk by lactating women, insisted that milk stations double as infant-care education centers. The CMC employed a woman to go door-to-door in all neighborhoods with milk stations to organize mothers' meetings. At these meetings women learned of the stark differences between bovine and human milk; why, if they gave cows' milk to their babies, it was essential that it be "good" cows' milk; how to care for milk in the home; and where to get medical care for their children. CMC workers urged the mothers who came to meetings to share their new knowledge with family, friends, and neighbors. During the commission's second summer, workers held mothers' meetings in African American churches and at settlement houses where women continued to learn about the importance of breast-feeding, clean milk, and how to use the four milk formulas sold or given away at milk stations.[90]

The CMC diligently educated dairy farmers as well as mothers. By the summer of 1904, 130 dairy farmers had filed requests with the CMC for inspection and instruction in sanitary practices. CMC physicians made regular, unannounced visits to all their certified farms. They toured the farms, noting, for example, how many feet the manure pile stood from the dairy, how often the stable's interior was whitewashed, whether the hairs around cows' udders were clipped, and how long milk spent in transit from farm to railroad. With preprinted CMC forms in hand, no detail escaped these inspectors.[91]

Initially, the cost of certified milk in Chicago presented no problem to the consumer. When milk stations opened in 1903, some customers paid one cent a bottle for modified milk and three cents a pint for pasteurized whole milk. Others paid nothing at all. Wanting to make the milk readily available even to the poorest Chicagoans, the CMC executive committee mandated that certified milk be distributed to the poor at a price "formerly paid for an inferior quality." But reality soon struck. It cost the CMC $10,276.65 to operate thirty-one stations during the summer of 1903, and the organization received only $7,000 from donations and $2,400.89 from milk sales.[92]

When the CMC ran out of money at the end of November 1903, board members opted to shut down until the organization was out of debt. The board did not make the decision lightly. Members recorded the move as a particularly harsh blow to the milk stations' primary beneficiaries, the infants of poor working mothers. Mrs. George Moulton mourned the closures as "the only thing to do for the creditors but a more heartless piece of business for the infants and their mothers would be hard to conceive." Infants, temporarily rescued from "whiskey, beer, etc.," would once again be forced to consume "the blue dirty milk of the corner grocery, or else their whiskey and beer."[93]

The CMC executive committee reluctantly reevaluated their milk prices. When milk stations reopened in June 1904, prices were double and, in some cases, triple those of the previous summer. The new prices were prohibitive to many, and it was not long before Harriet Fulmer, the superintendent of the Chicago Visiting Nurse Association (VNA), appealed to the CMC to provide milk to VNA patients for free. The CMC agreed and, in return, VNA nurses worked occasionally for the commission, explaining to mothers why clean milk was important and how to care for milk at home.[94]

Pricing milk out of the reach of the families who needed it most was only one of many problems faced by the CMC. In 1903 milk stations were staffed by volunteers who did not have the expertise to advise mothers on the appropriate formula for their babies. The CMC replaced these volunteers with paid employees who learned to follow strict rules. They were not permitted to give a mother an infant formula or switch a baby to another formula without a written order from a doctor.[95] In the fall of 1909, however, CMC directors discovered that workers at milk distribution stations prescribed an infant formula whenever a mother complained that the milk ordered by her infant's physician disagreed with her baby. CMC directors ordered CMC workers not to deviate from doctors' orders for any reason and to tell mothers to take their babies back to the doctor for an examination and a new written order if feeding problems occurred.[96]

Other difficulties surfaced. In 1908, Isaac Abt began to fret over the quality of CMC milk. Abt pointed out that pathogenic bacteria occasionally entered CMC milk from the well water used to wash milking utensils. He therefore cautioned that analysis of milk and inspection of barns and cows were no guarantee that certified milk was safe. He also noted with dismay that despite all of the CMC's publicity, raw milk—not certified, pasteurized, or modified milk—remained the infant food used by most women who fed their babies artificially. A disgusted Chicago Medical Society editorialized in 1909, "We even incline to the opinion that the babies and children would get along very nicely if the entire milk supply, whether pasteurized or not, were shut off entirely and permanently." The Chicago Department of Health responded to the disquiet by paying ten physicians to work three hours each day at CMC stations, examining babies whose mothers came to the stations for milk.[97]

But physicians long instrumental in the CMC's work remained troubled. At a May 1910 CMC meeting one doctor worried that they were making it too easy for a mother "to shirk her obligations" and bottle-feed her baby. CMC superintendent Minnie Ahrens assured him that CMC workers emphasized breastfeeding "wherever possible."[98]

In response to doctors' anxiety, the CMC instructed its workers to keep detailed feeding records for each infant served, including the formula prescribed, who prescribed it, how much of it was distributed to a mother and when, and when and why a baby stopped consuming it. The CMC also instituted a new requirement: any mother receiving a CMC formula had to bring her baby to the station weekly to be weighed. If she failed to do so even once, workers denied her more formula. If a baby lost weight, the milk

Table 6.1 Modified Milk Formulas Available at CMC Milk Stations, Summer 1903

Formula	Recommended Age of Child	Fat (%)	Milk Sugar (%)	Proteids (%)
Number 1	Sick infants under 3 months	1.5	5	.5
Number 2	Healthy infants 1 to 4 or 5 months	3	6	1
Number 3	Healthy infants 5 to 10 months, older sick babies	3.5	6	1.5
Number 4	Healthy infants 1 year to 18 months, older sick children	4	7	2

Source: "Minutes of Milk Commission July 7, 1903," Infant Welfare Society Papers.

station notified the baby's doctor immediately. To achieve even tighter control over their stations, CMC directors voted unanimously in December 1910 to limit the milk stations to ten, down from twenty-two the previous summer.[99]

A subsequent four-month study conducted by Ahrens confirmed the medical community's worst fears. Ahrens admitted that the personnel at CMC milk stations had been lax, commonly selling milk to mothers without also instructing them in proper feeding methods. Worse, she wrote, the very presence of a milk station in a neighborhood was indeed "apt to encourage artificial feeding when there should be breastfeeding." Ahrens suggested that caring for breastfed babies and teaching pregnant women about the importance of breastfeeding become an integral part of milk stations' activities.[100]

The CMC board acted on Ahrens's recommendations immediately, changing the name of the organization to the Infant Welfare Society (IWS) to reflect a much broader range of concerns than the distribution of clean milk. Admitting that the manner in which the CMC had issued milk not only discouraged breastfeeding but also encouraged mothers to wean babies unnecessarily—"to some extent . . . unknowingly"—the IWS replaced every milk station with an infant welfare station. The new stations, as Ahrens suggested, coupled the medical supervision of pregnant women—"in order that they may nurse their babies"—with the care of breastfed babies. "Under this plan," wrote CMC directors, "the educational work will be of more value than the distribution of milk."[101]

The IWS continued to provide milk to the mothers who insisted on using artificial food, rationalizing that the practice was for babies' sake. Unlike the CMC, however, the IWS did not consider milk distribution to be the primary purpose of infant welfare stations, and milk was difficult to obtain from the IWS. Mothers had to present a milk card signed by an IWS physician. Women needed a good excuse not to breastfeed, and the IWS required its doctors to state the reason a baby was not breastfed in a baby's medical record. Nor did the IWS publicize its certified milk and formula service.[102]

While certified milk stations might have benefited some individuals, their existence did not markedly alter infant mortality from diarrhea. Diarrheal deaths did not lower appreciably between 1902, just before the opening of the first CMC milk station, and late 1910, when the CMC became the IWS (see appendixes B.1 and B.2). In Chicago, as in most other cities, the certified milk movement gave way to the infant welfare movement.[103] A primary mission of the infant welfare movement was to convince more mothers to breastfeed their babies and to breastfeed them for longer periods of time. The distribution of clean milk became a sideline.

The Chicago Medical Society Milk Commission: "To Encourage the Production of Certified Milk"

By 1908 the CMC service was so popular that some milk dealers began selling false certified milk to unwitting customers. Wanting to quash the charlatans, Chicago Health Commissioner Walker Evans asked the CMC to organize one legitimate certifying body for the entire city.[104] CMC board members, already thinly stretched and beginning to doubt the value of their work anyway, declined. Instead, members of the Chicago Medical Society agreed to certify milk for the city. In early 1909, a board of seven physicians—elected to three-year terms by Chicago Medical Society members—began operating the Chicago Medical Society Milk Commission (CMSMC). Isaac Abt and Frank Spooner Churchill, two of the CMC's original executive committee members, were members of the first board.[105]

The Chicago Medical Society attempted to thwart corrupt dealers by sealing its CMSMC milk bottles with a copyrighted insignia and instructing the public to look for the distinctive logo when buying milk.[106] By the end of 1909, three dairies had signed with the Chicago Medical Society: the Arcady Farm in Lake Forest, Illinois, the Sedgley Farm in Hinsdale, Illinois, and the Edgewood Farm in Pewaukee, Wisconsin.[107] By 1914 the CMSMC oversaw milk production at thirteen farms and certified ten thousand quarts of milk daily.[108]

Beginning in 1912, physicians from the CMSMC gave monthly physical examinations to every certified dairy employee. These doctors wielded considerable power; when smallpox appeared in a small town housing a certified dairy farm, the Chicago Medical Society fired every dairy employee refusing vaccination.[109] During the 1918 influenza epidemic the CMSMC stepped up its physicals.[110]

Certified milk commissions, however, were never more than a stopgap measure in any city. In Chicago, the CMSMC was even less successful than the CMC because most of its milk was unpasteurized. This made it somewhat cleaner than raw milk but did not, as one CMSMC doctor admitted, mean that their certified milk never had a bacterial count over ten thousand. Rather, it meant that any certified dairy farm whose milk had a count over ten thousand could be decertified within ten days of notification unless they cleaned up their milk. "Our object is to encourage . . . the production of certified milk," the doctor told a group of Illinois physicians in 1914, "and were we, or any other commission, to stop certification merely because of a count of fifty or even a hundred thousand [bacteria] per c.c . . . there would probably be no certified milk in the United States."[111]

Bowman Dairy: "A Safe Supply of Pure Country Milk"

Milk laboratories and certified milk stations were not the only purveyors of clean milk in the early twentieth century. There were also reputable dairies. Although dairies did not intend that their product be used primarily by infants, before the 1940s most babies who were not breastfed consumed unmodified cows' milk or canned milk. By the early 1920s an estimated two-thirds of children under the age of one, even breastfed children, drank at least some cows' milk daily.[112] Dairies not connected with a milk laboratory or a milk station were the source of most of that milk.

The Bowman Dairy Company, whose founders made clean milk their primary goal from the dairy's inception in the 1870s, was the largest and, with their milk wagons pulled by trademark black horses, the most visible dairy in Chicago. In 1917 Bowman had 900 horses and 795 routes covering fifty miles from north to south and twelve miles from east to west.[113] By the late 1930s, when Bowman's home delivery service reached its apex with 2,000 routes and 2,400 black horses, the company produced an average of one million pounds of milk each day, one-quarter of Chicago's daily milk supply.[114]

J. R. Bowman and his two brothers started the dairy in St. Louis in 1874. Cognizant of "very poor traditions in the business," they advertised their ware as "A Safe Supply of Pure Country Milk" and worked hard to make it so. In 1885 the brothers abandoned the St. Louis operation and moved to the faster-growing Chicago market, purchasing nine milk routes from urban dairyman M. A. Devine. That same year Dr. Comfort E. Peck, husband of the Bowman brothers' sister Kate, joined the family business. Peck, whose medical background made him a natural for handling the sanitary end of the business, was largely responsible for the dairy's fanatic focus on cleanliness. The Bowmans boasted of their company's storage room, "the sanitary condition of which is perfect in every way," and "fully equipped" laboratory. In the laboratory Peck analyzed random samples of milk for signs of skimming, watering, and adulteration. When Peck's son David, also a physician, joined the business in 1900 he took charge of an additional laboratory that inspected milk for signs of bacterial contamination. Bowman inspectors occasionally called on customers to ascertain customer satisfaction with the product and to bring back still more samples to the laboratory.[115]

Bowman Dairy's innovations were legion. They operated their own laboratories for the daily examination of milk samples from each of their bottling stations. They began pasteurizing all their milk in 1905, eleven years before they were required to do so by law. Bowman was the first dairy in the city to use refrigerated freight cans for milk shipment. The company also developed its own farm inspection system.[116]

Bowman took advantage of all the municipal and philanthropic warnings about milk, touting their innovations to an edified public. Chicagoans learned from Bowman Company pamphlets that Bowman inspected each of its two thousand supplying dairies at least once a month to ensure hygienic milking practices; that Bowman pasteurized all the milk they sold; and that Bowman bottled and sealed milk in the country, not the city, to reduce chances for contamination. Bowman bragged that they packed milk bottles in crushed ice, shipped the bottles in refrigerated cars, unloaded them directly onto waiting delivery wagons at the city's railroad stations, and delivered them straight to customers. When families returned milk bottles, the Bowman Company soaked the bottles in one tank filled with cleaning solution, brushed them in a second tank, rinsed them with hot water in a third, and steam sterilized them in a fourth. The safeguards meant Bowman milk was not cheap; in 1917 it cost the consumer twelve cents a quart. But Bowman—touting their attention to hygiene to a public now loaded with savvy—urged consumers not to be penny wise and pound foolish.[117]

Although the Bowman Dairy Company never appealed specifically to the mothers of infants, by 1915 Bowman advertised its milk alongside pictures of babies. The words "Pure!" or "Safe!" or the slogan "Me for Bowman Milk" accompanied the infants' photos. Bowman ads informed mothers that "If Your Baby Could Talk—he or she would say 'Give me Bowman's Milk.'" In

1924 Bowman distributed manuals to their drivers—who doubled as salesmen, receiving a base salary plus commissions on the butter and milk they sold—explaining how to increase sales. Capitalizing on the contemporary concern over the differences in baby's "natural food" and cows' milk, Bowman subtly equated the two. The manual offered drivers a catchy slogan: "First in Mother Nature's plan, Comes good Milk as food for man."[118] Nature's product was still the most desirable for babies. The public perception of exactly what constituted the natural, however, was changing. If it was not tainted by carelessness, dirt, long train trips, deliberate adulteration, rides on the milk wagon in the hot sun, and the countless other evils of urban living, cows' milk was now as "natural" for human babies as human milk.

Bowman milk ads reflected the tenor of the times in other ways as well. Exploiting the public's newfound knowledge of communicable disease and their respect for preventive medicine, Bowman not only guaranteed that its milk was free of pathogenic bacteria, but also hinted that it had medicinal properties. "PHYSICIANS prescribe BOWMAN'S MILK because it is rich and pure," and "It gives the little tot strength to ward off illness" were typical messages. Bowman's milk, mothers learned, "works miracles."[119]

By 1940 Bowman Dairy advertisements read, "Three generations of mothers have safely given Bowman's to their babies."[120] But the company also warned salesmen to recommend cows' milk only for older babies. They suggested having this kind of conversation with mothers: "Mrs. Jones, you have wonderfully fine children; we want to keep them that way. The diet of this little six months old fellow is under the direction of your doctor isn't it? That's the doctor's responsibility and we all know that your doctor's instructions should be followed carefully without any change. But the diet of these older youngsters is pretty much up to you; that's your responsibility."[121]

By the late 1920s, Bowman and other reputable dairies did not hesitate to evoke the blessing of the medical community when they peddled their wares. The Milk Foundation sponsored a twice-weekly radio program on health featuring Chicago Health Commissioner Herman Bundesen. In 1930 Bowman sent a pamphlet to all Chicago-area physicians outlining the great strides taken by "modern science" to perfect the distribution "of Nature's most nearly perfect food." When Bowman introduced vitamin D milk in 1934, they sent a letter to physicians thanking them for their "wide spread acceptance."[122] In the face of so many artificially fed babies and the growing purity of cows' milk, physicians' advice that mothers breastfeed was becoming less insistent and their support of bottle-feeding more commonplace.

♦

In 1908 one doctor wrote, "There was a time not so long ago when not a few physicians honestly believed that cows' milk, properly modified, could be made interchangeable with breast milk. . . . The effect of this superstition, while it lasted, was a remarkable falling off in the percentage of nursing mothers."[123] His words proved prophetic. Worried that their nerves, uncontrollable emotions, improper diets, and inability to exercise daily might taint their own milk, mothers gladly embraced the newly sanctified cows' milk. Their reluctance to breastfeed no longer portended disaster.

Cities, charities, medical milk commissions, canned milk companies, dairies, and doctors now guaranteed that cows were clean and healthy and "free from nerves." The very different milk of a very different species was beginning to seem like the safer and surer "natural" choice. Even as physicians continued to invoke nature as the ideal, they managed to change the definition of nature markedly. For the many babies with no access to human milk, cows' milk was fast becoming, in the words of Dr. John Kellogg, "a priceless boon . . . the choicest product of nature's laboratory."[124]

Epilogue

"A Matter of Nursery Routine": Infant Feeding since the 1930s

The Sheppard-Towner Maternity and Infancy Protection Act, enacted by the United States Congress in late 1921 and repealed in 1929, led to the last concerted, albeit scattered, breastfeeding campaigns in the United States. Congress hoped that the federal money provided by Sheppard-Towner, to be matched by each state (Illinois was one of three states that refused the funds),[1] would improve maternal and infant health mainly via education. The act paid for visiting nurses to dispense pre- and postnatal care to women in their homes, clinics to counsel mothers on infant care, and pamphlets to advise mothers how best to improve and maintain their own and their children's health. Forty-three of the participating states also used some of their Sheppard-Towner funds to encourage mothers to breastfeed.[2] These breastfeeding campaigns took a variety of forms—from visiting nurses stressing to mothers the importance of breastfeeding, to the distribution of breastfeeding literature, to lectures and conferences on the importance of human milk to infants' health. States reported varying success with the crusades. In New Hampshire in 1928, 57 percent of mothers breastfed their newborns, although less than half those women (24.8 percent) were still breastfeeding at three months. In South Carolina in 1928, on the other hand, at least 90 percent of mothers breastfed their newborns.[3]

Despite the effort represented by these latter-day campaigns, however, few doctors continued to exhibit much concern about low breastfeeding rates. By the late 1920s, compared to twenty years earlier, artificial food posed little overt danger to babies. Doctors trained in the 1930s and after were largely indifferent to bottle-feeding since clean water, pasteurized milk, refrigerated railroad cars, and iceboxes in every home now alleviated the most immediate and recognizable side effects of artificial feeding. Mothers

187

were similarly reassured. No longer faced with virtually certain difficulties if they did not breastfeed, "their consciences [were] . . . at rest" knowing that their babies would likely "do well on the bottle."[4]

Troubled public health nurses noted this marked change in mothers' and doctors' attitudes as early as 1931. Instead of advising that mothers breast-feed if at all possible, physicians now promised women that artificial food posed little, if any, threat to their babies' health.[5] As some doctors observed, the campaigns for a wholesome milk supply had succeeded in making artifi-cial feeding "unduly safe and easy." At long last, one relieved physician noted in 1935, pediatricians could concentrate on "pediatric problems" rather than endless infant-feeding controversies.[6]

Even workers at Chicago's medical charities—long among the most adamant proponents of breastfeeding, especially for the poverty-stricken populace they served—now expressed gentle amusement when any of their largely foreign-born clientele artificially fed a baby. Bottle-feeding, appar-ently, had become a symbol of successful assimilation. In 1939, the Infant Welfare Society proudly reported one Polish mother's philosophy of proper infant care, gleaned from the doctors and nurses at her local infant welfare station: "American babies sleep alone; my babies too. No coffee for American babies; Pulaski babies drink [cows'] milk. . . . America good place."[7] The Vis-iting Nurse Association's public health nurses, who traditionally "insist[ed] upon breast feeding," were equally tolerant of bottle-feeding by the early 1940s. One nurse, called to help a woman with a broken arm unable to care for her two month old, reported matter-of-factly that she "spent most of her morning [t]here, giving the baby his feeding and putting him to bed in his crib."[8] In 1950, another visiting nurse recalled her futile attempt to explain the benefits of breastfeeding to a Chinese woman who spoke no English. The nurse recounted approvingly that the woman's husband interrupted the interaction to explain that in China, where no alternative to breastfeeding existed, mothers had no choice but to nurse their babies. In the United States, however, he and his wife wanted their babies to have what American chil-dren enjoyed—bottled cows' milk.[9]

The transition from physicians primarily advising their patients to breastfeed to virtually always sanctioning artificial food was nevertheless slow and by no means seamless. Even many doctors who lauded the new safety of artificial food continued to tell mothers that "with all the advances in artificial feeding, breastfeeding still remains the simplest and safest way to nourish an infant."[10] Disagreement was most evident between longtime pediatricians and the newest generation of doctors. Older doctors still urged breastfeeding, not only because human milk remained the easiest substance for an infant to digest, but because they had observed during their many decades of medical practice that human milk protected babies from illness.[11] One Illinois doctor, noting that during a recent measles epidemic artificially fed babies suffered severe illness and occasional death, while breastfed babies had only mild cases of the illness if they sickened at all, urged colleagues in 1934 to consider not only the nutritive properties of breast milk but its "immunizing qualities" as well.[12] The vast majority of older pediatricians thus remained human milk devotees long after artificial food was the norm.

Chicago pediatrician Joseph Brennemann was typical of this group. He blamed parents as well as physicians for mothers' dependence on and love affair with artificial food. He described one "intelligent, medically educated young mother" whose fourteen month old suffered from chronic diarrhea. When Brennemann asked her what she fed her son, "she handed me a table showing the number of grams of fat, carbohydrate and protein the infant was getting, together with the number of calories per kilogram of body weight daily." Brennemann expressed tremendous frustration with this "more active, more evident and more voluminous 'scientific' treatment" of babies and urged a "laissez faire therapy" in its place. In 1930, as the newly installed president of the American Pediatric Society, he subtitled a speech "A Plea for the More Extended Use of Conservatism and of Common Sense in the Practice of Pediatrics" and urged colleagues to remember that "nature is a potent factor in restoring the pathologic to the normal and . . . it is . . . common sense not only to recognize and utilize that force more freely and frankly than is done in the practice of medicine, but perhaps, even more, not unwisely to run counter to that force."[13]

But as Brennemann well knew, parents and younger doctors no longer quite trusted what they deemed the antiquated theories and methods of older pediatricians, especially when it came to infant feeding. At a 1952 testimonial dinner for pediatrician Julius Hess, admirers staged a skit that poked good-natured fun at Hess's dogmatism about breastfeeding.

PATIENT: My hair hurts.
J.H.H. [Julius H. Hess]: Which one?
PATIENT: The middle one.
J.H.H.: Breast milk is what you need.[14]

Now that breastfeeding had ceased being *the* factor guaranteed to increase the odds of infants surviving their first year, many doctors simply stopped making the extra effort to push human milk.[15] As one doctor explained, "The mother who refuses to nurse her infant when she is capable of it is probably injuring herself more than she is the child if only by her failure to establish the proper relationship between them."[16] W. McKim Marriott, a St. Louis physician, assured colleagues that all the old fears about cows' milk as a food for infants—that it would cause diarrhea, infectious disease, decayed teeth, bowed legs, and mental deficiency, for example—were outdated, particularly for babies under a doctor's supervision. "However true these . . . [worries] may [still] be for babies improperly fed on unsuitable proprietary foods and improperly constructed formulas, they do not apply to babies who are fed according to the underlying principles of infant nutrition which are now well understood." In justifying his support of artificial food Marriott contended, "There is nothing mysterious or sacred about breast milk. It is just a food."[17]

The doctors who never saw an infant die from causes attributable to artificial food and seldom saw one sicken hinted that artificial food was not only on a par with human milk, it was, just possibly, better. "Except for conferring certain immunity," one physician explained, "all other requirements for feeding the baby are more easily met by a formula than by breast feeding." Unlike his predecessors—who spent decades writing prescriptions for formulas so that each of their infant patients could enjoy a unique version of cows' milk as personal need ostensibly dictated—this physician contended that the beauty of formula lay in its immutable nature. "Many uncontrollable factors enter into breast feeding," he argued, while formulas remained steadfastly and precisely the same. Thus, only a formula could be counted on to "produce consistently normal growth and development."[18] Even doctors working for the Chicago Board of Health, whose breastfeeding campaigns between 1908 and the 1920s had been tireless, noted in their 1951 annual report that "fortified" infant formula had a higher vitamin and mineral content than breast milk. Perhaps, the report implied, this bonus made artificial food better.[19] Some board of health doctors expressed doubt that breast milk had value even for premature babies. They cautioned, "The question as to whether the premature infant should be fed breast milk, which is claimed by many to be more digestible but of lower mineral content than artificial mixtures, is one that as yet has not been answered with unanimity."[20]

Some older physicians blamed younger doctors' medical education for the changing attitudes. Henry Niblack, chief of the Bureau of Child Welfare for the Chicago Board of Health, explained in 1936 that interns and student nurses "are not trained to teach mothers the art of breast feeding; they are not led to have any strong conviction in the matter; they go out to practice; may become, in turn, members of the hospital staff, responsible for the training of following groups of interns and nurses; thus a vicious circle is created." Niblack urged the doctors and nurses who worked in hospitals to learn about human milk: "If every one in the institution believes in breast feeding, talks breast feeding, and if breast feeding is actually carried out, the mother develops the same spirit and enthusiasm."[21]

In an era when infant-care experts urged mothers to rely on doctors for infant-feeding advice, younger doctors' growing ignorance of lactation and the benefits of human milk portended the almost complete abandonment of breastfeeding. A mother anxious about her breastfed infant now had difficulty finding an expert sympathetic to and knowledgeable about breastfeeding. As one mother warned in a letter to an infant-care magazine in 1938, "Don't count too heavily on nursing your baby. . . . Even if you are breast-feeding you may be ordered by your doctor to give him supplementary feedings by bottle, so it is fairly safe to count on bottles and their attendant equipment."[22]

Lack of faith in the efficacy of breastfeeding among the majority of mothers and doctors became the rule. One doctor explained in 1961 that mothers' trepidation about breast milk quantity, especially in the first few days after birth, usually prompted physicians to urge weaning—"the easiest and quickest way" of alleviating mothers' worries, not to mention their own— before a mother had even established a milk supply. Other doctors recommended supplementary bottle-feedings for breastfed babies right after birth "in misguided apprehension about the baby's weight." Nor did physicians customarily explain to breastfeeding mothers the difference between the thick, yellow colostrum produced immediately after birth and the thin, bluish liquid produced a few days later. According to one doctor, "Many women view the change with dismay, assuming that their milk is deteriorating." The lethal combination of mothers' alarm and doctors' growing ignorance of lactation physiology and breastfeeding management led more times than not to a mother abandoning breastfeeding.[23]

Early weaning and early mixed feeding among breastfeeding mothers, as I have explained, was fairly common even at the end of the nineteenth century. By the 1930s, however, the majority of women never even initiated breastfeeding. This was due not only to younger doctors' ignorance of breastfeeding and the relative safety of artificial food, but to formula companies' new, aggressive sales techniques. Rima Apple points out that by the 1930s, in order to make themselves indispensable to mothers, some physicians collaborated with infant food manufacturers to have instructions removed from infant formula cans and made available only through physicians.[24] Mothers flocked to doctors' doors.

Infant formula manufacturers also perfected their sales calls. In early 1929, Brennemann gave unwitting credence to the lofty claims of evaporated milk salesmen in an article he authored for the *Journal of the American Medical Association* summing up the results of a six-month study at Children's Memorial Hospital in Chicago. The study showed that babies did equally well on evaporated milk as on acid or sour milk.[25] The latter was, at the time, preferred by physicians over evaporated milk.[26] In triumph, Pet Milk salesmen called on doctors with Brennemann's study in hand, only to be rebuffed. Fretting that "doctors are allergic to salesmen," Pet executives responded by opening a medical relations department whose staff approached physicians as ostensible medical specialists, not as salesmen. By 1940, fifty-five men worked in medical relations for Pet. Their job was to convince doctors that Pet Milk was a viable food for newborns. By 1962, Pet employed "a nationwide force of full-time medical detail men."[27]

One retired Chicago obstetrician who delivered babies from 1947 to 1988 recalled that the sales calls he received from representatives of infant formula companies were numerous and persuasive. He admitted, "They gave you a long line about how their formula was better than mothers' milk. . . . Perhaps that swayed me." He also recalled the many lavish vacations he enjoyed paid for by a formula company. "They paid fantastic amounts of money for doctors to go on their trips. . . . We had nice, beautiful accommodations, all of us . . . always the best." The only condition of the sponsored trips was that doctors spend one of their evenings viewing a film or listening to a lecture about the sponsor's product.[28]

The new custom of infant formula companies calling on physicians coincided with a dramatic increase in hospital births. Formula companies now had not only an audience of amenable physicians to play to, but a congregation of hospitalized mothers as well. In 1900, virtually all births took place at home. By 1926, 55.1 percent of mothers in Chicago gave birth in hospitals. By 1930, 68 percent did. In the United States as a whole, 88 percent of births took place in hospitals by 1950. By 1960, virtually all births did.[29]

In hospitals, where women customarily remained for six to ten days after a normal vaginal birth, mothers found themselves more reliant on physicians' advice and more uncertain about their own abilities to mother than they might have been if they had birthed at home. One woman with many younger siblings had plenty of experience caring for infants before she gave birth to her first child in 1943, but the rigid scheduling inherent in hospital life and the authoritative hospital personnel undermined her confidence. "The baby didn't belong to me . . . the hospital owned him," she complained. As a result, her first few weeks of motherhood were filled with tension and insecurity.[30] The Chicago Board of Health was one of many health authorities that encouraged mothers' dependence on hospital staff. In its 1931 regulations for maternity wards and infants' nurseries the Board warned, "A mother does not instinctively know how to care for her infant. A knowledge of the modern methods of infant care, as suggested by her physician, will help her keep the infant well and strong."[31]

This missive posed a special problem for mothers wanting to breastfeed. Rarely did they receive support, encouragement, and guidance from the hospital staff. As one doctor explained in 1953, "An insecure mother with a sleepy baby in a hospital that discourages nursing will be an entirely different problem in management from an insecure mother with a sleepy baby in a hospital sympathetic to breast feeding."[32] Another doctor lamented in 1961 that "the hospital environment—hospital arrangements, routines and, above all, staff attitudes and expectations—often spells the difference between . . . [breastfeeding] failure and success."[33]

Unsurprisingly, companies like Pet Milk did well in this milieu. They proudly described their involvement with hospital nurseries:

> The expectant mother may first hear about PET milk when learning about formula preparations in the hospital's orientation class. She and her husband may select the baby's name from a list supplied by a company medical relations representative. The name card on her baby's crib in the hospital nursery might bear the PET insignia. Most important, her baby's first bottle of formula may very well be made with PET brand evaporated milk. These "little things" add up to a convincing acceptance of the PET brand.[34]

Rigid hospital routine also affected infant-feeding practices. Immediately after a birth, nurses hustled babies off to hospital nurseries. As long as mothers remained hospitalized they saw their infants only at infrequent and prearranged times. At Chicago's Michael Reese Hospital, for example, nurses did not permit mothers to breastfeed until six hours after giving birth. After that initial feeding, nurses brought babies to their mothers only once every four hours, but never more than five times in twenty-four hours.[35] Thus, nurses commonly gave even breastfed infants artificial food in the nursery. Artificial food received medical sanction in hospitals while mothers' milk supplies languished.[36]

That the women who gave birth in the hospital in the 1930s and early

1940s had a profoundly different experience with breastfeeding than many of the women who continued to birth at home is corroborated by Josephine Sobolewski, a longtime Chicago public health nurse. While Sobolewski was a nursing student in the early 1930s, she observed new mothers, mostly middle- and upper-class, breastfeeding in the hospital. Shortly after, as a visiting nurse, she cared for hundreds of women postpartum, mostly working-class, who had given birth at home attended by a Chicago Maternity Center physician.[37] Women who gave birth in the hospital normally did not see their babies for twelve to twenty-four hours after giving birth and only infrequently after that. "So," Sobolewski recalled, "that breast starts to get engorged and it gets hard and the baby has trouble nursing and then they tried to pump on the mother." The problem invariably worsened during the course of a woman's hospital stay. "Oh, it used to be a mess . . . you'd feel sorry for them," Sobolewski lamented. "And then they'd go home like that." Discouraged, the women who had given birth in the hospital often ended up bottle-feeding their babies. The mothers who gave birth at home attended by maternity center physicians had a different experience. They breastfed their babies soon after birth. "You see the baby was right there with mama," Sobolewski explained, "and if the baby . . . started to cry, the babies would be put to that breast. . . . And so they didn't have the problems . . . she'd feed it whenever the baby wanted to eat."[38]

Clifford Grulee first noticed a rash of breastfeeding failures among mothers who gave birth at Chicago's Presbyterian Hospital in 1930. Like the women Sobolewski was observing, the women giving birth at home with the aid of Presbyterian's outpatient maternity service did not evidence any problems with lactation. Grulee investigated reasons for the discrepancy and discovered that in hospital nurseries, formula was often given to breastfed babies by "the nurse who looks at the weight curve, holds up her hands in holy horror and immediately tries to have something more given to the child."[39] At Grulee's behest, Presbyterian Hospital halted this practice. Presbyterian's breastfeeding rate at discharge went from 40 percent in 1930 to 85 percent by 1936.[40]

Grulee was not the only experienced Chicago pediatrician who noticed that switching babies to artificial feeding was becoming the routine, not the aberration, in hospital nurseries. When the Chicago Board of Health demanded to know in 1936 why so many of the newborns that their doctors examined at infant welfare stations were bottle-fed, station physicians invariably contended, "The baby was put on the bottle in the hospital and so discharged; when the baby is registered [for care at the infant welfare station] he is already in the habit of having a bottle, and the mother of giving it."[41] Like Grulee, Julius Hess blamed hospital neonatal nurses for the trend, charging that bottle-feedings were "a matter of nursery routine, often without consultation with the obstetrician or the pediatrician." Nurses, he complained, often worried that a newborn's weight loss in the days after birth was a "dangerous adventure" to be prevented. "This unjustifiable fear," he argued, "is responsible for many artificially fed infants." He explained that the "easy flowing content from the bottle" required little work on the baby's part; thus a newborn given the choice between breast and bottle "becomes lazy and refuses to help his mother stimulate her breasts to meet his needs. There in lies the cause of a high percentage of babies being discharged from our hospitals on unnecessary bottle feedings."[42]

Mothers' experience in the hospital proved equally pivotal to breast-feeding failures. Nurses imposed the hygienic rituals necessary to make artificial feeding safe even on lactating women. Bottles and rubber nipples needed sterilization before going into a baby's mouth, now human nipples did too. Although the Chicago Board of Health Revised Code of 1931 continued to laud human milk, advising that "ALL MOTHERS SHALL BE IMPRESSED CONSTANTLY WITH THE IMPORTANCE OF BREAST FEEDING" and "the breast-fed baby is the best-fed baby," the code also required rituals that likely made many lactating mothers uneasy. Board guidelines for the city's maternity wards recommended that all nursing mothers wear a "suitable jacket" while breastfeeding because "unless a suitable jacket is worn, the breasts are easily contaminated." Guidelines also suggested that nurses thoroughly cleanse mothers' nipples before permitting mothers to breastfeed "to keep infection from the infant."[43]

That their own nipples might pose a health threat to their babies was probably frightening to new mothers. As Brennemann put it, "She is afraid of the consequences if she does not learn . . . the mystic contents of the boric acid jar." Brennemann, who advised toning down the cleansing rituals lest they intimidate mothers, reminded his colleagues of the "well-known effect of nervousness and worry on the supply of milk . . . quite familiar to the dairyman."[44] Despite such pleas, however, most physicians continued to advise that "prior to nursing, the mother washes her hands or cleanses them with an antiseptic aqueous solution of benzalkonium . . . chloride (1:1000) and cleanses the nipples and breasts with isotonic sodium chloride solution. These solutions and cotton balls for their application are kept at the bedside at all times in small sterile containers."[45] This "atmosphere of ritualism," Brennemann complained, made "a deep and often ineffaceable impression on the mother," contributing to many breastfeeding failures.[46] And one can only imagine how a human nipple covered in isotonic sodium chloride solution must have tasted to babies, most likely discouraging many an infant from relishing, or even beginning, a meal.

The messages doctors conveyed personally to new mothers might have been as intimidating to women as hospital ritual. Even a doctor as convinced of the efficacy of maternal nursing as Clifford Grulee occasionally offered anxiety-producing advice. In 1930 Grulee treated the baby of a woman from Atlanta who had given birth at Chicago's Presbyterian Hospital. The new mother apparently feared that she did not have enough milk for her baby and discussed her concern with Grulee. He gave the woman a set of complicated instructions allegedly designed to increase her milk supply, keep her baby well, and allay her fears. Nurse the baby for twelve minutes exactly, he ordered the mother. Then lay the baby down and pump any milk left in the breasts. Pour the pumped milk into a bottle and feed it to the baby. If the baby still appeared hungry after consuming mother's milk via breast and bottle, he advised that she bottle-feed again, this time with Mead Johnson and Company powdered protein milk. Despite the mammoth ritual Grulee expected this conscientious mother to implement, he was privately pessimistic about the outcome and warned the woman's doctor in Atlanta: "I am inclined to think that she will not be able to nurse the baby very long, but have prolonged the period of nursing in order to give the child breast milk at the time when, in my opinion, he most needs it."[47] When the woman returned home a few weeks later, she did not see her own doctor for several additional weeks because he was out of town. Finally away from the stress of the hospital and doctors' complicated, time-consuming instructions, she and the baby evidently did much better. The woman's doctor wrote to Grulee six weeks later, "I found the child in excellent condition. He is gaining steadily on the mother's milk exclusively—her supply evidently having increased considerably after she came home."[48]

By the 1940s, doctors recommended that solid foods be made part of a baby's diet early in life, thus dissuading even the few women who breastfed from doing so for long. In 1955 Julius Hess estimated that 90 percent of pediatricians recommended giving a baby solid foods at three months of age or younger; sixty-six percent urged introducing solid foods at two months of age or younger. Hess complained, "The fact that most infants accept and tolerate such foods is a credit to both the human structure and the manufacturers' ability but it does not prove that the practice is necessarily good."[49]

Younger pediatricians protested that it was mothers who insisted on giving their two or three month olds solid food. Mothers, these doctors charged, competed obsessively with friends and neighbors for the fattest baby. Hess agreed that the urge to cater to a mother's desires was a problem all pediatricians faced. Pediatricians were reluctant to disagree with a mother, he complained, because she "begins to wonder whether he is uptodate and there is nothing more damaging to the career of the young pediatrician these days than to be considered old-fashioned."[50]

Not until the late 1970s, with the advent of "natural childbirth" and "family-centered" birthing rooms in hospitals, did breastfeeding rates begin an ascent. The social activism of the 1960s and early 1970s gave rise to both environmental and feminist movements that worked in tandem to advocate the natural in both childbirth and infant feeding. Activists encouraged women to learn about and trust their bodies, take responsibility for their own health, and wrest women's medical care away from "condescending, paternalistic, judgmental and non-informative" physicians.[51] Unmedicated birth and breastfeeding were two ways, feminists argued, to take from the largely male medical profession what should have been the sole prerogative of women all along.

The return to breastfeeding was also due in part to La Leche League, a voluntary organization that originated in a Chicago suburb in 1956. Convinced that "feeding a baby was not a medical matter; it was a maternal matter,"[52] seven women who had breastfed their babies successfully organized a mothers' group in their neighborhood to dispense advice to friends and neighbors who wanted to breastfeed.[53] From an initial meeting of twelve women in 1956, La Leche League support groups grew to 43 in 1961, 430 in 1966, 1,260 in 1971, and 3,000 in 1976.[54] The organization reached an even wider audience via its book, *The Womanly Art of Breastfeeding,* first published in 1958. A second revised edition of the book in 1963 sold 1,172,200 copies. La Leche League published the sixth revised edition of their bestseller in 1997.[55]

Reminiscent of late nineteenth- and early twentieth-century public health authorities, the League has called breastfeeding "God's plan for mothers and babies."[56] This rhetoric, and the mother-to-mother support and solid advice that has accompanied it, helped increase breastfeeding rates in the United States from 22 percent of newborns in 1972 to 62 percent in 1982. Breastfeeding rates began another decline in 1982, leveling off at 52 percent in 1989.[57] The rate began to rise again in 1991, reaching 57.4 percent in 1994.[58]

These statistics are deceptively high, however, for they represent only the percentage of mothers who leave the hospital breastfeeding and include babies fed human milk supplemented with artificial food. Exclusive breastfeeding rates are much lower than these figures indicate. Prolonged breastfeeding rates are lower still; barely 20 percent of *all* babies are still nursing at six months and only 5.6 percent continue to nurse until their first birthday.[59] Moreover, certain women are much less likely to breastfeed at all than others. Today the least likely women to breastfeed are teenagers, women with low levels of education, women with low income, and unmarried women. African American and Mexican-American women are much less likely to nurse their babies than Anglo-American women.[60]

In December 1997, to encourage more mothers to initiate breastfeeding and to increase exclusive breastfeeding and breastfeeding duration rates, the American Academy of Pediatrics (AAP) issued a policy statement, "Breastfeeding and the Use of Human Milk," which outlined new breastfeeding standards. The media widely reported the new guidelines. The AAP advised mothers to breastfeed their babies exclusively for six months (in an attempt to discourage early weaning and mixed feeding), to continue to breastfeed for an additional six months while the baby is introduced to other foods, and to keep on breastfeeding (that is, mixed feeding) "thereafter for as long as mutually desired."[61]

In their statement the AAP also called for changes in hospital routines that undermine breastfeeding. They recommended that babies remain with their mothers throughout postnatal recovery and that babies breastfeed within one hour after birth. The AAP also called for an abandonment of any rigid scheduling of infant feeding. They urged mothers to nurse their newborns at least eight to twelve times every twenty-four hours and to do so at their babies' first sign of hunger, that is, whenever their babies exhibited "increased alertness or activity, mouthing, or rooting." The AAP cautioned that crying was an infant's last, frantic resort to let a mother know of hunger.[62]

In November 2000 in another widely publicized initiative, the Department of Health and Human Services (HHS) issued the "HHS Blueprint for Action on Breastfeeding," which they touted as "a comprehensive breastfeeding policy for the nation." Calling breastfeeding "one of the most important contributors to infant health," HHS decried the low number of breastfed babies in the United States, particularly at six months postpartum, and urged the nation to "address those low breastfeeding rates as a public health challenge." For the first time since the 1910s and 1920s, when municipal, state, and national health agencies treated low breastfeeding rates as an urgent public health crisis and designed dramatic public health messages accordingly, a federal agency is calling for "national, culturally appropriate strategies to promote breastfeeding."[63] Babies' consumption, or nonconsumption, of human milk is once again on the table as a health issue that should concern us all.

♦

The AAP and HHS statements informed the American public that despite the medical community's ability to rescue virtually all artificially fed babies from the most obvious and immediate consequences of artificial feeding—via electrolyte therapy, antibiotics, and childhood inoculations—low breastfeeding rates continue to constitute a nationwide health problem. Preventing illness is still preferable to curing it and contemporary evidence corroborates the impression of nineteenth-century doctors. Breastfed infants *are* better able to fight disease than artificially fed babies. Human milk not only contains certain static anti-infection factors, but is, in the words of one doctor, "a living, dynamic secretion" whose antibodies are constantly changing in response to health threats in the environment.[64]

To illustrate only one facet of the capacity of human milk: a mother's body, unlike her infant's, has accumulated years of experience fighting all sorts of infections. Lying in the plasma cells of an adult's small intestine is the know-how to battle each gastrointestinal pathogen ingested in a lifetime. The plasma cells and their immunological memory remain in a woman's small intestine throughout her life, fighting invading viruses and bacteria. They move from that spot only if a woman lactates, when some plasma cells migrate to the mammary glands and are passed on to the woman's baby in her milk. Breastfed babies essentially share their mothers' time-honored immune systems.[65]

Breastfed infants enjoy not only better short-term health than artificially fed babies, but, many pediatricians suspect, far better long-term health as well. Human milk not only reduces the afflictions of childhood thought to be "normal" ever since artificial feeding became predominate practice—like respiratory infections and middle-ear infections—but also offers possible protection from much more serious illnesses like bacterial meningitis, insulin-dependent diabetes, lymphoma, leukemia, and assorted allergic diseases.[66] The medical community is just beginning to document the many serious diseases that breastfeeding might prevent both short- and long-term. Recently, researchers in Sweden demonstrated that human milk kills cancer cells in the laboratory. Their discovery has led to speculation that breastfed babies have considerably fewer cases of childhood cancers than bottle-fed babies because human milk kills errant cells before they become cancerous.[67] Even breastfeeding mothers (that is, the mothers who breastfeed according to the AAP guidelines) enjoy long-term health benefits, including improved bone strength, meaning fewer hip fractures after menopause, and reduced risk of both ovarian cancer and premenopausal breast cancer.[68]

The health benefits of prolonged breastfeeding are not widely known among the laity, however. Despite a rash of well-publicized health crises among children—epidemics of ear infections, asthma, and food allergies as well as frightening tales of bacterial meningitis, for example—breastfeeding is rarely, if ever, mentioned as a preventive of these illnesses.[69] On an October 9, 1999, *Today Show* segment a pediatrician explained to parents how to prevent children's ear infections. She advised parents to maintain smoke-free, well-ventilated homes, to avoid dairy (presumably cows' milk) in their children's diets, and to teach children how to blow their noses properly. But she did not mention breastfeeding, despite the fact that the connection between breastfeeding and lowered rates of otitis media is indisputable.[70] Similarly, on a *Good Morning America* segment in June 2000, physician-journalists Timothy Johnson and Nancy Snyderman reported an epidemic of life-threatening food allergies among children. They agreed, "We don't know why" there are so many more allergies, and so many more severe allergies, among children today. Neither physician mentioned that full breastfeeding can prevent food allergies, and concomitantly, minimal breastfeeding offers little, if any, protection.[71]

When breastfeeding is mentioned at all by the media it is most often in conjunction with health threats. Before the AAP issued its breastfeeding guidelines in 1997, the most recent national publicity given to breastfeeding was in 1994 when newspapers and television news shows reported that several breastfed babies almost died from dehydration. A few suffered permanent disability from their ordeal. Although one pediatrician said of the tragedies, "[I]nsufficient intake is rare . . . and there's no reason it should undermine any mother's plan to breast-feed," the reports were terribly alarming, reminiscent of the late nineteenth-century warnings that breast milk could be quite harmful.[72]

More recently, the ABC newsmagazine show *20/20* ran a story on February 26, 1999, about Tabitha Walrond, a teenage New York mother, charged with murdering her newborn son, Tyler. She exclusively breastfed Tyler and, at seven weeks of age, he died of starvation. Cynthia McFadden, narrator of the segment, explained, "What Tabitha thought was Tyler's healthy appetite was actually the baby struggling to get enough milk to survive. There is no question that Tyler Walrond starved to death." Tabitha Walrond tearfully assured McFadden, "He was . . . on my breast all the time." Not until more than halfway through the story did McFadden explain that Walrond had breast reduction surgery when she was fifteen and her past and present doctors had failed to warn her that the surgery might prohibit her from successfully breastfeeding.[73] Indeed, the casual listener might have missed that crucial tidbit altogether. The print media ran similar accounts. Not until the tenth paragraph in the *New York Times*'s version of the story did the reporter mention that "at age 15, she had breast reduction surgery, which experts say greatly increases the chances of insufficient breast milk."[74] Other details of the tragedy surfaced. Walrond, who was enrolled in Medicaid, had tried repeatedly to have her son examined by a doctor but was rebuffed because her son had not yet been assigned a Medicaid number.[75]

Soon after the Walrond story broke, *Newsweek* jumped on the bandwagon. Under the heading "Nursing Trouble," the first paragraph of a story warning women about the dangers of insufficient breast milk ended with one tearful mother alerting other mothers, "I couldn't believe I was starving my baby and didn't know it."[76] At least two television dramas—*Chicago Hope* (on October 21, 1998) and *Law and Order* (on February 9, 2000)—subsequently featured storylines in which a mother, driven by unrelenting pressure to breastfeed, inadvertently killed her baby because she had inadequate breast milk.

The Tyler Walrond tragedy could have provoked many national debates: about the inadequacy and inefficiency of Medicaid; about the inherent injustice in our medical system's distribution of health care; about poor communication between doctors and patients; about teen pregnancy and motherhood; about inadequate preparation for parenthood; about how important it is for patients to do their own homework and not rely wholly on their doctor for critical information; about a downside to breast reduction surgery; about the nonexistent public support network for pregnant and nursing mothers in the United States, support that mothers in other western industrialized countries can take for granted. Instead, the story sounded a quite different alarm—the foolhardiness of blindly breastfeeding a baby without considering artificial food supplements.

That breastfeeding can be a difficult, even impossible, undertaking, and that human milk is prone to inadequacy and that inadequate breast milk can on occasion harm, even kill, are notions that began in the late nineteenth century and have now risen to the level of cultural truths.[77] Today we learn from news shows, television dramas, news magazines, and newspaper headlines that breastfeeding is so difficult, unreliable, and mysterious that you can starve your baby and not even know it until he is dead. The consensus seems to be that the Walrond baby died, not from public and private neglect and ignorance, but because, in the words of one on-line magazine, he was "nursed to death."[78]

Contemporary tales like the dehydration and starved-to-death disasters garner enough publicity to quash any public discussion on the health benefits of breastfeeding for children and women. We are in much the same place as in 1908 when one angry doctor called the American notion of preventive medicine "twisted" because doctors and assorted reformers scurried to organize milk commissions so mothers would have palatable cows' milk to give their babies "while we have no similarly organized body devoting its attention to the many perplexing problems of the human milk supply."[79] This irate doctor would probably voice similar concerns today. Most physicians remain woefully ignorant of lactation and how to aid the women who come to them with breastfeeding questions. Thus, although members of the medical community pay lip service to the importance of breastfeeding, they do not actively promote the practice. Rather, pediatricians prescribe antibiotics to cure babies' ear infections, infections that might have been prevented by breastfeeding. Obstetricians urge postmenopausal women to take estrogen to prevent osteoporosis, a disease that can be prevented or diminished in severity by breastfeeding.

Women have been instrumental in shaping infant-feeding practices over the last 120 years. As this book demonstrates, however, health choices are rarely completely voluntary and medical recommendations are rarely wholly dispassionate. Then, as now, society limits women's choices and shapes physicians' medical advice. Breastfeeding advocates can tout the social, economic, health, immunological, cognitive, developmental, and psychological benefits of breastfeeding loud and long. But just as posters trumpeting the detrimental effects of artificial food were insufficient to change mothers' habits in the 1910s, publicizing the many benefits of breastfeeding today will not be sufficient to increase breastfeeding rates in the twenty-first century. Mothers are still constricted in their infant-feeding choices by the demands of work outside the home, lack of paid maternity leave, lack of on-site day care, lack of facilities to pump and store milk at work, and general discomfort with breastfeeding in public and, in some instances, with breastfeeding at all. Medical students learn little, if anything, about lactation physiology, breastfeeding management, and the relationship between human milk and human health in medical school, and consequently as physicians they are ill-equipped to advise lactating mothers and to discuss infant-feeding choices with women. According to one large national survey, more than half of all residents and more than 30 percent of physicians could not describe the correct clinical management of common breastfeeding problems. Today, the effectiveness and accuracy of physicians' breastfeeding advice has little to do with their medical school education or with the knowledge gained through clinical practice, and much more to do with their private experience. Whether the physician herself or the physician's wife breastfed is currently the most important factor influencing a physician's ability to diagnose and treat lactation-related ailments and to make accurate recommendations about infant feeding options.[80]

Contemporary views of breastfeeding and human milk have been long in the making and will not easily be altered. The transformation in infant-feeding practice that began in the United States in the nineteenth century is a dramatic and complex story, driven by a change in attitude toward some of our most important institutions: marriage, motherhood, and medicine. Mothers' decisions then, as today, are also influenced by views of time, efficiency, self-control, nature, health, the human body, and what constitutes "normal" interaction with babies—all concepts deemed so important by Americans that each generation foolishly thinks of them as eternally static. History, however, enables us to see more clearly the origins of these attitudes and, hopefully, can aid us in making breastfeeding more the public health matter that it should be and less the activity tainted by preconceived fears of inadequacy and notions of propriety that it has become.

APPENDIX A.1

Deaths from Diarrhea under Two Years of Age in Chicago per 100,000 Live Births, 1877 to 1925

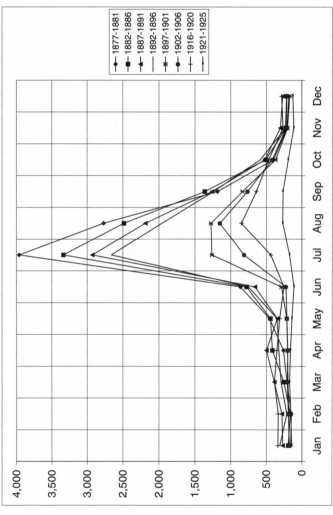

Source: Annual Reports of the Department of Health of the City of Chicago.

Note: I was unable to find the city's monthly breakdown for diarrheal deaths for the years 1907–1915. Also, the diarrheal deaths represented on this graph are from Chicago's original statistics and do not represent the way I totaled diarrheal deaths in Appendix B.1 and Appendix B.2.

APPENDIX A.2

Deaths from Diarrhea under Two Years of Age in Chicago,
1877 to 1925

Year	Jan.	Feb.	Mar.	Apr.	May	Jun.	Jul.	Aug.	Sept.	Oct.
1877	18	12	20	36	29	58	386	269	142	53
1878	11	10	21	20	17	23	366	238	109	28
1879	12	10	20	16	23	117	409	292	97	31
1880	23	22	19	18	52	185	449	256	97	47
1881	27	36	43	53	162	141	661	541	218	62
1882	40	27	37	40	41	79	393	496	268	86
1883	20	13	47	52	57	129	602	331	173	60
1884	26	24	32	108	88	130	668	419	256	103
1885	28	28	27	74	131	140	567	379	174	64
1886	46	44	66	67	47	163	481	380	231	103
1887	24	51	117	47	53	268	728	366	224	78
1888	44	35	45	101	53	112	685	548	250	89
1889	47	27	42	46	68	75	745	583	412	147
1890	151	169	108	107	94	179	692	607	303	127
1891	89	86	174	360	179	141	650	579	368	220
1892	159	76	78	139	132	214	702	635	337	151
1893	79	63	146	124	94	144	995	802	495	199
1894	75	63	129	114	129	223	1108	712	531	287
1895	71	74	74	53	108	334	877	556	486	184
1896	142	90	73	117	131	381	844	607	252	175
1897	121	89	79	80	73	94	638	622	315	191
1898	79	106	129	119	110	88	455	492	334	138
1899	56	84	92	99	102	235	702	502	344	134
1900	77	63	55	70	95	92	447	571	398	177
1901	59	63	70	74	88	117	473	562	421	157
1902	75	77	85	79	84	119	419	593	302	141
1903	84	96	95	100	113	123	408	542	312	168
1904	84	91	97	100	106	102	343	467	363	205
1905	83	98	120	96	103	101	424	638	451	257
1906	113	116	119	126	124	113	413	608	470	265
1916	206	209	279	201	192	132	444	743	426	260
1917	185	171	191	178	177	150	197	542	463	267
1918	170	154	226	211	167	121	247	517	387	359
1919	198	213	200	201	183	183	235	349	277	219
1920	198	197	201	206	172	136	113	255	266	221
1921	132	142	159	131	134	101	212	248	212	130
1922	83	101	109	123	83	76	95	169	149	98
1923	66	82	87	79	74	55	66	133	160	143
1924	71	69	84	60	75	41	58	90	106	97
1925	67	57	63	73	43	49	71	137	140	84

Source: Annual Reports of the Department of Health of the City of Chicago.
Note: I was unable to find the city's monthly breakdown for diarrheal deaths for the years 1907–1915. Also, the diarrheal deaths in this table are Chicago's original statistics and do not represent the way I totaled diarrheal deaths in Appendix B.1 and Appendix B.2. Births 1879–1897 estimated based on 2.6% birth rate. Births 1877, 1878, and 1898–1920 estimated by the Chicago Department of Health. All others are actual births reported.

Nov.	Dec.	Year Total	Population	Births	% Diarrheal Deaths/Births	Births/Pop. (%)
19	21	1,063	430,000	7,443	14.28	1.73
13	13	869	436,731	11,152	7.79	2.55
21	16	1,064	491,516	12,779	8.33	2.60
30	18	1,216	503,185	13,083	9.29	2.60
41	39	2,024	540,000	14,040	14.42	2.60
33	21	1,561	560,693	14,578	10.71	2.60
35	47	1,566	580,000	15,080	10.38	2.60
48	32	1,934	629,885	16,377	11.81	2.60
42	39	1,693	665,000	17,290	9.79	2.60
25	38	1,691	703,715	18,297	9.24	2.60
55	30	2,041	760,000	19,760	10.33	2.60
43	28	2,033	802,651	20,869	9.74	2.60
85	78	2,355	935,000	24,310	9.69	2.60
75	56	2,668	1,099,850	28,596	9.33	2.60
129	170	3,145	1,148,795	29,869	10.53	2.60
79	99	2,801	1,199,730	31,193	8.98	2.60
69	55	3,265	1,253,022	32,579	10.02	2.60
97	75	3,543	1,308,682	34,026	10.41	2.60
79	70	2,966	1,366,813	35,537	8.35	2.60
72	70	2,954	1,427,527	37,116	7.96	2.60
87	76	2,465	1,490,937	38,764	6.36	2.60
96	78	2,224	1,557,164	43,132	5.16	2.77
91	76	2,517	1,626,333	43,901	5.73	2.70
94	79	2,218	1,698,575	44,842	4.95	2.64
75	60	2,219	1,751,968	46,076	4.82	2.63
120	149	2,243	1,801,255	47,192	4.75	2.62
96	81	2,218	1,850,542	48,299	4.59	2.61
101	82	2,141	1,899,829	49,395	4.33	2.60
112	87	2,570	1,949,116	50,482	5.09	2.59
123	127	2,717	1,998,403	51,556	5.27	2.58
150	187	3,429	2,517,172	56,416	6.08	2.24
158	166	2,845	2,569,755	56,574	5.03	2.20
203	198	2,960	2,622,338	56,732	5.22	2.16
130	148	2,536	2,674,921	56,893	4.46	2.13
120	118	2,203	2,728,022	57,000	3.86	2.09
80	74	1,755	2,780,655	56,543	3.10	2.03
68	91	1,245	2,833,288	56,724	2.19	2.00
86	64	1,095	2,886,971	55,935	1.96	1.94
49	76	876	2,939,605	58,900	1.49	2.00
42	61	887	2,995,239	59,693	1.49	1.99

APPENDIX B.1
Percentage of Deaths under Age One in Chicago by Cause, 1897 to 1939

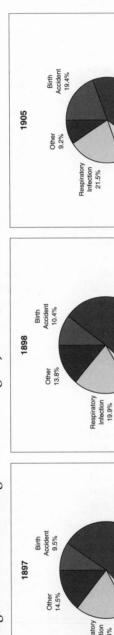
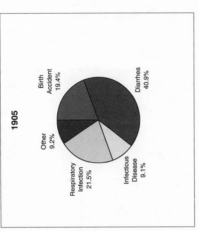
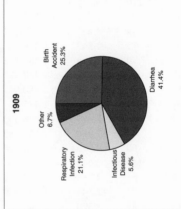
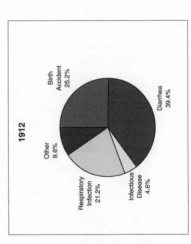
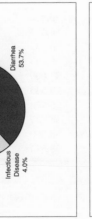
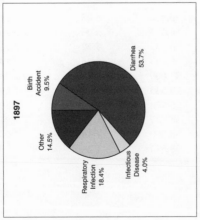
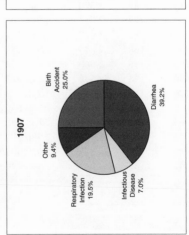

1897
Birth Accident 9.5%
Diarrhea 53.7%
Infectious Disease 4.0%
Respiratory Infection 18.4%
Other 14.5%

1898
Birth Accident 10.4%
Diarrhea 51.2%
Infectious Disease 4.7%
Respiratory Infection 19.9%
Other 13.8%

1905
Birth Accident 19.4%
Diarrhea 40.9%
Infectious Disease 9.1%
Respiratory Infection 21.5%
Other 9.2%

1907
Birth Accident 25.0%
Diarrhea 39.2%
Infectious Disease 7.0%
Respiratory Infection 19.5%
Other 9.4%

1909
Birth Accident 25.3%
Diarrhea 41.4%
Infectious Disease 5.6%
Respiratory Infection 21.1%
Other 6.7%

1912
Birth Accident 25.2%
Diarrhea 39.4%
Infectious Disease 4.6%
Respiratory Infection 21.2%
Other 9.6%

APPENDIX B.1 *(continued)*
Percentage of Deaths under Age One in Chicago by Cause, 1897 to 1939

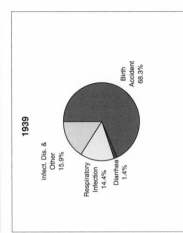

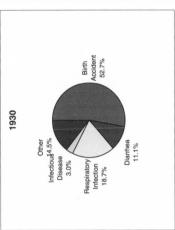

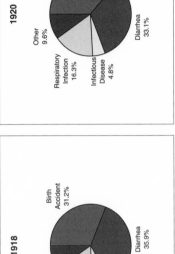

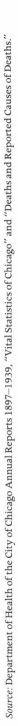

Source: Department of Health of the City of Chicago Annual Reports 1897–1939, "Vital Statistics of Chicago" and "Deaths and Reported Causes of Deaths."

APPENDIX B.2

Deaths under One Year of Age in Chicago by Select Causes, 1897 to 1939

Disease	1897	1898	1905	1907	1909
Infectious Diseases					
Diphtheria	39	32	24	42	49
Influenza	2	36	19	9	15
Measles	43	16	48	58	46
Meningitis			166	132	77
Scarlet fever	4	38	5	33	25
Tb meningitis			43	41	41
Tb pulmonary	44	22	39	38	38
Whooping cough	98	112	187	114	65
Birth Accidents					
Atelectasis	26	36	59		
Birth injury	40	37	54	200	365
Congenital defect	183	194	593	740	618
Congenital syphilis	46	37	80	85	106
Premature birth	248	260	343	647	622
Diarrheal Diseases					
Cholera infantum	721				
Cholera morbus	2	5			
Convulsions	619	547	476	468	28
Marasmus	693	697			
Intestinal inflammation	408	436	5		
Infantile diarrhea	111				
Gastritis	77	69	65	103	18
Diarrhea	17	563	538		
Gastro-enteritis	412	439	837		
Enteritis			442		
Dysentery	19	15	22	28	13
Diarrhea & enteritis				2,025	2,583
Respiratory Infections					
Bronchitis	486	496	401	354	56
Pneumonia	567	583	851	949	1,289
Other					
Brain inflammation	222	254	1		
Homicide	1	1	3	34	40
Lack of care					
Rickets	16	13	34		
Spinal cord disease	102	74			
Total[a]	5,246	5,012	5,335	6,100	5,998
Total[b]	5,735	5,415	5,831	6,699	6,384
Population	1,490,937	1,557,164	1,949,116	2,047,690	2,146,264
Births[c]	38,764	43,132	50,482	52,625	54,729

Source: "Vital Statistics of Chicago" and "Deaths and Reported Causes of Deaths," Department of Health of the City of Chicago Annual Reports 1897–1939.

APPENDIX B.2 (*continued*)

1912	1916	1918	1920	1924	1930	1939
59	40	41	38	17	15	2
10	24	275	99	25	15	14
32	42	22	17	21	2	—
49	21	21	20	13	9	11
23	5	2	5	2	1	—
41	34	37	20	14	8	3
21	31	22	11	16	12	8
73	56	87	62	60	32	17
164	186	161	168	165	64	85
229	249	237	251	266	340	254
476	537	528	574	516	385	235
100	81	59	71	52	43	10
715	1,004	1,084	988	1,054	802	463
40	8	6	—	7	14	
				15	16	
2,596	2,890	2,374	1,880	745	313	22
47	144	209	215	137	45	20
1,373	837	849	708	693	536	201
6	6	3	6	10	8	3
4	24	13	12	—	—	—
24	49	27	46			
6,082	6,268	6,057	5,191	3,962	2,670	1,350
6,689	6,907	6,636	5,674	4,528	3,103	1,533
2,301,946	2,517,172	2,622,338	2,728,022	2,939,605	3,392,700	3,607,000
56,397	56,416	56,732	57,000	58,900	58,083	49,055

[a]Not all causes of death listed here. Numbers in this row represent the total deaths listed on this table only.
[b]Total deaths of all infants who died in Chicago under one year of age.
[c]Births 1898–1920 estimated by the Chicago Department of Health. 1897 births estimated based on 2.6% birth rate. All others are actual births reported.

APPENDIX C
What Chicago Mothers Fed Their Newborns, 1911–1933

Reporting Agency	Date	Total Surveyed	% Breastfed	% Partially or Wholly Artificially Fed	% Artificially Fed or "Bottle-Fed"
IWS stations[a,b]	1911	2,798	35.5	64.5	14.2
DoH field nurses[c]	1911	23,960	73.4	26.6	26.6
IWS stations[d]	March 1912	1,246	39.9	60.1	0.0
DoH field nurses[c]	1912	30,901	38.6	61.4	24.6
IWS stations[e]	1913	3,678	45.3	54.7	42.0
DoH field nurses[c]	1913	19,319	38.1	61.9	16.1
DoH field nurses[c]	1914	23,326	33.9	66.1	22.2
DoH stations[f]	1914	5,423	32.9	67.1	2.7
IWS stations[g]	1915	9,313	46.9	53.1	41.3
DoH field nurses[c]	1915	20,622	38.8	61.2	28.5
DoH stations[h]	1915	1,596	37.8	62.2	4.9
IWS stations[i]	1916	9,927	46.0	54.0	45.0
DoH field nurses[c]	1916	27,023	39.3	60.7	32.4
DoH stations[f]	1916	1,254	54.9	45.1	25.2
DoH field nurses[c]	1917	26,542	36.1	63.9	36.9
DoH stations[f]	1917	998	58.9	41.1	27.6
DoH field nurses[c]	1918	17,795	38.2	61.8	34.7
DoH stations[f]	1918	1,333	55.4	44.6	18.8
DoH stations[j]	1919	8,395	42.1	57.9	30.6
DoH field nurses[k]	Summer 1919	10,951	27.1	72.9	19.8
DoH stations[j]	1920	1,781	66.5	33.5	13.6
DoH stations[l]	1921	3,401	45.1	54.9	9.3
DoH field nurses[m]	1922	4,472	56.0	44.0	12.3
DoH stations[j]	1922	4,431	56.0	44.0	12.2
DoH stations[j]	1923	8,485	61.2	38.8	14.3
DoH stations[j]	1924	11,465	57.7	42.3	26.7
DoH stations[j]	1925	14,310	57.2	42.8	30.1
DoH field nurses[n]	1925	46,427	91.9	8.1	8.1
DoH stations[o]	1926	14,484	59.9	40.1	25.5
DoH stations[o]	1927	15,406	56.8	43.2	26.4
DoH stations[o]	1928	14,804	53.5	46.5	27.4
DoH stations[o]	1929	13,626	49.9	50.1	29.7
DoH stations[o]	1930	14,926	44.5	55.5	33.8
DoH stations[p]	1933	15,171	43.4	56.6	36.0

Key: IWS = Infant Welfare Society; DoH = Chicago Department of Health
Note: Some infants were apparently placed in multiple categories, which is why totals exceed 100%. Mixed-fed infants evidently account for this phenomenon. The numbers listed next to DoH field nurses represent mothers with newborns visited by DoH nurses. The health department chose the mothers to interview by dividing the city into forty-acre tracts and then targeting districts from the most congested areas of the city as determined by the U.S. Census. The numbers listed next to

APPENDIX C (*continued*)

	Partially or Wholly Artificially Fed						
	Cow's Milk						
% Mixed Feeding	Pasteurized (%)	Raw (%)	Boiled (%)	Modified (%)	Home Modified (%)	Laboratory Modified (%)	Allait Mix (%)
27.4	0.0	0.0	0.0	0.0	22.7	0.3	0.0
0.0	0.0	0.0	0.0	0.0	0.0	0.0	0.0
28.5	0.0	0.0	0.0	0.0	19.7	0.6	11.4
17.9	0.0	18.9	0.0	0.0	0.0	0.0	0.0
0.0	0.0	0.0	0.0	0.0	0.0	0.0	12.7
27.8	0.0	18.0	0.0	0.0	0.0	0.0	0.0
20.6	0.0	23.4	0.0	0.0	0.0	0.0	0.0
44.8	0.0	19.7	0.0	0.0	0.0	0.0	0.0
0.0	0.0	0.0	0.0	0.0	0.0	0.0	11.7
28.7	0.0	4.0	0.0	0.0	0.0	0.0	0.0
32.8	11.3	13.1	0.0	0.0	0.0	0.0	0.0
0.0	0.0	0.0	0.0	0.0	0.0	0.0	9.0
25.5	0.0	2.8	0.0	0.0	0.0	0.0	0.0
17.9	0.0	2.0	0.0	0.0	0.0	0.0	0.0
25.6	0.0	1.3	0.0	0.0	0.0	0.0	0.0
13.5	0.0	0.0	0.0	0.0	0.0	0.0	0.0
26.2	0.0	0.9	0.0	0.0	0.0	0.0	0.0
17.0	0.0	8.9	0.0	0.0	0.0	0.0	0.0
27.3	0.0	0.0	0.0	0.0	0.0	0.0	0.0
16.6	22.5	0.7	11.2	2.1	0.0	0.0	0.0
19.8	0.0	0.0	0.0	0.0	0.0	0.0	0.0
18.1	27.5	0.0	0.0	0.0	0.0	0.0	0.0
31.8	0.0	0.0	0.0	0.0	0.0	0.0	0.0
31.7	0.0	0.0	0.0	0.0	0.0	0.0	0.0
24.5	0.0	0.0	0.0	0.0	0.0	0.0	0.0
15.6	0.0	0.0	0.0	0.0	0.0	0.0	0.0
12.7	0.0	0.0	0.0	0.0	0.0	0.0	0.0
0.0	0.0	0.0	0.0	0.0	0.0	0.0	0.0
14.6	0.0	0.0	0.0	0.0	0.0	0.0	0.0
16.8	0.0	0.0	0.0	0.0	0.0	0.0	0.0
19.0	0.0	0.0	0.0	0.0	0.0	0.0	0.0
20.4	0.0	0.0	0.0	0.0	0.0	0.0	0.0
21.6	0.0	0.0	0.0	0.0	0.0	0.0	0.0
20.7	0.0	0.0	0.0	0.0	0.0	0.0	0.0

IWS and DoH stations represent mothers who brought their babies voluntarily to either IWS or DoH infant welfare stations, respectively. Either the charity or the city supplied free medical care at these stations. Thus, virtually all of the babies represented in this appendix probably were born to poor or working-class mothers.

[a]"Report, November 13th, 1911," IWS Papers. These records are inexplicably contradictory. In the previous months there were reports of babies fed laboratory modifications, but not in this tally.

(*continued*)
Here babies are reported as breastfed, bottle-fed, on a mixed diet, or being fed by a "mother doing home modification."

[b]"The Month of December 1911," IWS Papers.

[c]"Infant Welfare Service," 1919, 567.

[d]Minnie Ahrens, "To the Board of Directors of the Infant Welfare Society A Report of Work for January, February, March," IWS Papers.

[e]"Infant Welfare Society of Chicago," 1913 pamphlet, IWS Papers.

[f]"Infant Welfare Service," 1919, 573.

[g]"Annual Report of the Infant Welfare Society of Chicago for the Year Ending December 31st, 1915," p. 22, IWS Papers.

[h]"Infant Welfare Station Work," 1916.

[i]"Report of Work for the Year 1916," IWS Papers.

[j]"Kind of Feeding," 1926.

[k]"Summer Infant Welfare Field Work," 1922.

[l]"Infant Welfare Work," 1922, 127.

[m]"Field Nurses," 1923.

[n]"Report of Health Department Infant Welfare Stations," 1926.

[o]"Feeding of Babies," 1931.

[p]"Feeding of Infants," 1934.

Notes

Introduction

1. Preston and Haines, 1991, 77. U.S. vital statistics are sketchy before the late 1890s. Preston and Haines base their estimate on the answers to two questions for women in the 1900 U.S. census: "Mother of how many children?" and "Number of these children living?" "For estimates of infant mortality given social, racial, ethnic, regional, and economic differences, see ibid., 49–176. In Chicago, 81,896 babies were born in 1897 and 1898 and 11,150 of them died before age one. Since Chicago began to correlate cause of death with age at death in 1897, the medical community could note with authority for the first time that an overwhelming number died of diarrhea. ("Deaths 1897," 1899, 222–59; "Deaths 1898," 1899, 252–59.)

2. Fisher, 1910, 39–40.

3. Davis, 1910, 2. This 15:1 death rate is the Department of Health's figure. However, if about 40 percent of babies were exclusively breastfed in Chicago, as field surveys indicate, the mortality rate relative to the number of bottle-fed vs. breastfed babies was actually 10:1, not 15:1.

4. *Bulletin Chicago School of Sanitary Instruction,* 1910d, 4; 1911c, back page.

5. Apple, 1987. For other physician- and proprietary-food-centered explanations of the move from breast to bottles, see Cone, 1976; Levenstein, 1983; and Meckel, 1991.

6. The "second summer" custom was especially telling. Most babies' deaths occurred during the summer, when food spoiled quickly, particularly during the first summer that they were exposed to any food other than mother's milk, customarily their second summer. For more on infant feeding during the colonial era, see Caulfield, 1952; Schnucker, 1974; Treckel, 1989; and Salmon, 1994.

7. Halpern, 1988, 63.

8. Abt, 1944, 43.

9. Aldis, 1913, 10.

10. Chicago, of course, is not illustrative of every single American city. Milwaukee mothers, for example, did not follow the infant-feeding patterns prevalent in Chicago, Philadelphia, Boston, and New York. Judith Walzer Leavitt infers that in Milwaukee in 1900, because the ward-level correlation between diarrhea and under-age-one mortality was *not* statistically significant, the great majority of Milwaukee's babies likely still enjoyed extended breastfeeding (Leavitt, 1996a, 31–32).

11. Madden-Lunsford, 1999.

12. These states currently include Alaska, California, Connecticut, Delaware, Florida, Idaho, Illinois, Iowa, Michigan, Minnesota, Nevada, New Jersey, New York, North Carolina, Pennsylvania, Rhode Island, Texas, Utah, Virginia, and Wisconsin.

13. For example, the Florida legislature has amended sections 800.02 (unnatural and lascivious acts), 800.03 (exposure of sexual organs), and 800.04 (lewd, lascivious, or indecent assault or act upon or in the presence of a child) of the state's laws to ensure that breastfeeding does not violate these sections. The Florida legislature has also had to exclude breastfeeding from being defined as "harmful to minors," "nudity," "obscene," and "sexual conduct" in section 847.001. Florida is not alone. Alaska, Illinois, Michigan, Nevada, Rhode Island, and Utah also amended obscenities statutes to exclude breastfeeding.

14. See, for example, Helliker, 1994; Bernstein, 1999c; and Greenberg, 1999.

Chapter 1

1. Letter from Nettie F. McCormick to Carthy, 31 July 1873, Nettie Fowler McCormick Papers.

2. Salmon, 1994.

3. "Decline," 1889, 111; Allen, 1889, 112–13; "Care of Infants Historical," 1912, 542.

4. John C. Cook, M.D., unpublished, untitled 1904 manuscript, Infant Welfare Society Papers (hereafter cited as IWS Papers).

5. "Talks with the Doctor," 1907.

6. Chapin, 1902, 194.

7. Quoted in Ladd-Taylor, 1994, 27.

8. Reilly, 1897, 112.

9. Wells, 1907.

10. "Notes from a Talk Given by Mrs. Welles President of the Auxiliary of Infant Welfare Society," July 1915, IWS Papers.

11. Abt, 1944, 123–24.

12. Letter from Martha Luey Parish to Lestern, Annie and Father, 2 November 1884, Parish Family Letters; Josephine K. Laflin Diary 1903–1907, 31 March 1903 entry, Laflin Family Papers; Katherine Shedd Bradley Diaries, Diary 1918–1922, selected entries from April and July 1920.

13. See, for example, Rotch, 1896, 209.

14. Earle, 1892, 472.

15. Churchill, 1896, 102.

16. "Mother's Parliament," July 1885, 246; "Nursery Problems," December 1892, 17.

17. Handwritten notes entitled "Dr. Fenger," 1890; Letter from Miss Hammond to Nettie Fowler McCormick, 29 August 1890; Letter from Miss Hammond to Nettie Fowler McCormick, 4 September 1890; Diary 1891, 1 January 1891 to 1 July 1891 diary entries, all in the Anita McCormick Blaine Papers.

18. Josephine K. Laflin Diary 1903–1907, 15 January 1903 and 31 March 1903 entries, Laflin Family Papers.

19. Letter from Katharine Kerr Moore to May Walden Kerr 19 April 1922, May Walden Kerr Papers.

20. Allen, 1908, 496; Earle, 1891, 442.

21. "Mothers' Department," 1883.

22. "Mothers' Department," 1881; Penfield, 1894; Hirshberg, 1909a; Dodson, 1911.

23. See entries from 13 April 1913 to 13 April 1914, Katherine Shedd Bradley Diaries; Sterling Morton, "On the Spanish Main," Sterling Morton Papers.

24. L. E. Laflin, Sr. Diary 1887, 19 January 1887 entry, Laflin Family Papers; Vinton, 1893; Josephine K. Laflin Diary January–May 1898, 21 March 1898 and 14 May 1898 entries, Laflin Family Papers.

25. Abt, 1944, 43.

26. The Chicago Department of Health, for example, distributed *Our Babies,* an infant-care manual, in English, Bohemian, Croatian, German, Italian, Lithuanian, Polish, Serbian, Swedish, and Yiddish. Posters displayed throughout the city advising women to breastfeed likewise appeared in whatever language(s) predominated in a particular neighborhood.

27. "Infant Welfare Service 1909–1910," 1911, 179. I have not found any information that would shed light on the infant-feeding practices of specific ethnic groups in Chicago. Preston and Haines, on the basis of studies in other cities, suggest that immigrants breastfed their babies in larger numbers than American-born women, and among immigrants, Italians, Poles, and Jews breastfed more commonly than women from other ethnic groups. A lower infant mortality rate among Jewish babies in particular, they argue, was likely due to the common practice among Jewish mothers of extended breastfeeding. Preston and Haines, 1991, 28.

28. "Infant Welfare Field Work," 1919.

29. Hatfield, 1891, 430–31.

30. Mrs. Geo. M. Moulton, "Report of the Milk Commission of the Children's Hospital Society of Chicago for the Period from June 2 1903 to June 31 1904"; and Mary Plummer, unpublished 1904 manuscript, IWS Papers.

31. *Babyhood,* September 1887.

32. "Diarrhea in Infants," 1911, 69.

33. Wile, 1909, 146.

34. A. Belcham Keyes, "The Intelligent Care of Infants in Summer," 1904, IWS Papers.

35. Mrs. Geo. M. Moulton, "Report of the Milk Commission of the Children's Hospital Society of Chicago," IWS Papers.

36. "Jewish Women," 1912.

37. Quoted in Ladd-Taylor, 1986, 148–49.

38. See, for example, Chicago Department of Health, *Our Babies,* undated circa 1917, p. 20. This pamphlet was published in English, Bohemian, Croatian, German, Italian, Lithuanian, Polish, Serbian, Swedish, and Yiddish. I was unable to find an English edition of this early version of the booklet and I am grateful to Herbert S. Wolf for translating a German copy.

39. "Diarrhea in Infants," 1911, 69.

40. Acker, 1915, 9–10. Preston and Haines point out that in Baltimore at the end of the nineteenth century the infant mortality rate was 59 percent above average among babies whose mothers worked outside the home and 5 percent below average

among babies whose mothers worked for pay inside the home. They contend that "almost certainly" this reflected the fact that mothers who worked at home breast-fed. Preston and Haines, 1991, 27.

41. "Miss Ahrens report," undated circa 1912, in "Minutes of Meetings Milk Commission Sept. 16, 1908 to Jan. 12, 1911," IWS Papers.

42. Ibid.

43. *Bulletin Chicago School of Sanitary Instruction,* 1912a, 21; "Little Mothers' Clubs," 1923.

44. "Report of the Social Service Department Central Free Dispensary for the Year of 1927," Central Free Dispensary Papers.

45. Leavitt, 1986.

46. Ulrich, 1990, 192–93, 196.

47. Quoted in Theriot, 1996, 64. For an analysis of how the mother-daughter relationship lay at the heart of the female world in the nineteenth century, see Smith-Rosenberg, 1985, 53–76.

48. Brumberg, 1997, 13–16. Brumberg argues that this seeming negligence on the part of mothers was not an abdication of responsibility, but a way of protecting daughters who were menstruating earlier and marrying later than previous generations. Brumberg writes, "Because knowledge about menstruation was considered the first step on the slippery slope to loss of innocence, many Victorian mothers simply avoided the subject altogether, believing it was in the best interest of their daughters."

49. L. Gordon, 1990, 150. The latest research shows that the decline in fertility was not limited to white, middle-class urban women but included African Americans, ethnic minorities, and rural women as well. Theriot, 1996, 40–41.

50. D'Emilio and Freedman, 1997, 73–84.

51. Quoted in ibid., 76.

52. Letter to "My darling, my love, my life" from Frederick 6 December 1897; letter to "My dear, dear wife" from Frederick 13 February 1901, Gookin Family Papers.

53. Sears, Roebuck and Co., 1969, 459.

54. Letter from The Madame Mozelle Compound Bust Developing Treatment to Miss A. I. Camp, Chicago, 14 December 1912, Health Fraud and Alternative Medicine Collection. The Madame Mozelle company sent this letter to Camp in response to her letter complaining "My chest is so very flat." The letter to Madame Mozelle was likely a ruse—Camp being either a pseudonym for Arthur J. Cramp, head of the Bureau of Investigation of the American Medical Association, or a female relative of Cramp.

55. 1914 pamphlet by Pauline Turner Co., Health Fraud and Alternative Medicine Collection.

56. "Nursery Problems," 1886b; "Nursery Problems," 1888.

57. Tomes, 1998, 135–54.

58. *Bulletin Chicago School of Sanitary Instruction,* 1911e, 216; 1912c, 80.

59. Tomes, 1998, 136–82; Meckel, 1990, 92–158. For more on the pressure put on women by public health authorities and Americans' growing obsession with cleanliness, see also Tomes, 1990; McClary, 1980; and Hoy, 1995.

60. Stephens, 1897.

61. "Nursery Problems," 1886c.

62. Letter from Mathilda Barchet to *The Alumnae,* April 1905, 68.

63. Wallace, 1914.

64. Ladd-Taylor, 1994, 27.

65. "Baby Saving," 1912.

66. Kober, 1908, 97.

67. Reilly, 1897, 112, 116.

68. Many contemporary studies address this complaint and they provide at least some insight into women's inability to breastfeed one hundred years ago. Tully and Dewey argue that what is now called "Insufficient Milk Syndrome" is a cultural construct fomented by the "breakdown of traditional patterns of social support for breastfeeding" (Tully and Dewey, 1985). One psychologist, who devoted the bulk of her career to the study of the psychology of breastfeeding, argues that a mother's attitude toward breastfeeding is directly related to whether or not she is able to successfully lactate (Newton and Newton, 1950). For more on a woman's social milieu and its effect on her ability to breastfeed, see Brack, 1975; Matich and Sims, 1992; Baranowski, et al., 1983; Kearney, 1988; Peterson and DaVanzo, 1992; and Marchand and Morrow, 1994.

69. "Breast Feeding," 1926, 232.

70. "Mother's Parliament," 1886b. I borrow the phrase "gospel of germs" from Nancy Tomes (Tomes, 1998).

71. Allen, 1889, 112–13.

72. Abt, 1904.

73. Levenstein, 1983, 89.

74. "Mother's Parliament," 1887.

75. 1902 Nutrolactis leaflet; letter from Dr. Paul S. Martins to *JAMA,* 16 May 1910, both in Health Fraud and Alternative Medicine Collection.

76. "Society Proceedings," 1891; Moody, 1899.

77. Quoted in Salmon, 1994, 256; "Mothers' Department," 1881; Mason, 1886; Hogan, 1892; Bundesen, 1926.

78. Holt, 1914, 46; Hess, 1928, 43.

79. Brennemann, 1911.

80. "Our Babies," undated circa 1916, p. 12.

81. Holt, 1914, 47, 49.

82. Hamilton, 1913; Hamilton, 1916.

83. This information is now common in breastfeeding advice literature. See, for example, Pryor, 1973, 35; Eigher and Olds, 1987, 146–47; Gaskin, 1987, 108–10; and La Leche League International, 1997, 137–43.

84. One anthropologist has charged that the breastfeeding problems addressed historically in U.S. pediatric literature are "culture-specific." She argues that the problems are "to some degree . . . a product of pediatric breastfeeding regimens themselves." She views the "factory model" of infant care as a particular impediment to breastfeeding. Millard, 1990, 211–12, 214.

85. Christopher, 1892, 727. Other physicians recognized this phenomenon as well. See, for example, Southworth, 1902, and Ostheimer, 1909, 520.

86. "Youngest Member," 1889; Eaton, 1909, 41.

87. Hill, 1923, 109; "Abstract of Discussion," 1922, 270; Grulee, 1934, 289; Letter from Katharine Kerr Moore to May Walden Kerr, 7 November 1921, May Walden Kerr Papers.

88. Mellin's Food Company, 1907, 45–46.

89. Letters from Katharine Kerr Moore to May Walden Kerr, 21 July 1921 and 1 March 1923, May Walden Kerr Papers.

90. Wood-Allen, 1895, 14; Wood-Allen, 1896, 181. The quote in brackets is also from Wood-Allen, 1896, 181.

91. For a history of child-rearing theories and techniques, see Grant, 1998. Grant argues that child-rearing theories in the United States swing continually between the Rousseauian concept of respecting a child's "innate nature" and the Lockean concept of relentlessly taming children so that they fit seamlessly into the adult world.

92. "Baby's Habits," 1884.

93. "Our Babies," undated circa 1916, p. 12.

94. Grulee, 1914, 90.

95. "Abstract of Discussion," 1909.

96. Davis, 1910, 2.

97. Letters from Katharine Kerr Moore to May Walden Kerr, 23 March 1917, 14 June 1921, 16 July 1921, 28 January 1921, and 18 February 1921, May Walden Kerr Papers.

98. *Bulletin Chicago School of Sanitary Instruction,* 1907a, 4.

99. "How to Keep the Baby Well," undated circa 1915–16, IWS Papers.

100. *Bulletin Chicago School of Sanitary Instruction,* 1912h, 109; 1913b, 118; 1919, 116.

101. Sullivan-Fowler, 1995.

102. For more on the dangerous urban food supply, see Duis, 1998, 113–44. For more on cholera, see Rosenberg, 1962. For more on typhoid, see Leavitt, 1996b.

103. Walls, 1909, 75; Eaton, 1909, 41.

104. Brennemann, 1928, 456; Educational Health Service Review, *Everybody's Baby,* vol. 1, May 1928, 11–12, Health Fraud and Alternative Medicine Collection.

105. MacDonald, 1920.

106. Sedgwick, 1920, 279.

107. Hess, 1928, 35–36; Hess, 1925.

108. "Baby's First Month," 1929.

109. Abt, 1904; Abt, 1944, 109.

110. "Abstract of Discussion," 1922; Hess, 1925, 718.

111. "Mothers' Parliament," 1887, 387–88.

112. "Mothers' Parliament," 1889.

113. "Decline," 1902, 6–7.

114. "Parents' Problems," 1906; "Parents' Problems," 1914.

115. Grulee, 1914, 19; Bundesen, 1925a, 25.

116. Dorothy Smith Dushkin Diary, 8 October 1932 entry, Dorothy Smith Dushkin Papers.

117. Abt, 1944, 109.

118. Rima Apple has described scientific motherhood as the late nineteenth/ early twentieth-century belief that mothers, in order to rear healthy children, had to rely on expert advice (Apple, 1995). Kathleen Jones argues that because of their experiences with charity patients, early pediatricians came to focus on problems inside the home as the cause of infants' health problems. They formed an alliance with mothers to mix mother-love with science—scientific motherhood was the result (Jones, 1983).

119. Grulee, 1934, 289.

120. Abt, 1944, 109.

Chapter 2

1. Wile, 1909, 139; Taylor, 1909, 67.

2. "Stop the Bogus Milk Traffic," 1892.

3. "Infant Welfare Service 1909–1910," 1911, 177. We do not know precisely what infants died from and in what numbers they died before the late nineteenth century. The current definition of infant mortality rate—the number of deaths before 1 year of age per 1,000 live births—was not even formulated until the 1880s. See Brosco, 1999.

4. Rosenberg, 1962, 5.

5. Duffy, 1990, 175.

6. When some human populations domesticated large mammals, highly communicable "crowd diseases" gained entry to the human community. Cows, for example, passed smallpox, measles, and tuberculosis to humans; influenza came from pigs and chickens. Crosby, 1986, 31.

7. Meckel, 1990, 26–27.

8. For more on the international efforts to lower infant mortality, see Koven and Michel, 1990. Alisa Klaus argues that a declining birth rate and the threat of war in Europe caused the French to think of infant welfare programs in a quite different light than Americans, who were beset with nativism and racism. The French needed healthy citizen-soldiers, while Americans were troubled by issues like "race degeneracy," which dissuaded them from focusing on universal aid for mothers and their babies (Klaus, 1993). See also Zelizer, 1985, who discusses the cultural factors that contributed to the redefinition of the value of children's lives.

9. Every big city had similar clean-milk crusades. Milwaukee's is described in Leavitt, 1996a, 156–89. New York City's is described in Meckel, 1990, 62–91.

10. Meckel, 1990, 5–6; Melvin, 1983.

11. Contemporary scholars agree that the pasteurization of milk and the use of dried, condensed, and evaporated milk as an infant food in lieu of raw cows' milk coincided with dramatically lowered infant mortality (Beaver, 1973). Preston and Haines contend that by the middle of the nineteenth century a new understanding of infectious disease led to a concerted effort to protect water, milk, and food from contamination (Preston and Haines, 1991, 20–21). These hypotheses suggest that the practice of feeding infants something other than human milk long before artificial food was safe was fairly routine.

12. Jelliffe, 1894; "Report of the Sanitary Milk Commission," 1907, 5.

13. "Chicago Medical Society Proceedings," 1892.

14. Miller, 1996, 64; Mayer and Wade, 1969, vii; "Vital Statistics of Chicago," 1899, 251; "Vital Statistics," 1906, 259; Holli, 1984, 462. For a description of living conditions in Chicago at the end of the nineteenth century, see Duis, 1998.

15. Buder, 1967, 4–5; Mayer and Wade, 1969, 176; Preston and Haines, 1991, 20–21.

16. These deaths hint at mothers' prevailing infant-feeding practices in Chicago. In Philadelphia, seasonal deaths from diarrhea were equally high for infants and one year olds until 1865 when deaths of one year olds began a dramatic decline. Rose Cheney attributes this to mothers' move away from extended breastfeeding and toward the early weaning of babies. Infants, Cheney argues, were now subjected to the stresses of weaning well before their first birthday. By 1865, however, children who survived their first year benefited from a cleaner water supply, regular garbage removal, and ice boxes in homes (ice cutting was first mechanized in 1855). The infant death rate in Philadelphia did not begin to decline until between 1910 and 1920, after the Philadelphia Board of Health gained control over the quality of the city's milk (Cheney, 1984).

17. Edson, 1885.

18. Fisher, 1910, 39–40.

19. Booker, 1901, 7, 13.

20. Rothman, 1994, 86.

21. Brodie, 1994, 13, 15, 47.

22. Booker, 1901, 11; Potter, 1833, 104; "Mortality for 1872," 1874.

23. Waugh, 1894; Van Derslice, 1911, 23–30.

24. Abt, 1944, 43.

25. Yale, 1885.

26. "Vital Statistics of Chicago: 1893," 1894.

27. "Diarrheal Diseases," 1909; "Diarrhea in Infants," 1911, 67.

28. Potter, 1833, 111–12; Earle, 1891, 439–40.

29. Doering, 1891, 433.

30. Kee and Chapell, "Facts Worth Knowing, gathered during Twelve Years' Experience, or, Points on Milk" (Chicago, 1885), 17, 25–30, Bowman Dairy Company Papers.

31. "Chicago Milk," 1892; "Stop the Bogus Milk Traffic," 1892.

32. Long, 1886.

33. "Will Have Pure Milk," 1892.

34. "Scarcely Any Pure Milk," 1892.

35. "They Water and Color the Milk," 1894.

36. "To Secure Pure Milk," 1894; "Report," 1895, 146.

37. Pooler, 1886, 471–72.

38. Kee and Chapell, "Facts Worth Knowing," 17, 14.

39. Edson, 1887.

40. Kee and Chapell, "Facts Worth Knowing," 17, 14; Edson, 1887.

41. Van Doozer, 1876.

42. Kee and Chapell, "Facts Worth Knowing," 17, 40.

43. "Edict Against Slop," 1892; "Will Sue Milkman Ryan," 1892.

44. "Report" 1906; "Dairy Inspection," 1907, 25; *Bulletin Chicago School of Sanitary Instruction,* 1910b, 3.

45. Yale, 1893; "Milk and Food Inspection," 1892.

46. Kee and Chapell, "Facts Worth Knowing," 17; Abt, 1908, 44.

47. *Bulletin Chicago School of Sanitary Instruction,* 1914d, 193; 1921, 36.

48. Ibid., 1912e, 86.

49. Ibid., 1912j, 123; "Country Dairy Inspection," 1919.

50. *Bulletin Chicago School of Sanitary Instruction,* 1912k, 126.

51. Kennicott, 1919, 146–47, 154–55; Kerr, 1909. Contagious diseases that had to be reported by law were Asiatic cholera, croup, diphtheria, measles, membranous croup, scarlet fever, smallpox, typhoid fever, typhus fever, "or any other contagious or infectious disease." The "card" the milk dealer feared was a notice of quarantine on his home and business.

52. Kee and Chapell, "Facts Worth Knowing," 17, 36–37.

53. *Bulletin Chicago School of Sanitary Instruction,* 1911d, 223; 1907b, 5.

54. *Report of the Department of Health of the City of Chicago for the Years 1907, 1908, 1909, 1910, 1911,* 102.

55. Merki, 1878.

56. "Slaughter of the Innocents," 1892.

57. Doering, 1891, 433; "Adulterated Milk," 1892; "Adulteration of Milk," 1892; "Look After the Milk," 1892.

58. "Its Effects Too Slow," 1893; "Improved in Quality Milk," 1892.

59. "Bureau of Milk Inspection," 1894, 11.

60. "Commissioner's Summary Report," 1906; "Its Effects Too Slow," 1893; "Methods," 1895.

61. "Our Milk Is Good," 1892; "Its Effects Too Slow," 1893.

62. Biehn, 1906; "New Milk Law in Effect," 1904.

63. "Chicago Milk," 1892; Kennicott, 1919, 150–56; "Will Have Pure Milk," 1892; "Our Milk Is Good," 1892.

64. Kennicott, 1919, 150–56.

65. Ibid.

66. "Its Effects Too Slow," 1893.

67. Kennicott, 1919, 145.

68. "Test the Milk," 1907.

69. "Report," 1895, 145.

70. Biehn, 1906, 7.

71. "Dairy Inspection," 1907; Biehn, 1906, 11–12.

72. "Milk Inspection and Dairy Inspection," 1911.

73. Biehn, 1906, 3–5.

74. Ibid., 12.

75. *Bulletin Chicago School of Sanitary Instruction,* 1910a, 3.

76. Ravenel, 1908; Letter from dairy farmer E. G. Harvey to Chicago Dr. Frank Churchill, 3 August 1903, Infant Welfare Society Papers (hereafter cited as IWS Papers); John C. Cook, unpublished, undated manuscript circa 1904, IWS Papers.

77. "Second Session," 1908.

78. Robertson, 1919, xv; *Bulletin of the Dairy Research Bureau,* 19 (8 May 1914): 53, Bowman Dairy Company Papers.

79. "State of Chicago's Health," 1910c; *Bulletin Chicago School of Sanitary Instruction,* 1911a, 3.

80. Erdman, 1921, 26.

81. *Bulletin Chicago School of Sanitary Instruction,* 1912g, 99; 1912j, 118; "Current Comment," 1912, 657.

82. *Bulletin Chicago School of Sanitary Instruction,* 1912i, 118; "Current Comment," 1912, 657.

83. *Bulletin Chicago School of Sanitary Instruction,* 1912k, 125.

84. *Bulletin Chicago School of Sanitary Instruction,* 1912f, 89; 1912i, 117.

85. "Medical News," 1912; *Bulletin Chicago School of Sanitary Instruction,* 1912i, 118–19; "Country Dairy Inspection, 1919, 903–7; "An Ordinance Regulating the Production, Transportation and Sale of Inspected and Pasteurized Milk in the City of Chicago and Repealing Sections 1273 and 1274 of the City Code of 1911 Passed by the City Council of the City of Chicago August 14, 1912," Bowman Dairy Company Papers; "Principal Health Ordinances," 1919.

86. *Bulletin Chicago School of Sanitary Instruction,* 1912l, 153.

87. Ibid., 1914b.

88. Ibid., 1912d, 84.

89. Ibid., 1914b, 78.

90. Lintner, 1927.

91. "Concerning Pasteurization," 1921.

92. "Report of the Sanitary Milk Commission," 1907.

93. "State of Chicago's Health," 1910a, 2.

94. Freeman, 1910; Howe, 1921; Kellogg, 1921; Moak, 1915.

95. "Important Experiments," 1893.

96. Moak, 1915, 147–48.

97. Ibid., 148.

98. "State of Chicago's Health," 1910a, 2.

99. *Bulletin Chicago School of Sanitary Instruction* 1912b, 64; 1912k, 126.

100. *Department of Health Weekly Bulletin,* 1928, 25; Robertson, 1919, xv–xvi.

101. Park and Holt, 1903, 891.

102. "Country Dairy Inspection," 1919, 911.

103. "Requirement," 1919.

104. "City Milk Inspection," 1922.

105. Wolcott, 1925, 4–6.

106. Ibid., 6–17.

107. Sedgwick, 1915, 161.

108. "State of Chicago's Health," 1909.

109. On the definition of the "average" American woman, see Scanlon, 1995, 197–98. As women's magazines proliferated they became extremely influential. See White, 1970, 58–92, and Zuckerman, 1998, 1–23. A single magazine—the *Ladies' Home Journal*—was the best-selling magazine in the United States within a few years of its initial appearance in 1883. By the 1910s, 20 percent of American women read the *Journal* (Damon-Moore, 1994, 1).

110. Articles on women's treatment of milk in the home include "Preservation of Milk," 1897; Coit, 1894; and McBride, 1897. Yale discusses how to recognize clean milk in Yale, 1898. Discussion of how to "humanize" clean cows' milk appears in Rorer, 1899; Coolidge, 1903; and Scovil, 1902.

111. "State of Chicago's Health," 1910a, 2.

112. *Bulletin Chicago School of Sanitary Instruction,* 1911b, 4.

113. Jelliffe, 1894, 296; "Talks," 1907.

114. *Bulletin Chicago School of Sanitary Instruction,* 1909, 2.

115. Ibid., 1912e, 86.

116. Ibid., 1915, 116.

117. "Mothers' Parliament," 1889, 219.

118. "Questions and Answers," 1924.

119. McBride, 1897, 85.

120. Coit, 1895.

121. *Bulletin Chicago School of Sanitary Instruction,* 1911b, 4.

122. *Report of the Department of Health of the City of Chicago for the Years 1919, 1920 and 1921,* 1923, 18, 338.

123. *Bulletin Chicago School of Sanitary Instruction,* 1922, 109.

124. "Child Welfare," 1931.

125. 1931 Pamphlet, Bowman Dairy Company Papers.

126. Bowman Dairy newspaper ad, 30 September 1921, Bowman Dairy Company Papers.

127. "Milk—Magic Ration," 1918.

128. Tobey, 1928.

129. Kegel, 1927.

130. Bundesen, 1925b.

131. Robertson, 1919, xvi.

132. "Long Arm," 1921.

133. Kegel, 1929.

134. "The best milk for the family," 1924, National Dairy Council Archives. The 1919 remark is quoted in Erdman, 1921, 7.

135. Mary R. Plummer, 1904 unpublished manuscript, IWS Papers.

136. Chapin, 1917, 132–33, 135. Doctors made these comments in a discussion following the presentation of Chapin's paper.

137. Bowman Milk Ads, 2 and 30 September 1921, Bowman Dairy Company Papers.

138. Vaughan, 1923, 145.

Chapter 3

1. Julius H. Hess, "A Half-Century of Infant Feeding," typed manuscript, undated circa 1954, Julius Hess Papers.

2. That was the general assumption in the United States. Breastfeeding customs varied from country to country, from region to region within countries, and among social classes. In Germany, for example, where infant-feeding habits varied by region, women in some southern areas did not breastfeed and fed their infants

pap instead. The few who did breastfeed in those districts were ridiculed and threatened. In other areas of Germany extended breastfeeding was the norm (Watkins, 1991, 267–68). Infant-feeding habits were so uniform within regions in Germany that infant mortality did not vary even between classes. At least one demographer has argued that this identical infant mortality rate among socioeconomic groups in certain regions of Germany suggests that infant-feeding method was a key, if not the key, determinant of infant death (Knodel, 1988, 447).

    3. Wet nursing was never a perfect solution in the absence of mother's milk. Death rates among babies who were wet-nursed were higher than among babies breastfed by their own mothers, although they did die in lower numbers than artificially fed babies (Golden, 1996). In France, where rural wet nurses took in urban infants, lack of parental supervision likely increased the mortality of nurslings (Sussman, 1982).

    4. "Decline," 1902, 6.

    5. Meigs, 1884, 217.

    6. Meigs, 1889, 71.

    7. Physicians defined complementary feedings as bottle feeding a baby immediately after breastfeeding and supplementary feedings as wholly replacing a breastfeeding session with the bottle.

    8. Snyder, 1908, 1213.

    9. Hirshberg, 1909b.

    10. Holt, 1914, 43–44.

    11. Earle, 1892, 472.

    12. Brennemann, 1908, 101.

    13. Denny, 1906, 1905; Denny, 1908, 625–26; Taylor, 1909, 73.

    14. Coit, 1912, 128–30, 135.

    15. These three studies cited in Taylor, 1909, 67–69.

    16. Hirshberg, 1909a; Walls, 1909, 80–81; Hess, 1923, 149. Contemporary studies corroborate these physicians' observations. See Cunningham, 1981; Arnold and Larson, 1993; Goldman, 1993; Garofalo, 1999.

    17. "Discussion of Papers," 1908. After the presentation of several papers on infant feeding, Jacobi reminisced about his experiences almost forty years prior.

    18. Chapin, 1908, 150.

    19. Churchill, 1896, 113; Abt, 1944, 111.

    20. Jacobi, 1882.

    21. Acker, 1915, 15.

    22. "Abstract of Discussion on Papers of Drs. Snyder, Davis, Pisek, Jacobi and Southworth," 1908, 1222

    23. For a sampling of some of the disagreements, see the theories presented in Southworth, 1908.

    24. Helmholz, 1910, 113. Jacobi made his remarks following the presentation of Helmholz's article.

    25. Abt, 1912, 116, 120.

    26. Walls, 1909, 70–73.

    27. Helmholz, 1910, 107.

28. Rotch, 1896, 189.

29. Brennemann, 1908, 104–5; Van Derslice, 1911, 34; Abt, 1912, 122.

30. Koplik, 1899, 114–16; Sedgwick, 1917, 417; Dietrich, 1922, 270. Abt made his comments in a discussion after Dietrich presented his paper.

31. Hess, 1923, 152–54.

32. Meigs, 1885, 14.

33. Meigs, 1884, 223; Meigs, 1889, 71.

34. Parvin, 1884, 243.

35. Meigs, 1884, 223.

36. "Mothers' Department," 1881.

37. Meigs, 1885, 28; Chapin, 1903, 49–57.

38. Meigs, 1889, 72–75.

39. Dietrich, 1920, 278. This is well known by lactation specialists today. See Riordan, 1999, 130.

40. Eiger and Olds, 1987, 20.

41. Meigs, 1885, 29. Thomas Rotch discusses the same phenomenon in Rotch, 1890, 90.

42. Meigs, 1885, 74, 87.

43. Ibid., 95.

44. Veeder, 1938, 50.

45. Meigs, 1889, 77–80.

46. Rotch, 1896, 231.

47. Ibid.

48. Rotch, 1896, 164; "The Chicago Medical Society Proceedings," 1897, 431; Chapin, 1899, 225 (Rotch made his remark during a discussion following the presentation of Chapin's paper); Rotch, 1908, 107.

49. Although historian Harvey Levenstein argues that percentage feeding was used most extensively by East Coast doctors and was limited everywhere only to the well-to-do families who could afford its high cost (Levenstein, 1983, 81–84), Chicago pediatricians made percentage feeding accessible even to Chicago's poorest residents via these philanthropic milk laboratories. I describe these activities in chapters 4 and 6.

50. Brennemann, 1908, 101.

51. Churchill, 1896, 103.

52. Ladd, 1907, 101.

53. "Abstract of Discussion on Papers of Drs. Snyder, Davis, Pisek, Jacobi and Southworth," 1908, 1222.

54. "The Chicago Medical Society Proceedings," 1897, 429.

55. Rotch, 1896, 276.

56. Rotch, 1896, 271–74; Rotch, 1904, 50–51; Rotch, 1910.

57. Holt, Courtney, and Fales, 1915.

58. Dunn, 1907, 62–63; Ladd, 1907, 101–3.

59. For an example of calories being taken into consideration when feeding by percentages, see Holt, 1911.

60. Van Derslice, 1907, 474–76.

61. Allen, 1907, 242–43.

62. Allen, 1908, 501. This formula, which is representative of infant-feeding formulas of the era, is incomprehensible. I provide it here only so the reader has a better understanding of what Joseph Brennemann meant in the following paragraphs when he complained of infant feeding calculations becoming "terrifyingly like treatises on mathematics or higher astronomy."

63. Brennemann, 1908, 104–5.

64. Rotch, 1908, 117. I have found no clinical data of Rotch's to support his contention that "some foods agree with babies better than others." I assume he is speaking only from personal experience.

65. Pisek, 1908, 1214.

66. Jacobi, 1908, 1218–19. Jacobi's comment was not immediately embraced. Boston physician John Lovett Morse responded, "We should feed them with brains and with mathematics." See "Abstract of Discussion on Papers of Drs. Snyder, Davis, Pisek, Jacobi and Southworth," 1908, 1222.

67. Rotch, 1908, 118. Jacobi said this in a discussion after Rotch presented his article.

68. Brennemann, 1938, 65.

69. Rotch, 1907, 532; Walls, 1909, 80.

70. Apple, 1995.

71. Allen, 1908, 497–99, 503.

72. See, for example, Ostheimer, 1909; Grulee, 1914, 92; Grulee, 1934, 291.

73. Ostheimer, 1909, 522.

74. Taylor, 1909, 66–67.

75. I borrow the phrase "information environment" from Joan Jacobs Brumberg, who contends that anorexia nervosa became a "communicable" disease in the 1980s after it was paraded endlessly in magazines and on television before "a reservoir of susceptible young women" (Brumberg, 1992, 141).

76. Apple, 1987, 53–94.

77. Abt, 1944, 41–49.

78. Van Derslice, 1907, 472.

79. For more on the eugenics movement, see Pernick, 1996, and Pernick, 1997.

80. Kellogg, 1921, 332–33. Kellogg was an ardent eugenicist and a featured speaker at the 1914 Race Betterment Conference (Pernick, 1997, 1768).

81. Pernick, 1997, 1767–72; Pernick, 1996, 23.

82. Abt, 1915, 281; Holt, 1914, 47; Newell, 1908, 533, 537–38; Wood-Allen, 1907.

83. "Mother's Parliament," 1886b; Sterling Morton Diary, 27 January 1912, Sterling Morton Papers.

84. "Decline," 1902, 6–7.

85. Clarke, 1873.

86. Newman, 1901, 459–62.

87. For a discussion of the notion of "civilization" as a threat to long-term human health and strength, see Rosenberg, 1998.

88. Churchill, 1897, 408.

89. Rotch, 1890, 88; Rotch, 1896, 188.

90. Rotch, 1890, 91–92; Rotch, 1896, 156.

91. Colostrum is the milk produced by the mammary gland immediately after birth. Thicker than mature milk and available only in minute quantity, it is exceptionally rich in antibodies to protect the newborn from disease. Nineteenth-century physicians had no knowledge of the antibodies in colostrum, and many were alarmed at its strange appearance and minuscule quantity as compared to that of mature milk.

92. Rotch, 1896, 166. The worry that colostrum could harm a baby had a long history. Until the late 1600s authorities on infant care warned against putting a baby to the breast immediately after birth. They feared that colostrum was poisonous, thus new mothers commonly employed wet nurses for the first two to three weeks after birth until their milk was no longer "toxic." Women who could not afford a wet nurse usually relied on a lactating neighbor. By the mid-eighteenth century women abandoned the practice of denying babies colostrum, having learned from William Cadogan's 1748 "Essay upon nursing" that colostrum prevented illness and death among babies (Treckel, 1989, 27–28).

93. Rotch, 1896, 181.

94. Jacobi, 1882, 79.

95. Davis, 1908, 1212; Davis, 1911, 4; Dietrich, 1922, 269; Brennemann, 1928, 455.

96. Hess, 1928, 36.

97. DeLee, 1920, 39.

98. Koplik, 1899, 118–19.

99. There were many methods of human milk analysis. In Chicago, the St. Luke's Training School for Nurses offered a class on laboratory diagnosis which included lessons, not only on blood and urine analysis, but also on how to examine cows' milk for chemical and bacterial contamination and human milk for its composition ("Course in Laboratory Diagnosis," 1914). A Chicago physician recommended two "quick and simple" methods for ascertaining the amount of fat in milk. One was to use the Feser lactoscope. The system was tricky, the doctor reminded his colleagues, as "there is a margin of 1 percent between the point where the lines are first seen and where they become distinctly visible." He warned that to get accurate results "one must have a good deal of experience with the method." The second method used centrifugal force to separate a mix of milk and sulphuric acid. After separation, physicians added hot water and once again applied centrifugal force. The fat that rose to the top of the bottle could then be "estimated in accordance with the already determined value of the scale" on the outside of the bottle (Whitman, 1905).

100. Riordan, 1999, 40, 126–33.

101. Churchill, 1896, 102–3, 106; "The Chicago Medical Society Proceedings," 1892; Jacobi, 1908, 1217.

102. Rotch, 1904, 42; Churchill, 1897, 409.

103. Churchill, 1898, 205–8; Churchill, 1896, 104.

104. For more on Sedgwick and his Breast Feeding Investigation Bureau of the Department of Pediatrics of the University of Minnesota, see Wolf, 1999.

105. Ostheimer, 1909, 520. Sedgwick made his comments after Ostheimer presented his paper.

106. Rotch, 1896, 271–74; Rotch, 1904, 50–51; Rotch, 1910.

107. Southworth and Schloss, 1908. Abt and others made these comments after presentation of the Southworth and Schloss paper.

108. Van Derslice, 1911, 25–26; Dietrich, 1922, 271 (Dr. George E. Baxter made this comment after Dietrich presented his paper); Brennemann, 1929, 365.

109. Rotch, 1890, 94–95; Rotch, 1896, 189.

110. Rotch, 1890, 88; Rotch, 1896, 188.

111. Rotch, 1896, 155, 165, 187.

112. Jacobi, 1874, 10–11.

113. Quoted in Walker, 1885, 8.

114. Churchill, 1898, 207–8.

115. Hess, 1928, 38, 40, 41.

116. Churchill, 1898, 206.

117. Grulee, 1914, 97; Rotch, 1896, 209.

118. Churchill, 1897, 411–12.

119. Van Derslice, 1911, 24.

120. Abt, 1944.

121. Rotch, 1896, 158.

122. Jacobi, 1896, 4.

123. Brennemann, 1938, 63–64.

124. Halpern, 1988, 45–46.

125. Rotch, 1983, 98.

126. Letter from Clifford G. Grulee to Dr. Norbert D. Gannon, 10 May 1930, Clifford Grulee Papers.

127. Brennemann, 1932, 153.

128. Grulee, 1936.

129. Garland and Rich, 1930, 1279.

130. Holmes, 1927, 335.

131. Poncher, 1936, 261.

132. Tow, 1934, 407.

Chapter 4

1. For more on mothers in Illinois and reformers' efforts to influence their health and infant-care practices, see Curry, 1999.

2. For more on the rise and fall of medical charities in Chicago, see McCarthy, 1982.

3. As John Duffy has pointed out, it was a terrible shock to many to learn that microbes did not respect wealth and that even the upper class was dependent on the health and well-being of everyone else (Duffy, 1971; Duffy, 1990, 93–109). See also Rosen, 1993, 270–471.

4. "Editorial. Preventive Medicine," 1891.

5. From the early nineteenth century until at least the 1920s, urban medical dispensaries—free-standing, outpatient clinics—were virtually the only vehicles for providing health care to the urban poor. Dispensaries also served as training grounds

for medical students. Created as an alternative to hospitalization—originally the only source of health care for the poor and a near-sure death sentence—most dispensaries existed on charitable contributions and physicians' volunteer labor. See Rosenberg, 1974.

6. *Visiting Nurse Association of Chicago Thirty-second Annual Report for Year Ending December 31, 1921,* inside front cover.

7. "Special Committee on Program and Policies Summary of First Meeting May 26th, 1924," Infant Welfare Society Papers (hereafter cited as IWS Papers).

8. "Infant Welfare Stations Established," 1923; "Visiting of New-Born Babies," 1926.

9. Edna L. Foley, "Helping and Healing," unpublished manuscript, 22 June 1932, Visiting Nurse Association of Chicago Papers (hereafter cited as VNA Papers).

10. *Bulletin Chicago School of Sanitary Instruction,* 1910d, 3–4.

11. Ibid., 1911c, back page.

12. Brennemann, 1911.

13. "Our Babies," undated circa 1916, 12. Translated from the German version.

14. See Klaus, 1993, 48–50. Nancy Pottishman Weiss argues that rather than work to guarantee a pure milk supply, health care professionals sought to regulate mothers' behavior, making the feeding question a moral issue rather than a public health issue. Weiss, 1978, 36–38. I contend, however, that health professionals were instrumental in the drive for a pure milk supply and that the medical community employed a moral tone when discussing breastfeeding precisely because they deemed it such a serious public health issue.

15. *Bulletin Chicago School of Sanitary Instruction,* 1911c, back page.

16. Ibid., 1912e, 85.

17. Hatfield, 1891, 431.

18. Reilly, 1897, 112.

19. For more on the design of breastfeeding surveys and how that design reflected and legitimated mothers' infant-feeding practices, even as public health workers tried to change these practices, see Wolf, 1999.

20. "First Annual Report Augusta Memorial Visiting Nurses," 1888; Letter to Miss Foley from Anna T. Dudley, November 25, 1920; "Work of the Visiting Nurses," 30 October 1929, all in the VNA Papers. "Visiting Nurses' Association of Chicago," 1901, 883; Fulmer, 1907, 22.

21. Tenney, 1909.

22. *Visiting Nurse Association of Chicago Thirty-first Annual Report,* 1921, inside front cover.

23. Letter to Mrs. Theodore Sheldon from Edna L. Foley, 12 January 1924, VNA Papers.

24. "Theory and Practice," 1906, 822.

25. Aldis, 1912, 5.

26. Reynolds, 1895, 26.

27. "Letter to Miss Helen V. Drake from Superintendent Foley," 27 March 1918, VNA Papers.

28. Foley, 1922, 27; King, 1922, 16.

29. The quote is from Gray, 1900, 15. Foley, 1914, explains a nurse's prenatal and postpartum duties.

30. "Rules," 1901, 10; "Some General Rules," 1905; "General Information," 1904.

31. Gray, 1900, 15; Foley, 1914, 9.

32. Fulmer, 1904, 17–18; Foley, 1914, 40.

33. Fulmer, 1910, 41.

34. Cudahy, 1929, 11–14; Foley, 1914, 65.

35. Foley, 1914, 42, 64.

36. Aldis, 1913, 10.

37. Cudahy, 1929, 11–14; Foley, 1914, 65.

38. Stickel, 1906, 81.

39. Foley, 1919, 18.

40. "New Effort," 1906.

41. Allin, 1910.

42. Allin, 1910; "Baby Tent Report," 1914.

43. Ibid.

44. "New Effort," 1906, 84.

45. "Infant Welfare Service 1909–1910," 1911, 180.

46. "Baby Tent Report," 1914, 35; Fulmer, 1908, 31–32.

47. Allin, 1910; "Baby Tent Report," 1914, 35.

48. Fulmer, 1911, 37; "Infant Welfare Service 1909–1910," 1911, 170–77.

49. Foley, 1917, 37.

50. *The Visiting Nurse Association of Chicago Thirty-eighth Annual Report,* 1928, 54.

51. "Radio Broadcast WLS Sunday June 20, 1937," VNA Papers.

52. "A Typical Day for One of Our Nurses," undated circa 1938, VNA Papers.

53. Sydney Halpern argues that preventive pediatrics had its origin in this urban movement to uplift the children of the poor but, ironically, its principal adherents were eventually middle-class women. "The result," Halpern contends, "was less social control of the poor than professional validation of the affluent" (Halpern, 1988, 153). Jeffrey Brosco argues that because public health reformers in the United States chose a hundred years ago to focus so much attention on the health of poor immigrant children, children's health became a matter of welfare rather than the public health matter it is in most other countries (Brosco, 1999, 478–85).

54. Ahrens, "To the Board of Directors of the Infant Welfare Society A Report of Work for January, February, March," undated but appears to be 1912, IWS Papers.

55. F. S. Churchill, "Infant Mortality," *Studies in Chicago Philanthropy* 1 (undated circa 1913 to 1916): 1, 4, IWS Papers.

56. "Board of Directors Meeting Held May 15, 1914," IWS Papers.

57. Sara B. Place, "The Work of the Infant Welfare Society," 1931; "To the Members of the Board of Directors of the Infant Welfare Society," undated but appears to be the 1912 Infant Welfare Society Annual Report; "Infant Welfare Society of Chicago," 1913, List of Stations, undated but circa 1915 to 1916, all in the IWS Papers.

58. "Miss Ahrens Report," undated but evidently read at the January 1912 annual meeting; "Superintendent's Report September 19, 1913; "Infant Welfare Society of Chicago," undated but contains report of the work done in 1911 and 1912, so

probably distributed in early 1913; "Infant Welfare Society of Chicago History," 1937, all in IWS Papers.

59. "Annual Report of the Infant Welfare Society of Chicago for the Year Ending December 31st, 1911," 18; "Infant Welfare Society of Chicago," undated pamphlet circa 1913 to 1916, both in the IWS Papers.

60. Assorted Infant Welfare Society cards, including milk card and physicians' record cards; "Report of the Laboratory Committee of the Infant Welfare Society March 9, 1911"; "Miss Ahrens Report"; "Superintendent's Report September 19, 1913," all in the IWS Papers.

61. "Miss Ahrens Report."

62. "Report for July 1911," IWS Papers.

63. "Miss Ahrens Report."

64. Weed, 1915.

65. "Miss Ahrens Report"; "Superintendent's Report September 19, 1913," both in the IWS Papers.

66. "Miss Ahrens Report."

67. "Infant Welfare Society of Chicago History," 1937, IWS Papers. Part of the reason for this startling difference was that few babies were cared for at IWS stations during the first few weeks of their lives, so the deaths of premature infants and infants with congenital defects were probably not part of IWS statistics. Nevertheless, the numbers were impressive.

68. In keeping with the era's nativism, reformers alleged that some ethnic groups had significantly less effective infant-care practices than others. Doctors maintained, for example, that Chicago had a higher infant death rate than New York City because Chicago's foreign-born population was largely Polish and New York's largely Italian (F. S. Churchill, "Infant Mortality," *Studies in Chicago Philanthropy* 1 [undated circa 1913 to 1916]: 1, 4, IWS Papers). In Chicago, the IWS noted that infant welfare stations that cared for babies with mostly Slavic mothers had higher death rates ("Annual Report of the Infant Welfare Society of Chicago for the Year Ending December 31st, 1915," 20, IWS Papers).

69. Helmholz and Hoffman, 1916.

70. This requirement was almost certainly related to breastfeeding because doctors did not ask a mother if she worked *inside* the home, taking in laundry or cooking meals for single men. Rather, they were concerned about the mothers who left home to work. Mothers who worked at home likely breastfed, while mothers who worked outside the home could not exclusively breastfeed. This was an important medical fact. Infant mortality was much higher than normal among babies whose mothers worked outside the home, while infant mortality was lower than normal among babies whose mothers worked *at* home, suggesting that a mother's working per se had little to do with infant death. Rather, breast milk deprivation seems to be the important factor. See Preston and Haines, 1991, 27–29.

71. Assorted Infant Welfare Society cards, including milk card and physicians' record cards; "Report of the Laboratory Committee of the Infant Welfare Society March 9, 1911"; "Miss Ahrens Report"; "Superintendent's Report September 19, 1913," all in the IWS Papers.

72. "1913 Annual Report"; "Baby Week To Help Chicago's Tenement Babies April 19 to 25, 1914," both in the IWS Papers.

73. "The First Ten Years of the Woman's Auxiliary of the Infant Welfare Society of Chicago," undated pamphlet, probably printed in 1923, 12–22; Mrs. L. H. Freer, "A History of the Woman's Auxiliary of the Infant Welfare Society of Chicago"; "Report of work from January 1st to April 1st, 1913"; Minnie H. Ahrens, "To the Board of Directors of the Infant Welfare Society May 16th, 1913," all in the IWS Papers.

74. "The First Ten Years of the Women's Auxiliary"; Mrs. L. H. Freer, "A History of the Woman's Auxiliary."

75. "The First Ten Years of the Woman's Auxiliary," 13; "The Kenwood Social Service Club Interview with Ruth Rogers April 24, 1960," both in the IWS Papers.

76. "By-Laws To Be Substituted For By-Laws Now In Use. Woman's Auxiliary Of The Infant Welfare Society"; "Kenwood Centre of the Infant Welfare Society"; "The Winnetka Branch of the Infant Welfare Society"; "The First Ten Years of the Woman's Auxiliary," 12–20; Mrs. L. H. Freer, "A History of the Woman's Auxiliary," 2, all in the IWS Papers.

77. "History of Baby Week," 15 March 1924; Untitled, undated letter from Dr. W. A. Evans to Chicago's pastors concerning Baby Week in Chicago 1914, both in IWS Papers.

78. *Bulletin Chicago School of Sanitary Instruction,* 1914a, 70.

79. "The First Ten Years of the Woman's Auxiliary," 19; "Infant Welfare Society 'Baby Week' April 19th to 25th," 1914, both in IWS Papers.

80. "Infant Welfare Society 'Baby Week'"; Diary citation is from "The First Ten Years of the Woman's Auxiliary," 19.

81. "Baby Weeks," 1919.

82. "History of Baby Week," 15 March 1924, IWS Papers; Meckel, 1990, 200–203.

83. Quoted in Meckel, 1990, 200.

84. "Social Service Report July–September," 1918, 17.

85. "The First Ten Years of the Woman's Auxiliary," 13.

86. "Report, November 13th, 1911"; "The Month of December 1911"; "Miss Ahrens Report"; "Superintendent's Report September 19, 1913," all in IWS Papers.

87. *Bulletin Chicago School of Sanitary Instruction,* 1913c, 186; Robertson, 1919, xxi.

88. "Infant Welfare Work," 1922, 132.

89. "Syllabus of Courses," 1919.

90. Ibid.

91. "The Infant Welfare Society," 1926.

92. "Special Committee on Program and Policies Summary of First Meeting May 26th, 1924," IWS Papers.

93. Grulee, 1934, 288.

94. In an infant-feeding poll taken in Chicago in 1912, for example, infant feeding is categorized as "breast feeding," "artificial feeding," and "mixed feeding" among other categories (Table LXXI, 1919). See also "The American Pediatric Soci-

ety's Collective Investigation," 1898, 485–86, where "breast milk" is categorized either as "alone," "with raw milk and amylaceæ," or "with sterilized milk and amylaceæ," and McClanahan, 1918, 188, where cases are categorized as "breast fed," "art. fed," and "mix. fed."

95. For a discussion of breastfeeding rates, the pasteurization of milk, and consequent infant mortality in the early twentieth century, see Wolf, 1999. That pasteurization had an immediate effect on infant morbidity was noted by VNA baby tent nurses in 1916 (Foley, 1916, 37).

96. Reilly, 1897, 112.

97. "Infant Welfare Service," 1919.

98. "Infant Welfare Service 1909–1910," 1911, 177.

99. "State of Chicago's Health," 1908.

100. Ibid.

101. "Infant Welfare Service," 1919, 562.

102. Van Derslice, 1911, 24.

103. "State of Chicago's Health," 1909.

104. *Bulletin Chicago School of Sanitary Instruction,* 1910c, 3.

105. "State of Chicago's Health," 1910a.

106. "Infant Welfare Service 1909–1910," 1911, 170–77.

107. *Bulletin Chicago School of Sanitary Instruction,* 1911F, back page.

108. "State of Chicago's Health," 1910a.

109. Ibid., 1910b.

110. "Organization of Field Work," 1919.

111. "Scoring of Sanitary Conditions," 1919.

112. "Care of Infants by Health Department Nurses," 1919.

113. *Bulletin Chicago School of Sanitary Instruction,* 1911c, back page. This poster's illustration was not unique to Chicago; many cities in the United States used it in their baby-saving campaigns. The wording on the poster, however, varied from city to city. A copy of the poster, with wording that differs from Chicago's, is in Meckel, 1990, following p. 158.

114. "Infant Welfare Work," 1914; *Bulletin Chicago School of Sanitary Instruction,* 1914c, 103–4.

115. "Infant Welfare Stations," 1919; "Infant Welfare Work," 1926.

116. Ibid.; "Infant Welfare Physicians," 1919.

117. "Infant Welfare Work," 1922, 127. As noted before, the citywide statistics included deaths caused by premature birth and congenital defects, so they were bound to be higher than at the stations where babies were not examined until they were at least a few weeks old. Nevertheless, the difference in infant mortality is significant.

118. "Infant Welfare Work," 1926, 228.

119. "Infant Welfare Stations Established," 1923; "Visiting of New-Born Babies," 1926.

120. "Chicago Wins Fight to Save Lives of Babies," 1927.

121. Ibid.

122. "Mother's Milk," 1925.

123. "Visiting of New-Born Babies," 1926.

124. That African American women were more likely to breastfeed than white women was a consistent observation of Chicago's doctors. Preston and Haines contend, however, that the only ethnic groups in the United States that showed extremes in infant-feeding habits were Portuguese and French-Canadian mothers, who breastfed significantly *less* frequently than most other women, and Jewish, Italian, and Polish mothers, who breastfed significantly *more* frequently than most other women. Perhaps the observation of Chicago's doctors was based more on racist stereotype than reality. This would help explain the paradox of a supposed high incidence of breastfeeding among African American women and a very high infant mortality rate among their babies. Or, perhaps, African American women fed their babies foods in addition to breast milk as so many women from other ethnic groups did. Or maybe they did not breastfeed for long. See Preston and Haines, 1991, 28–29.

125. Niblack, 1936, 259–60.

126. "Infant Welfare," 1926; "Infancy Service," 1928; "Infant Welfare Stations," 1926.

127. Bundesen, 1925c.

128. "Chicago Wins Fight to Save Lives of Babies," 1927.

129. "Breast Feeding," 1926.

Chapter 5

1. "Abstract of Discussion on Papers of Drs. Snyder, Davis, Pisek, Jacobi and Southworth," 1908, 1224.

2. Abt, 1944, 111.

3. Caulfield, 1952, 677, 679.

4. Salmon, 1994.

5. For a general history of wet nursing through the ages, see Fildes, 1988. For a history of wet nursing in the United States, see Golden, 1996.

6. In European countries the demise of wet nursing played out differently. George D. Sussman has argued that in France, for example, wet nursing did not decline with the growing safety of artificial food but with the advent of World War I. Wet nursing was such an entrenched practice in France, Sussman contends, that it took World War I, which disrupted access to wet nurses, to demonstrate to families that improved artificial food could safely replace wet nurses (Sussman, 1982, 182–83).

7. With the advent of HIV, human milk and its donors are once again tainted and suspect. Because HIV can be transmitted through breast milk, many human milk banks in the United States closed. The few milk banks that remain test donors carefully. See Arnold, 1998. There is preliminary evidence, however, that the transmission of HIV from mother to baby might actually be lower among *exclusively* breastfed infants than among those fed formula exclusively. This discovery raises the possibility that HIV acquired during the birth process might be neutralized by immune factors in breast milk. See Coutsoudis, et al., 1999.

8. Janet Golden discusses the animosity inherent in the employment of wet

nurses and changing attitudes toward the purchase and use of human milk in Golden, 1996.

9. A rich source of one physician's personal experience with wet nurses is Isaac Abt's autobiography (Abt, 1944, 111). Infant-care books and pamphlets written as late as the 1920s mentioned wet nurses as an infant-feeding option. See, for example, U.S. Department of Labor Children's Bureau, 1927, 59–60.

10. "Mothers' Parliament," 1886a, 142.

11. Smith, 1889, 87–88; Joseph B. DeLee, "Motherhood, An Address before the Women's Society of Isaiah Temple," 4 January 1898, Joseph B. DeLee Papers.

12. "Abstract of Discussion on Papers of Drs. Sedgwick, Abt and Hoobler," 1917.

13. Smith, 1889, 87.

14. "God's Dealings," 1879.

15. "Fourth Annual Report," 1875, 14.

16. "God's Dealings," 1879.

17. "God's Dealings," 1882; "God's Dealings," 1883.

18. "Nursery Problems," 1886a; "Feeding of the Baby," 1910; U. S. Department of Labor Children's Bureau, 1927, 59–60.

19. Talbot, 1913, 324.

20. Abt, 1944, 94–95; Talbot, 1913, 324; Talbot, 1928, 610.

21. Meigs, 1889, 81; Smith, 1889, 88–89; Churchill, 1896, 109.

22. "Fourth Annual Report," 1875, 13.

23. Hess, 1928, 49; "News Items," 1899; "Influence of the Milk of Wet-Nurses," 1887, 372.

24. Grulee, 1914, 94–95; Cleveland, 1884b, 389.

25. Educational Health Service Review, *Everybody's Baby*, vol. 1, May 1928, 12, Health Fraud and Alternative Medicine Collection; Hess, 1928, 46; Allen, 1889, 112–13.

26. Westcott, 1907, 198. Dr. Cotton made this comment in a discussion following the presentation of Westcott's article.

27. Adams, 1885, 275, 278; Cleveland, 1884a.

28. Christopher, 1892, 727–28.

29. Hirshberg, 1909a.

30. Winters, 1886, 508–9. Winters was right about the excessive mortality among wet-nursed infants. However, he ignored the likeliest reasons for the phenomenon: (1) These babies were already terribly weak when they came under a wet nurse's care; and (2) these babies might have received inadequate attention from their resentful wet nurses, who often were told by private employers that if they wanted to work they had to place their own babies in foundling homes.

31. Cleveland, 1884a.

32. Coolidge, 1904.

33. "Nursery Problems," 1886a.

34. Westcott, 1906, 16.

35. "Mothers' Parliament," 1886a.

36. For more on mothers and wet nurses and the nursery as their "contested terrain," see Golden, 1987, 130.

37. "Influence of the Milk of Wet-Nurses," 1887, 372.

38. According to Golden, Workman was the wife of a physician and the daughter of a former Massachusetts governor at the time she wrote the letter to *Babyhood*. She eventually became an author and explorer, setting world records in mountain climbing. Golden, 1996, 159–60.

39. This and all following quotes from Workman in "Mothers' Parliament," 1886a.

40. "Nursery Problems," 1886a, 245; "A Defence of Wet-Nurses," 1887.

41. Both quotes from "The Mother's Parliament," 1887, 384.

42. "Influence of the Milk of Wet-Nurses," 1887, 372–73; Abt, 1917a, 418–19.

43. *The Chicago Daily Tribune,* 1885.

44. One private employment agency for wet nurses in New York, for example, routinely placed mothers in private homes to work as wet nurses and simultaneously placed their babies in foundling homes. Ninety percent of the babies placed in foundling homes died (Talbot, 1913, 325).

45. Smith, 1889, 87–88; Hess, 1928, 51; U.S. Department of Labor Children's Bureau, 1927, 59; Grulee, 1914, 95; Winters, 1886, 511, 513; "'Six Months Law'" 1925.

46. Cleveland, 1884b, 389; Grulee, 1914, 95.

47. In a series of eighteenth-century experiments in a Parisian hospital, syphilitic wet nurses given mercury by medical personnel breastfed babies with congenital syphilis in an effort to pass on the mercury to the babies through milk and cure the babies of the disease. During the course of the experiments, doctors observed that syphilis was easily transmitted from baby to wet nurse (many of the women who lived at the hospital had acquired syphilis in this manner) but very rarely from wet nurse to baby (Sherwood, 1995).

48. Grulee, 1914, 85.

49. Watson, 1906. This story might be inaccurate. The same doctor reported that the wet nurse's nine-year-old daughter contracted syphilis from kissing the baby.

50. Talbot, 1911; Grulee, 1916.

51. "Influence of the Milk of Wet-Nurses," 1887, 373; Abt, 1917a, 419; Grulee, 1914, 94–95.

52. Bonner, 1991, 136–37.

53. Burhans and Smith, 1923.

54. Hess, 1928, 47.

55. Westcott, 1906, 198; Snyder, 1908, 1214; Denny, 1909, 163.

56. "Experiment in Infant Feeding," 1914.

57. Golden suggests that as the use of wet nurses declined by the early twentieth century, women and physicians began viewing human milk as a commodity "identified by its value to those who received it rather than by the character of its producers" (Golden, 1996, 179).

58. Hoobler, 1917, 421–22.

59. "Annual Report of the Infant Welfare Society of Chicago for the Year Ending December 31st, 1911," 11, Infant Welfare Society Papers (hereafter cited as IWS Papers).

60. Philbin, 1926, 102.

61. "News Items," 1905.

62. Foley, 1914, 42.

63. Denny, 1909, 163.

64. "Abstract of Discussion on Papers of Drs. Sedgwick, Abt and Hoobler," 1917, 426.

65. Chicago Pediatric Society Proceedings, 19 November 1907, 17 December 1907, and 20 October 1908.

66. For a more detailed history of Boston's Wet Nurse Directory, see Golden, 1988, 589–605.

67. Talbot, 1911; Bedinger, 1915, 252.

68. Morse, 1918.

69. Talbot, 1911.

70. Ibid. The quote is from Morse, 1918.

71. Talbot, 1911.

72. Leavitt, 1986, 73–74, 87.

73. Talbot, 1911.

74. Talbot, 1927.

75. Holt, 1911, 281 (Churchill said this in a discussion following the presentation of Holt's paper); Grulee, 1916; Abt, 1917a, 418.

76. De Lee, 1903, 259–60. For more on DeLee's work, see Leavitt, 1988; Berkow, 1977, 167–81; and Baker, 1996, 76–77.

77. For more on the work of Julius Hess, see Baker, 1996, 168–74.

78. Julius Hess, "Watching the Premature Babies' First Years," undated typed manuscript, Julius Hess Papers; Hess and Lundeen, 1941, 153; Evelyn C. Lundeen, "History of the Hortense Schoen Joseph Premature Station," *The Voice of the Clinic* 2 (Fall 1937): 8, Michael Reese Hospital Papers.

79. For more on Sarah Morris Children's Hospital, which Abt founded, see Abt, 1944, 134–53 and S. Gordon, 1981, 62–93.

80. "Abstract of Discussion on Papers of Drs. Sedgwick, Abt and Hoobler," 1917.

81. Abt, 1917a.

82. Ibid.

83. Abt, 1921; Abt, 1923; Abt, 1926, 5, 7–8.

84. Churchill, 1914, 499–500. A few years earlier Churchill noted that wet nurses at Children's Memorial Hospital offered their milk to hospitalized babies in bottles to prevent infection passing from a sick baby to the wet nurse. See the discussion following Holt, 1911, 281. According to the 1914 article, however, it seems that this policy was dropped.

85. Churchill was speaking in a discussion after the presentation of Holt, 1911, 281.

86. Rohtge, 1914.

87. Abt, 1917b, 540.

88. "Social Service," 1914; Grulee, 1916, 10; "Social Service Report—October 1916," 1916; "United Report," 1918.

89. Grulee, 1916, 9; Bass, 1928.

90. Hess, 1916; Grulee, 1916, 11; Abt, 1944, 147.

91. Abt, 1944, 147.

92. Abt, 1917a, 419–20.

93. Ibid., 418–20.

94. Rohtge, 1914; Douglas, 1914; "Social Service Report," 1915a; "Social Service Report," 1915b; "Social Service Report, 1916; "Quarterly Report," 1916; "January Report," 1917.

95. "Social Service Report," 1916; "Quarterly Report," 1916; "Social Service Report," 1917.

96. Tobey, 1929, 1110.

97. Hoobler, 1927, 1787–88.

98. Hoobler, 1925.

99. Ibid.

100. Hoobler, 1927, 1786–88.

101. City of Chicago Employment History for Gertrude Plotzke.

102. Chicago Board of Health, 1931, 32; "Mothers' Breast Milk Station," 1941.

103. Mrs. Gertrude Rosenberger (nee Plotzke), interview by author, tape recording, Chicago, Illinois, 10 December 1996.

104. Ibid.

105. Ibid.

106. Mrs. Josephine Zuzak Sobolewski, interview by author, tape recording, Chicago, Illinois, 28 April 1997.

107. Golden, 1996, 179–201.

108. Hoobler, 1927, 1786–88.

109. Tobey, 1929, 1110.

110. Hoobler, 1927, 1787–88.

111. In Chicago human milk and race was never an issue. The Chicago Board of Health Mothers' Breast Milk Station was located in an African American neighborhood and most of the mothers who provided the station with milk were African American. According to Sobolewski, no Chicago mother whose baby used the milk asked about its source. She recalled, "That baby meant so much to that mother. She didn't care where that milk came from." Mrs. Josephine Zuzak Sobolewski, interview by author, tape recording, Chicago, Illinois, 28 April 1997.

Chapter 6

1. *Bulletin Chicago School of Sanitary Instruction*, 1914a, 70.

2. Treckel, 1989, 30.

3. Churchill, 1896, 103.

4. Earle, 1891, 441; Earle, 1892, 473.

5. Note that in the naming of the various brands of condensed and evaporated milks and in doctors' discussions, the term "condensed milk" is used even in reference to evaporated milk. Condensed milk seems to have been the generic phrase for all canned milk, condensed *and* evaporated. Unsweetened, *evaporated* milk was actually physicians' canned milk of choice for babies, but they usually

referred to it not as evaporated milk but as condensed milk, just as the Helvetia Milk Condensing Company did when they named their product Highland Brand Condensed Milk even though it was evaporated milk. Throughout, when doctors discuss the use of condensed milk (usually meaning evaporated) I quote what the doctors said in their journal articles, not what they probably meant.

6. Bell, 1962, 4, 11; Weaver, 1974, 27.

7. Heer, 1966, 28.

8. Bell, 1962, 27.

9. Heer, 1966, 34–42, 60–63, 67–75, 89.

10. Bell, 1962, 4, 11, 28, 34, 42; Heer, 1966, 66, 89; Weaver, 1974, 23.

11. Weaver, 1974, 11–24.

12. Ibid., 30; Undated Carnation milk ad circa 1912, Health Fraud and Alternative Medicine Collection.

13. Letter from Mahin Advertising Company, 4 September 1913; Letter from Harvey W. Wiley to Dr. George H. Simmons of *JAMA,* both in Health Fraud and Alternative Medicine Collection.

14. Jordan and Mott, 1910, 391, 395, 397–400.

15. Earle, 1891, 443; Van Derslice, 1911, 34; Grulee, 1914, 19; Brennemann, 1928, 456.

16. "Chicago Medical Society Proceedings," 1897, 429.

17. Mellin Food Company, "Historical," 1914 pamphlet, Health Fraud and Alternative Medicine Collection.

18. Scovil, 1902, 26.

19. Nestlé's Food ad, 1914; Lactated Brand Infant Food ad, 1907; Nestlé's Food ad, 1914.

20. At least some of the testimonials in these ads were likely apocryphal. One physician complained to the American Medical Association in 1915 that representatives of Nestlé's Food and Eagle Brand Condensed Milk Companies had approached some of his patients—who had healthy, wholly breastfed babies—to solicit photographs of the infants for their artificial food ads. The doctor asked the AMA to expose these companies for "misleading the Medical profession and defrauding the public." Letters from Dr. Paul Riche to the American Medical Association, 15 April 1915 and 7 August 1915, Health Fraud and Alternative Medicine Collection.

21. Mellin's Food ad, 1902.

22. Marion, 1980, 70.

23. Eskay's Food ad, 1905.

24. "Nursery Problems," 1889.

25. "Chicago Wins Fight," 1927.

26. Fyffe, 1897.

27. Mellin's Food Company, 1908, unnumbered front pages.

28. Ibid., unnumbered front pages, 8, 18, 30–179.

29. In 1903 two doctors examined the milk modified by mothers in their homes and by nurses in hospitals. These physicians argued that it was impossible for even the most careful nurse or mother to accurately modify milk because milk was more commonly mislabeled than not. Creams labeled 20 percent had a fat content as low

242 Notes to Chapter 6

242 Notes to Chapter 6

242 *242* ◆ Notes to Chapter 6

as 13 percent and as high as 26.5 percent. "Ordinary market milk" ranged from 2.5 percent to 8.8 percent fat. Moreover, they argued, inaccuracy in the home modification of milk was exacerbated further by complicated formula recipes that confused even "persons of the more intelligent classes" (Edsall and Fife, 1903, 59–61).

30. Mellin's Food Company, 1908, ii, vi, ix.

31. Edsall and Fife, 1903, 59–61.

32. Churchill, 1897, 410.

33. Rotch, 1893, 99; "The Chicago Medical Society Proceedings," 1896.

34. Rotch, 1896, 158. Rotch never established or invested in milk laboratories personally. "I as an individual exponent of a system of feeding, the product of which must be sold to the public," he wrote, "could not in any way be identified with a project of this kind financially" (Rotch, 1907, 535).

35. Rotch, 1907, 536.

36. Rotch, 1893, 100.

37. "News Items," 1908, 251.

38. Earle, 1892, 472, 474.

39. Churchill, 1897, 410.

40. Josephine K. Laflin Diary, January–May 1898, 21 March 1898, 1 May 1898, and 15 June 1898 entries, Laflin Family Papers.

41. J. Charless Cabanne, "A Bit of History," 17 October 1908, Bowman Dairy Company Papers.

42. "News Items," 1908.

43. "Milk Laboratory Exactness," 1895.

44. Wentworth, 1902a, 683–84; Wentworth, 1902b.

45. "Chicago Medical Society Proceedings," 1897, 430, 437.

46. Churchill, 1897, 410.

47. "Milk Station at Hull House," 1902.

48. F. X. Walls, untitled, unpublished manuscript, IWS Papers.

49. Talbot, 1911, 1717.

50. Quoted in Gordon, 1981, 87, 91.

51. Abt, 1944, 147.

52. "New Milk Laboratory Helps Babies," 1936.

53. "Bacteria Free Feedings," 1938.

54. The United States government credited European *consultation de nourrissons* for Coit's innovation (Kerr, 1909b, 89). In France, *consultation de nourrissons* were most often attached to maternity hospitals. They encouraged breastfeeding by offering food and money to mothers who breastfed. Like milk stations in the United States, however, *consultation de nourissons* also provided sterilized milk to women who fed their babies artificially.

55. "Milestones of Milk History," undated; *Bulletin of the Dairy Research Bureau* 19 (8 May 1940): 53, both in the Bowman Dairy Company Papers.

56. Coit, 1907, 10–13.

57. Coit does not mention his son's death in his accounts of the founding of the first medical milk commission, but that is apparently what precipitated his suggestion to the New Jersey State Medical Society. See Waserman, 1972, 361–62.

58. Coit, 1907, 10–13; McEwen, 1917, 166–67.

59. "Medical Progress," 1896.

60. Quoted in Waserman, 1972, 364. Coit's hope was characteristic of some pediatricians of the era. Russell Viner argues that early pediatricians in the United States, like Abraham Jacobi, saw pediatrics as a way to guarantee equality in American society. Improving child health, Jacobi argued, was necessary to democratize human progress (Viner, 1999, 232–34).

61. "Editorial. Certified Milk.," 1897.

62. "Members of the American Association of Medical Milk Commissions," 1907; Kerr, 1909b, 89.

63. Kerr, 1909b, 89; McCleary, 1904, 330–31; Wile, 1909, 148.

64. Howe, 1919, 203; Freeman, 1907, 17–18.

65. Abt, 1908, 44.

66. Howe, 1919, 204, 217–18.

67. Coit, 1907, 13–15.

68. Wile, 1909, 139–43.

69. One typical column is Griffith's, 1907. See discussion of traveling tips in "What Other Women Have Found Out," 1907.

70. Erdman, 1921, 37.

71. Waserman, 1972, 364–65.

72. Wile, 1909, 148.

73. Pearson, 1908, 71.

74. Van Derslice, 1915, 167–68; Howe, 1919, 202.

75. McCleary, 1904, 361.

76. "Historical Notes on Milk Commission of Chicago and Infant Welfare Society of Chicago"; A. Belcham Keyes, "The Reason Why the Milk Commission Exists," Summer 1904, both in the Infant Welfare Society Papers (hereafter cited as IWS Papers).

77. "The Milk Commission created by the Children's Hospital Society, June 2nd, Nineteen hundred and three"; "June 7th 1903 Minutes of Milk Commission," both in IWS Papers.

78. Mrs. Geo. M. Moulton, "Report of the Milk Commission of the Children's Hospital Society of Chicago for the Period from June 2 1903 to January 31 1904"; "The Milk Commission created by the Children's Hospital Society"; "The Reason Why the Milk Commission Exists," 1904; A. Belcham Keyes, "The Reason Why the Milk Commission Exists," Summer 1904; Mary R. Plummer, 1904 unpublished manuscript; Mary R. Plummer, "Speech Given Before the Chicago Pediatric Society," 19 April 1904; "Milk Deliveries," *The Chicago Medical Recorder* 25 (November 1903): 346, all in the IWS Papers.

79. Although Dr. Henry Koplik opened the first milk station in the United States in New York in 1889, philanthropist Nathan Straus fostered the practice nationwide. Straus and his brother were the owners of Macy's department store. In 1893 Straus opened his first pasteurized milk depot to provide clean, inexpensive milk to the poor. In addition to pasteurized whole milk for older babies, the Straus depots provided modified-pasteurized milk for infants. Initially, the milk at Straus's pasteurized milk

depots was sold—or given away—only to the poverty-stricken mothers of sick babies. Straus soon made pasteurized whole milk available to the general public and his depots became popular family haunts. Straus's work had tremendous impact in New York City and elsewhere. He urged municipal governments to supply their citizens with clean milk—after all, they already did just that with clean water—and hoped that his depots would spur government action. His tactic eventually worked. Following Straus's example, New York City opened fifteen of its own milk stations in 1911. In 1914 the city passed an ordinance requiring that all milk sold in the city be pasteurized. In 1916 city officials declared that universal pasteurization made milk stations obsolete and transformed the city's milk stations into child health centers. Miller, 1993, 159–84.

80. "Letter to Mrs. Plummer from Lina Straus May 20, 1903"; "Letter to Mrs. Geo. W. Plummer from Sylvester Byrnes (Straus's personal secretary) June 9, 1903"; "Telegram to Dr. I. A. Abt from Nathan Straus June 12, 1903"; "Letter to Dr. I. A. Abt from A. L. Kinkeod June 13, 1903," all letters addenda to "Minutes of the Chicago Milk Commission June 15, 1903," all in the IWS Papers.

81. "The Reason Why The Milk Commission Exists," 1904, IWS Papers.

82. Letter dated 4 November 1903 to Mrs. Flora G. Moulton from Arthur R. Reynolds, M.D.; Mary R. Plummer, "Speech Given Before the Chicago Pediatric Society," 19 April 1904, both in IWS Papers.

83. "Minutes. Milk Commission June 11, 1903," IWS Papers; "Sterilized Milk Station," 1903–4.

84. "The Reason Why the Milk Commission Exists," 1904; "Minutes of the Annual Meeting of the Milk Commission of Chicago Held Feb 2, 1909," both in IWS Papers.

85. "The Milk Commission created by the Children's Hospital Society"; "June 7th 1903 Minutes of Milk Commission"; Mrs. Geo. M. Moulton, "Report of the Milk Commission of the Children's Hospital Society of Chicago"; "The Reason Why The Milk Commission Exists," 1904; A. Belcham Keyes, "The Reason Why the Milk Commission Exists," Summer 1904; Mary R. Plummer, 1904 unpublished manuscript; Mary R. Plummer, "Speech Given Before the Chicago Pediatric Society," 19 April 1904, all in the IWS Papers.

86. "The Milk Commission created by the Children's Hospital Society," IWS Papers.

87. "Minutes of the Milk Commission July 17, 1903"; "The Milk Commission created by the Children's Hospital Society"; "Minutes of Milk Commission July 7, 1903"; Mary R. Plummer, 1904 unpublished manuscript, all in the IWS Papers.

88. "The Milk Commission," 1903.

89. "Minutes of Milk Commission July 7, 1903"; Mary R. Plummer, 1904 unpublished manuscript, both in the IWS Papers.

90. "Report of the Extension Work," October 1903; "The Milk Commission created by the Children's Hospital Society"; Julia W. Nicholson, "Report of the sub-committee of the Milk Commission in charge of education," all in the IWS Papers.

91. "The Reason Why the Milk Commission Exists," 1904; "The Full require-

ments for the production of Certified milk are as follows," 1903; "Gordon Valentine Farm Report of the Milk Commission of Chicago," all attached to the minutes of the 27 August 1903 CMC meeting; Mrs. Geo. M. Moulton, "Report of the Milk Commission of the Children's Hospital Society of Chicago"; "Minutes of Chicago Milk Commission July 28, 1903"; "Minutes of Chicago Milk Commission August 4, 1903," all in the IWS Papers.

92. "Historical Notes on Milk Commission of Chicago and Infant Welfare Society of Chicago"; "The Milk Commission created by the Children's Hospital," both in the IWS Papers.

93. Mrs. Geo. M. Moulton, "Report of the Milk Commission of the Children's Hospital Society of Chicago," IWS Papers.

94. Letter from Harriet Fulmer to Mr. Bicknell, read into the Minutes of the Milk Commission of the Children's Hospital Society August 12, 1904, IWS Papers.

95. "Infant Welfare Society of Chicago History," 1937, IWS Papers.

96. "Milk Commission of Chicago 946 Adams St.," 22 October 1909, IWS Papers; "News Items," 1909.

97. Abt, 1908, 41–43; "Editorial," 1909, 63; "State of Chicago's Health," 1909.

98. "Minutes of a meeting of the Milk Commission held May 3, 1910," IWS Papers. This controversy was not unique to Chicago. New York grappled with the same charge. In 1911, responding to the accusation that their work harmed babies by discouraging breastfeeding, the four operators of New York's sixty-nine milk stations—Nathan Straus, the New York Milk Committee, the New York City Department of Health, and the Diet Kitchen Association—agreed to require all mothers receiving modified milk to bring their babies in for weekly examinations by station doctors. If a mother failed to do so, station workers refused to give her milk ("Summer Milk Stations in New York," 1911). Physician Ira Wile urged colleagues at a meeting of the American Association for the Study and Prevention of Infant Mortality to require all milk station workers, who often supplied milk to pregnant women, to teach expectant mothers about breastfeeding. He also suggested that mothers not be given any modified milk unless they could prove that they were physically incapable of nursing their baby (Phillips, 1910, 86).

99. "Chicago Minimum," undated memo circa 1909–10; "Monthly Report of the Milk Commission of Chicago December 6, 1910," both in the IWS Papers.

100. Minnie H. Ahrens, "Superintendent's Report referred to in Monthly Report of December 6, 1910," IWS Papers.

101. "Infant Welfare Society of Chicago (formerly Milk Commission)," undated leaflet circa 1910–11; Untitled typed manuscript dated 5 January 1911, both in the IWS Papers.

102. Assorted Infant Welfare Society cards including milk card and physicians' record cards; "Report of the Laboratory Committee of the Infant Welfare Society March 9, 1911"; "Miss Ahrens Report," undated but evidently read at the January 1912 annual meeting, all in the IWS Papers.

103. Van Derslice, 1915, 167.

104. Abt, 1908, 46. "Minutes of the Board of Directors of the Milk Commission

of Chicago December 22, 1908"; "Minutes of the Board of Directors of the Milk Commission of Chicago and a Committee appointed by the Council of the Chicago Medical Society December 28, 1908," both in the IWS Papers.

105. "Doctors to Censor Milk," 1909.

106. Tuley, 1908, 65; Van Derslice, 1915, 168–69.

107. "Editorial. The Chicago Medical Society Milk Commission," 1909.

108. Ferguson, 1914, 579–80.

109. Ibid.

110. Campbell, 1921.

111. Ferguson, 1914, 581.

112. Erdman, 1921, 7.

113. "Memorandum," 10 December 1917, Bowman Dairy Company Papers. The Borden Dairy was a close second in size. Bowman, however, was "greatly larger" than any other dairy in the city except Borden.

114. "Conversation with Maurice R. De Baets at the Chicago Historical Society, April 29, 1982," Bowman Dairy Company Papers.

115. "Meeting Report December 13, 1943," 2–3; "Notes of Conversation with Mr. M. J. Metzger November 7, 1945"; Untitled Talk by Dr. David Peck, 29 July 1944; *Welcome: Your Job with the Bowman Dairy Company,* 1949; Bowman and Co., "A Safe Supply of Pure Country Milk," undated pamphlet but circa 1885; "The Flourishing Tree," 13–14, all in the Bowman Dairy Company Papers.

116. "Meeting Report December 13, 1943," 4, 9; *Welcome: Your Job with the Bowman Dairy Company,* 1949; "Protection of Milk from Cow to Consumer," undated pamphlet circa 1900–1915, all in the Bowman Dairy Company Papers.

117. "Safe Milk Bowman Dairy Company," 1915; "Protection of Milk from Cow to Consumer"; "Penny Wise or Pound Foolish Cheap Milk Means Letting Down the Bars Which Make Safe Milk," November 1917, all in the Bowman Dairy Company Papers.

118. Bowman Dairy Company, "Our Products From Farm to Customer in Words and Pictures," undated pamphlet circa 1900–1915; Bowman Dairy newspaper ad, 21 February 1922; H. T. Adamson memo, 6 April 1924; Memorandum, 10 December 1917; M. O. Maugham, *Manual for Milk Salesmen,* 1924, 55, all in the Bowman Dairy Company Papers.

119. Bowman Dairy newspaper ads, 20 March 1922, 22 March 1922, and 10 April 1922, Bowman Dairy Company Papers.

120. "What Bowman Does To Bring You The Milk of Superior Flavor," undated pamphlet circa 1925–40; full-page ad (in the *Chicago Tribune*) 12 September 1934, Bowman Dairy Company Papers.

121. "Suggestions To Help Sell Irradiated Vitamin-D Milk," undated manuscript circa 1934–40, Bowman Dairy Company Papers.

122. "Dr. Bundesen's Radio Inquiry, undated postal card; 1930 pamphlet to physicians from Bowman Dairy Company Chicago and Vicinity, front cover; letter sent to all doctors and dentists in Bowman Company territory and signed by B. Peck M.D., Vice-President, 16 June 1934, all in the Bowman Dairy Company Papers.

123. Snyder, 1908, 1213.

124. Kellogg, 1921, 332–33.

Epilogue

1. Massachusetts and Connecticut were the other two. Illinois refused the funds in part because the American Medical Association lobbied heavily against the act. Chicago is home to the AMA and the organization strenuously opposed the "state medicine" that Sheppard-Towner advocated. See Curry, 1999, 120–32.

2. For more on Sheppard-Towner, see Lindenmeyer, 1997, 92–108; Lindenmeyer, 1990; Ladd-Taylor, 1993; Ladd-Taylor, 1988; Meckel, 1990, 200–219.

3. Tonks and Enochs, 1931.

4. von Meysenbug, 1934–35, 738–39.

5. "Are Infant Feeding Methods Changing," 1931, 581; Armstrong, 1932, 426.

6. Snedeker, 1935, 648.

7. *The health of a people is really the foundation upon which all their happiness and all their power as a state depend,* 1939, Infant Welfare Society Papers.

8. Westphal, 1942, 10.

9. Westphal, 1950, 22.

10. Snedeker, 1935, 648.

11. Grulee, 1936.

12. "Discussion," 1934.

13. Brennemann, 1930, 1, 5–6, 16–17.

14. "The Spirit of '76 or The Story of a Pioneer, Julius H. Hess," typed, unpublished manuscript, 23 January 1952, Julius Hess Papers.

15. See, for example, Tow, 1934, 406.

16. Garland and Rich, 1930, 1279.

17. "Are Infant Feeding Methods Changing," 1931, 583.

18. Ibid., 582.

19. For more on the ramifications of Americans' love affair with vitamins, see Apple, 1996.

20. "Report of the Progress," 1952.

21. Niblack, 1936, 259.

22. Quoted in Apple, 1987, 126.

23. Stitt, 1961, 631.

24. Apple, 1980.

25. Acid or sour milk (the names were used interchangeably) was made from whole milk that was kept in a warm place until it thickened. Alternatively, to make it sour more quickly, living lactic acid bacilli was added to the milk. Acid or sour milk was similar to buttermilk, but buttermilk is made from churning sour cream then removing the butter, while acid or sour milk is made from sour whole milk, not cream. See Shaw and Williams, 1922. Shaw argued on p. 54 of the article: "The babies fed on acid milk mixtures . . . look healthier and thrive better on average than those fed on the regulation sweet milk formulas."

26. Brennemann, 1929. Feeding infants evaporated milk remained popular for decades after the publication of Brennemann's article. In 1955, 29.2 percent of one-week-old infants were breastfed, 4.1 percent consumed cows' milk, 23.2 percent consumed a formula, and 45.9 percent consumed evaporated milk. These numbers total

102.4 percent because the breastfed infants included infants who consumed artificial food in addition to breast milk (Martinez and Krieger, 1985, 1005).

27. Bell, 1962, 102–3.

28. Dr. David Turow, interview by author, tape recording, Winnetka, Illinois, 12 July 1996.

29. "Births in Hospitals Increase," 1931. The incidence of hospital births seems to have grown more rapidly in Chicago than in other locales. Neal Devitt estimates that 55.8 percent of births in the United States took place in hospitals in 1940 and 67.9 percent in 1942 (Devitt, 1977, 56).

30. Quoted in Apple, 1987, 159.

31. Chicago Board of Health, 1931, 28.

32. Barnes et al., 1953, 192.

33. Stitt, 1961, 630.

34. Bell, 1962, 102–3.

35. Julius H. Hess, "Breast Feeding," typed, undated, unpublished manuscript circa 1940, Julius Hess Papers.

36. Apple, 1994.

37. Joseph DeLee opened the Chicago Maternity Center, originally called the Maxwell Street or Chicago Lying-In Dispensary, in 1895. The dispensary provided trained physicians to attend the home births of poor women at no charge. The center closed in 1973. For more on the Maxwell Street Dispensary and the Chicago Maternity Center, see Berkow, 1977, 167–81.

38. Mrs. Josephine Zuzak Sobolewski, interview by author, tape recording, Chicago, Illinois, 28 April 1997.

39. Grulee, 1934, 292.

40. Poncher, 1936, 259.

41. Niblack, 1936, 260.

42. Hess, "Breast Feeding," Julius Hess Papers.

43. Chicago Board of Health, 1931, 25–26.

44. Brennemann, 1932, 156.

45. Barnes, 1953, 194.

46. Brennemann, 1932, 156.

47. Letter from Dr. Clifford Grulee to Dr. Hines Roberts, 11 January 1930, Clifford Grulee Papers.

48. Letter from Dr. M. Hines Roberts to Dr. Clifford G. Grulee, 27 February 1930, Clifford Grulee Papers.

49. Julius H. Hess, "The Danger of Taking the Infants Out of the Hands of the Pediatrician," 9 March 1955, typed unpublished manuscript, Julius Hess Papers.

50. Ibid.

51. Boston Women's Health Book Collective, 1976, 11.

52. Despite this rhetoric La Leche League (LLL) has always relied heavily on physicians' advice and approval. The LLL's founders allied themselves with physicians, albeit unconventional ones, from its very inception. Dr. Gregory White, husband of LLL cofounder Mary White, and his mentor, Dr. Herbert Ratner, physicians who encouraged home birth and breastfeeding, advised the organization from the

start. By 1973 LLL offered breastfeeding seminars to doctors which the American Medical Association and other medical organizations recognize for continuing education credit (Weiner, 1994, 1367, 1376). In her very interesting article Weiner argues that LLL offered "both prologue and counterpoint" to the women's movement. The league anticipated feminists' call for increased control of childbirth and infant care, only to eventually decry women's move into the workplace and away from the full-time care of their infants.

53. Rodkin, 1996.

54. Weiner, 1994, 1359.

55. La Leche League International, 1958, 1963, 1981, 1987, 1991, 1997.

56. Weiner, 1994, 1368.

57. Ryan, 1991; Peterson and DaVanzo, 1992, 431.

58. Rodkin, 1996, 22. See also Ross Laboratories, 1991.

59. Ibid.; Freed, 1993; Ryan 1997. Full breastfeeding (exclusive breastfeeding for six months followed by partial breastfeeding for at least one year), as currently defined by the American Academy of Pediatrics, is associated with the lowest illness rates among infants, as there is a dose-response relationship between breastfeeding and infant morbidity. Minimal breastfeeding is not protective (Raisler et al., 1999).

60. Wieman et al., 1998; Peterson and DaVanzo, 1992, 431; Baranowski, et al. 1983; Leary, 1988; Matich and Sims, 1992; Rassin et al., 1984. Blum, 1999, discusses why women from different ethnic and cultural backgrounds view breastfeeding differently, arguing that white, middle-class mothers are concerned about using the "best," most "natural" methods when caring for their babies. The "dominant perspective" long has considered the bodies of white working-class women "suspect" and Blum found that, accordingly, these women viewed their bodies and breasts as "one key site of failure." Blum also contends that African American women, with their legacy of slavery and sexual exploitation by slave owners, reject breastfeeding because of its quasi-sexual exposure and association with animal-like qualities.

61. American Academy of Pediatrics, 1997.

62. Ibid.

63. Department of Health and Human Services, 2000, 3.

64. Short, 1994, 263. See also Garofalo and Goldman, 1999; Buescher, 1994; Wold and Hanson, 1994; Arnold and Larson, 1993; Goldman, 1993; Duncan et al., 1993; Cunningham, 1991; Shortridge et al., 1990; Howie et al., 1990; Cunningham, 1981.

65. Short, 1994, 263.

66. For more on breastfeeding and the incidence of insulin-dependent diabetes mellitus, see Borch-Johnsen et al., 1984 and Mayer et al., 1988. For more on breastfeeding and the reduced risk of childhood leukemia, see Shu et al., 1999.

67. Radetsky, 1999, 68–75; Shu et al., 1999.

68. American Academy of Pediatrics, 1997.

69. The introduction of artificial food before four months of age is significantly associated with asthma development (Odd, 1999).

70. NBC News, *Today Show,* 9 October 1999; Duncan et al., 1993; Sheard, 1993.

71. ABC News, *Good Morning America,* 13 June 2000. Why artificially fed babies are prone to more allergies (and more severe allergies) than breastfed babies is still

the subject of debate, but many doctors believe that it is because the human infant is born with a porous gut, and if foreign proteins (like cows' milk) are made part of the baby's diet before the gut closes at around three months, these foreign proteins can enter the circulatory system and provoke an immune response (Short, 1994, 263).

72. Helliker, 1994.

73. ABC News, *20/20,* first aired 26 February 1999. A Bronx jury subsequently convicted Walrond of negligent homicide. Most convincing to the jury was a horrific photograph of Tyler's "skeletal corpse, eyes staring and mouth open." As one juror explained, "No matter what, she was the mother . . . she should have been strong enough to do more" (Bernstein, 1999c).

74. Bernstein, 1999a.

75. Bernstein, 1999b.

76. Greenberg, 1999.

77. Most American mothers who stop breastfeeding in the first days or weeks postpartum do so either because they find breastfeeding painful or because they fear they have insufficient milk. While mild nipple tenderness can occur during the first week postpartum, prolonged and severe soreness is abnormal. It is usually caused by improper positioning of the baby at the breast or an infection like candida. Both are easily remedied. Moreover, lactation specialists contend that milk insufficiency is almost always a perceived rather than an actual problem. If human milk insufficiency had occurred in even a small fraction of mothers in human history, they point out, humans would not have survived as a species (Riordan and Auerbach, 1999, 314–19).

78. Houppert, 1999. For more recent examples of the breast-is-best-but genre, see Dalmain, 2000; Verdon, 2000; Jameson, 2000.

79. Snyder, 1908, 1214.

80. Freed et al., 1995.

Works Cited

Archival Sources

The Alumnae: Official Organ of the Alumnae Association of St. Luke's Training School for Nurses. Rush-Presbyterian-St. Luke's Medical Center Archives, Chicago.

Blaine, Anita McCormick. Papers. State Historical Society of Wisconsin, Madison.

Bowman Dairy Company. Papers. Chicago Historical Society.

Bulletin Chicago School of Sanitary Instruction (1907–1924). Municipal Reference Collection. Harold Washington Library, Chicago.

Bradley, Katherine Shedd. Diaries. Newberry Library, Chicago.

Chicago Department of Health. Annual Reports (1870–1952). Municipal Reference Collection. Harold Washington Library, Chicago.

Central Free Dispensary Papers, Rush-Presbyterian-St. Luke's Medical Center Archives, Chicago.

The Chicago Foundlings Record. Chicago Historical Society.

Chicago Pediatric Society Proceedings. The Department of Special Collections. University of Chicago Library.

The Corpuscle: A Monthly Journal of Medicine and Surgery. Official Organ of the Alumni Association of Rush Medical College. Rush-Presbyterian-St. Luke's Medical Center Archives, Chicago.

DeLee, Joseph B. Papers. Northwestern Memorial Hospital Archives, Chicago.

Dushkin, Dorothy Smith. Papers. Sophia Smith Collection. Neilson Library, Smith College. Northampton, MA.

Faith's Record. Chicago Historical Society.

Gookin Family Papers. Newberry Library, Chicago.

Grulee, Clifford. Papers. The Department of Special Collections. University of Chicago Library.

Health Fraud and Alternative Medicine Collection. American Medical Association Archives, Chicago.

Hess, Julius. Papers. The Department of Special Collections. University of Chicago Library.

Hull House Bulletins (1896–1906). Special Collections. Richard J. Daley Library, University of Illinois at Chicago.

Infant Welfare Society Papers. Chicago Historical Society.

Kerr, May Walden. Papers. Newberry Library, Chicago.

Laflin Family Papers. Chicago Historical Society.

McCormick, Nettie Fowler. Papers. State Historical Society of Wisconsin, Madison.

Michael Reese Hospital. Papers. Chicago Jewish Archives, Spertus College, Chicago.

Morton, Sterling. Papers. Chicago Historical Society.

National Dairy Council Archives, Rosemont, IL.

Parish Family Letters. Newberry Library, Chicago.

The Presbyterian Hospital of the City of Chicago Bulletin (1909–1944). Rush-Presbyterian-St. Luke's Medical Center Archives, Chicago.

Visiting Nurse Association of Chicago. Annual Reports (1894–1952). Chicago Historical Society.

———. Papers. Chicago Historical Society.

Interviews

Rosenberger, Gertrude (née Plotzke). Interview by author. Tape recording. Chicago, 10 December 1996.

Sobolewski, Josephine Zuzak. Interview by author. Tape recording. Chicago, 28 April 1997.

Turow, David. Interview by author. Tape recording. Winnetka, IL, 12 July 1996.

Primary Sources

"Abstract of Discussion." *Journal of the American Medical Association* 53 (14 August 1909): 523.

"Abstract of Discussion." *Journal of the American Medical Association* 79 (22 July 1922): 270–71.

"Abstract of Discussion on Papers of Drs. Sedgwick, Abt and Hoobler." *Journal of the American Medical Association* 69 (11 August 1917): 427–29.

"Abstract of Discussion on Papers of Drs. Snyder, Davis, Pisek, Jacobi and Southworth." *Journal of the American Medical Association* 51 (10 October 1908): 1222–24.

Abt, Isaac A. "Domestic Science Conducted by the School of Domestic Arts and Science of Chicago Lesson No. 212—Milk Commission." *Chicago Tribune,* 24 April 1904, 16.

———. "Certified Milk." *Chicago Medical Recorder* 30 (January 1908): 41–46.

———. "Milk As a Food for Infants." *Chicago Medical Recorder* (March 1912): 115–22.

———. "Facts and Fallacies about Breast Feeding." *Saint Paul Medical Journal* (1915): 281–96.

———. "The Technic of Wetnurse Management in Institutions." *Journal of the American Medical Association* 69 (11 August 1917a): 418–20.

———. "The Technic of Wet-Nurse Management in Institutions." *The American Journal of Obstetrics and Diseases of Women and Children* 76 (September 1917b): 540–47.

———. "Human Milking Machine." *Transactions of the American Pediatric Society* 33 (1921): 344–46.

————. "Some Further Observations on the Electric Breast Pump." *Transactions of the American Pediatric Society* 35 (1923): 21–25.

————. "Observations on the Electric Breast Pump." *Alumni Bulletin: The Chicago Lying-In Hospital and Dispensary* (February 1926): 5–8.

————. *Baby Doctor.* New York, London: Whittlesey House, 1944.

Acker, George N. "Some Present Day Problems in Pediatrics." *Transactions of the American Pediatric Society* 27 (1915): 9–16.

Adams, Samuel S. "How Shall We Feed the Baby?" *Archives of Pediatrics* 2 (May 1885): 269–82.

"Adulterated Milk." *Chicago Tribune,* 1 October 1892, 4.

"Adulteration of Milk." *Chicago Inter Ocean,* 10 September 1892, 4.

Aldis, Mary. "President's Report." *Twenty-second Annual Report of The Visiting Nurse Association of Chicago for Year Ending December 31, 1911,* 1912, 5–9.

————. "President's Report." *Twenty-third Annual Report of The Visiting Nurse Association of Chicago for Year Ending December 31, 1912,* 1913, 8–15.

Allen, Nathan. "Laws of Maternity." *Babyhood* 5 (March 1889): 111–13.

Allen, Thomas Grant. "Methods of Calculating Proteid and Energy in Infant Feeding." *Chicago Medical Recorder* 29 (April 1907): 232–46.

————. "Some Observations Necessary to Successful Infant Feeding." *Chicago Medical Recorder* (September 1908): 496–503.

Allin, Frank W. "The Baby-Tent Idea." *Illinois Medical Journal* 17 (1910): 423–25.

American Academy of Pediatrics. "Breastfeeding and the Use of Human Milk." *Pediatrics* 100 (December 1997): 1035–39.

"The American Pediatric Society's Collective Investigation on Infantile Scurvy in North America." *Archives of Pediatrics* 15 (July 1898): 481–508.

"Are Infant Feeding Methods Changing." *Public Health Nursing* 23 (1931): 581–85.

Armstrong, Irene. "Breast Feeding for Infants: A Reestablishment Program." *Public Health Nursing* 24 (1932): 426–28.

Arnold, Lois D. W. "How to Order Banked Donor Milk in the United States: What the Health Care Provider Needs to Know." *Journal of Human Lactation* 14 (1998): 65–67.

Arnold, Lois D. W., and Elaine Larson. "Immunologic Benefits of Breast Milk in Relation to Human Milk Banking." *American Journal of Infection Control* 21 (October 1993): 235–42.

Babyhood 3 (September 1887): 319.

"Baby Saving." *Bulletin Chicago School of Sanitary Instruction* 15 (6 April 1912): 53–54.

"Baby's First Month." *Chicago's Health* 23 (12 November 1929): 154.

"The Baby's Habits." *Arthur's Home Magazine* 52 (November 1884): 654.

"Baby Tent Report for Summer 1913." *Twenty-fourth Annual Report of The Visiting Nurse Association of Chicago for Year Ending December 31, 1913,* 1914, 35–36.

"Baby Weeks." *Report and Handbook of the Department of Health of the City of Chicago for the Years 1911 to 1918 Inclusive.* Chicago, 1919, 575.

"Bacteria Free Feedings." *The Presbyterian Hospital of the City of Chicago Bulletin* 30 (May 1938): 2. Rush-Presbyterian-St. Luke's Medical Center Archives.

Baranowski, Tom, et al. "Social Support, Social Influence, Ethnicity and the Breast-feeding Decision." *Social Science and Medicine* 17 (1983): 1599–1611.

Barnes, George R., et al. "Management of Breast Feeding." *Journal of the American Medical Association* 151 (17 January 1953): 192–99.

Bass, Mrs. Perkins B. "Unified Annual Report." *The Presbyterian Hospital of the City of Chicago Bulletin* (January 1928): 8. Rush-Presbyterian-St. Luke's Hospital Archives.

Bedinger, George R. "The Wet Nurse Directory of Boston." *Transactions of the Annual Meeting of the American Association for the Study and Prevention of Infant Mortality* (1915): 252–54.

Bernstein, Nina. "Placing the Blame in an Infant's Death." *The New York Times,* 15 March 1999a, A21.

———. "At Trial, Mother Denies Intent to Starve Baby." *The New York Times,* 19 May 1999b, A24.

———. "Bronx Woman Convicted of Negligent Homicide in Starving of Breast-Fed Son." *The New York Times,* 20 May 1999c, A25.

Biehn, Joseph Favil. "Report of the Health Department Laboratories for 1905." *Biennial Report of the Department of Health of the City of Chicago for the Years 1904–1905,* Chicago, 1906, 13–18.

"Births in Hospitals Increase." *Report of the Department of Health of the City of Chicago for the Years 1926 to 1930.* Chicago, 1931, 243.

Booker, W. D. "The Early History of the Summer Diarrhoeas of Infants." *Transactions of the American Pediatric Society* 13 (1901): 7–35.

Borch-Johnsen, K., et al. "Relation between Breast-Feeding and Incidence of Rates of Insulin-Dependent Diabetes Mellitus." *The Lancet* (10 November 1984): 1083–86.

Boston Women's Health Book Collective. *Our Bodies, Ourselves: A Book by and for Women.* New York: Simon and Schuster, 1976.

Brack, D. "Social Forces, Feminism and Breastfeeding." *Nursing Outlook* 23 (1975): 556–61.

"Breast Feeding." *Report of the Department of Health of the City of Chicago for the Years 1923, 1924 and 1925.* Chicago, 1926, 231–32.

Brennemann, Joseph. "Remarks on the Feeding of the Healthy Infant." *Journal of the American Medical Association* 51 (11 July 1908): 101–5.

———. "Diarrheal Diseases." *Bulletin Chicago School of Sanitary Instruction* 14 (13 May 1911): 5.

———. "Prevention and Treatment of Neo-Natal Morbidity and Mortality." *Illinois Medical Journal* 54 (1928): 452–61.

———. "The Curd and the Buffer in Infant Feeding." *Journal of the American Medical Association* 92 (2 February 1929): 364–66.

———. "Vis Medicatrix Naturae in Pediatrics." *American Journal of Diseases of Children* 40 (July 1930): 1–17.

———. "Psychologic Aspects of Nutrition in Childhood." *The Journal of Pediatrics* 1 (August 1932): 145–71.

———. "Periods in the Life of the American Pediatric Society: Adolescence, 1900–1915." *Transactions of the American Pediatric Society* 50 (1938): 56–67.

Buescher, E. "Host Defense Mechanisms of Human Milk and Their Relations to Enteric Infections and Necrotizing Enterocolitis." *Clinics of Perinatology* 21 (June 1994): 247–62.

Bulletin Chicago School of Sanitary Instruction. 10 (17 August 1907a).

———. 10 (12 October 1907b).

———. 12 (26 June 1909).

———. 13 (1 January 1910a).

———. 13 (8 January 1910b).

———. 13 (2 July 1910c).

———. 13 (13 August 1910d).

———. 14 (8 April 1911a).

———. 14 (20 May 1911b).

———. 14 (3 June 1911c).

———. 14 (8 July 1911d).

———. 14 (22 July 1911e).

———. 14 (19 August 1911f).

———. 15 (10 February 1912a).

———. 15 (20 April 1912b).

———. 15 (18 May 1912c).

———. 15 (25 May 1912d).

———. 15 (1 June 1912e).

———. 15 (8 June 1912f).

———. 15 (22 June 1912g).

———. 15 (13 July 1912h).

———. 15 (27 July 1912i).

———. 15 (3 August 1912j).

———. 15 (10 August 1912k).

———. 15 (28 September 1912l).

———. 16 (1 June 1913a).

———. 16 (26 July 1913b).

———. 16 (22 November 1913c).

———. 17 (18 April 1914a).

———. 17 (2 May 1914b).

———. 17 (20 June 1914c).

———. 17 (21 November 1914d).

———. 18 (24 July 1915).

———. 21 (29 June 1919).

———. 23 (26 February 1921).

———. 24 (1 July 1922).

Bundesen, Herman N. *Our Babies.* Chicago: Department of Health, 1925a.

———. "Chicago, The Summer Resort: A Good Place to Spend a Vacation." *Chicago's Health* 19 (7 July 1925b): 704.

————. *Chicago's Health* (21 July 1925c): 715.

————. "Baby's First Month." *Chicago's Health* 20 (27 April 1926): 120.

"Bureau of Milk Inspection." *Annual Report of the Department of Health of the City of Chicago for the Year Ended December 31, 1893*. Chicago, 1894, 11–12.

Burhans, C. W., and D. N. Smith. "The Inorganic Constituents of Human Milk with Particular Reference to Racial Variations." *American Journal of Diseases of Children* 26 (October 1923): 303–8.

Campbell, Grace H. "Medical Inspection of Employees on Certified Farms." *Proceedings of the Fifteenth Annual Conference of the American Association of Medical Milk Commissions Held at Boston, Mass., June 6 and 7, 1921*, 413–17.

"Care of Infants by Health Department Nurses." *Report and Handbook of the Department of Health of the City of Chicago for the Years 1911 to 1918 Inclusive*. Chicago, 1919, 565–66.

"The Care of Infants: Historical Data." *Journal of the American Medical Association* 59 (17 August 1912): 542–43.

Chapin, Henry Dwight. "The Use of Gruels as Diluents of Cow's Milk." *Transactions of the American Pediatric Society* 11 (1899): 219–29.

————. *The Theory and Practice of Infant Feeding with Notes on Development*. New York: William Wood and Company, 1902.

————. "Principles of Infant Feeding as Based on the Evolution of Mammals." *Transactions of the American Pediatric Society* 15 (1903): 49–58.

————. "A Plan of Dealing with Atrophic Infants and Children." *Transactions of the American Pediatric Society* 20 (1908): 138–50.

————. "The Necessity of a Pure Raw Milk." *Proceedings of the Eleventh Annual Conference of the American Association of Medical Milk Commissions at Brooklyn, New York, June 1 and 3, 1917*, 124–37.

Chicago Board of Health. *Regulations for the Conduct of Maternity Hospitals, Maternity Divisions of General Hospitals, and Nurseries for the Newborn*. Chicago, 1931.

The Chicago Daily Tribune. Help wanted advertisement. 25 January 1885, 20.

Chicago Department of Health. *Our Babies*. Circa 1916, 1917.

"The Chicago Medical Society Proceedings." *Chicago Medical Recorder* 3 (August 1892): 500.

"The Chicago Medical Society Proceedings." *Chicago Medical Recorder* 10 (February 1896): 130.

"The Chicago Medical Society Proceedings." *Chicago Medical Recorder* 12 (June 1897): 429–37.

"Chicago Milk." *Chicago Inter Ocean*, 30 September 1892, 4.

"Chicago Wins Fight to Save Lives of Babies." *Chicago's Health* 21 (8 and 15 February 1927): 38–41.

"Child Welfare." *Report of the Department of Health of the City of Chicago for the Years 1926 to 1930 Inclusive*. Chicago, 1931, 248–49.

Christopher, W. S. "Feeding the Healthy Infant." *Chicago Medical Recorder* 3 (November 1892): 726–32.

Churchill, Frank Spooner. "Infant Feeding." *Chicago Medical Recorder* 10 (February 1896): 102–14.

———. "Substitute Feeding in Infancy." *Chicago Medical Recorder* 12 (June 1897): 408–13.

———. "The Management of Breast Feeding." *The Corpuscle: A Monthly Journal of Medicine and Surgery. Official Organ of the Alumni Association of Rush Medical College* 7 (January 1898): 205–11, Rush-Presbyterian-St. Luke's Medical Center Archives, Chicago.

———. "The Wet Nurse in Hospital Practice." *American Journal of Obstetrics and Diseases of Women and Children* 70 (1914): 499–501.

"City Milk Inspection." *Report of the Department of Health of the City of Chicago for the Years 1919, 1920 and 1921.* Chicago, 1922, 324.

"City Milk Inspection." *Report of the Department of Health of the City of Chicago for the Years 1923, 1924 and 1925.* Chicago, 1926, 519.

Clarke, Edward H. *Sex in Education; or, A Fair Chance for Girls.* Boston: James R. Osgood & Co., 1873.

Cleveland, Clement. "The Wet-Nurse vs. the Bottle." *Archives of Pediatrics* 1 (May 1884a): 346.

———. "Some Observations upon the Feeding of Infants." *Archives of Pediatrics* 1 (June 1884b): 389–90.

Coit, Henry L. "The Proper Care of Milk." *Babyhood* 10 (July 1894): 230–32.

———. "Axioms with Respect to Milk." *Babyhood* 11 (May 1895): 169.

———. "The Origin, General Plan, and Scope of the Medical Milk Commission." *Proceedings of the First Annual Session of the American Association of Medical Milk Commissions, Atlantic City, June 3, 1907,* 10–17.

———. "The Effects of Heated and Superheated Milk on the Infant's Nutrition (Recent Investigations)." *Transactions of the American Pediatric Society* 24 (1912): 128–38.

———. "Essential Factors in the Scientific Substitute Feeding of Infants." *Report of the Proceedings of The English-Speaking Conference on Infant Mortality Held at Caxton Hall, Westminster, on Aug 4 and 5, 1913,* 302–8.

"Commissioner's Summary Report." *Biennial Report of the Department of Health of the City of Chicago for the Years 1904–1905.* Chicago, 1906, xiii–xiv.

"Concerning Pasteurization." *Bulletin Chicago School of Sanitary Instruction* 23 (11 June 1921): 94.

Coolidge, Emelyn Lincoln. "The Baby from Birth to Three." *Ladies' Home Journal* 19 (February 1903): 38.

———. "The Young Mother's Calendar." *Ladies' Home Journal* 21 (September 1904): 36.

Cotton, A. C. "Baby's Milk." *Bulletin Chicago School of Sanitary Instruction* 14 (13 May 1911): 7.

"Country Dairy Inspection." *Report and Handbook of the Department of Health of the City of Chicago for the Years 1911 to 1918 Inclusive.* Chicago, 1919, 910–11.

"Course in Laboratory Diagnosis for Nurses. Subjects Taught." *The Alumnae: Official Organ of the Alumnae Association of St. Luke's Training School for Nurses* 12 (November 1914): 5, Rush-Presbyterian-St. Luke's Medical Center Archives, Chicago.

Coutsoudis, Anna, et al. "Influence of Infant Feeding Patterns on Early Mother-to-Child Transmission of HIV-1 in Durban, South Africa: A Prospective Cohort Study." *Lancet* 354 (7 August 1999): 471–76.

Cudahy, Jean M. "President's Report." *The Visiting Nurse Association of Chicago Thirty-ninth Annual Report for Year Ending December 31, 1928,* 1929, 11–14.

Cunningham, Allan S. "Breast-Feeding and Morbidity in Industrialized Countries: An Update." *Advances in International Maternal and Child Health* (1981): 128–68.

————, et al. "Breast-Feeding and Health in the 1980s: A Global Epidemiologic Review." *The Journal of Pediatrics* 118 (May 1991): 659–66.

"Current Comment." *Journal of the American Medical Association* 59 (1912): 657.

"Dairy Inspection." *Annual Report of the Department of Health of the City of Chicago for the Year 1906.* Chicago, 1907, 21–25.

Dalmain, Melissa. "Is Breast Always Best?" *Parents* (June 2000): 191–92.

Davis, Effa V. "The Quantity and Quality of Breast-Milk during the First Two Weeks of the Puerperium." *Journal of the American Medical Association* 51 (10 October 1908): 1209–12.

————. "Breast Feeding." *Bulletin Chicago School of Sanitary Instruction* 13 (18 June 1910): 2.

————. "Care of the New-Born Baby." *Bulletin Chicago School of Sanitary Instruction* 14 (13 May 1911): 4.

"Deaths and Reported Causes of Deaths: 1897." *Biennial Report of the Department of Health of the City of Chicago for the Years 1897 and 1898.* Chicago, 1899, 222–29.

"Deaths and Reported Causes of Deaths: 1898." *Biennial Report of the Department of Health of the City of Chicago for the Years 1897 and 1898.* Chicago, 1899, 252–59.

"The Decline of Suckling Power among American Women." *Babyhood* 5 (March 1889): 111–15.

"The Decline of Suckling Power among American Women." *Babyhood* 19 (December 1902): 5–8.

"A Defence of Wet-Nurses." *Babyhood* 3 (September 1887): 352.

DeLee, Joseph B. "Infant Incubation, with the Presentation of a New Incubator and a Description of the System at the Chicago Lying-In Hospital." *Quarterly Bulletin of Northwestern University Medical School* 5 (September 1903): 252–64.

————. "The Prophylactic Forceps Operation." *American Journal of Obstetrics and Gynecology* 1 (October 1920): 34–44.

Denny, Francis P. "Value of Small Quantities of Human Milk in the Treatment of Infantile Atrophy and the Infections of Infants." *Journal of the American Medical Association* 47 (8 December 1906): 1904–9.

————. "The Use of Human Milk in Typhoid Fever to Increase the Bacteriolytic Power of the Blood." *Boston Medical and Surgical Journal* 158 (7 May 1908): 625–30.

————. "Human Milk in the Treatment of Various Infections." *Boston Medical and Surgical Journal* 160 (11 February 1909): 161–63.

Department of Health and Human Services Office on Women's Health. "HSS Blueprint for Action on Breastfeeding." Washington, D.C.: U.S. Department of Health and Human Services, Office on Women's Health, 2000.

Department of Health Weekly Bulletin 22 (7 February 1928).

"Diarrhea in Infants." *Report of the Department of Health of the City of Chicago for the Years 1907, 1908, 1909, 1910.* Chicago, 1911, 67–69.

"Diarrheal Diseases." *Bulletin Chicago School of Sanitary Instruction* 3 (20 February 1909): 6.

Dietrich, Henry. "The Food Requirement of the Breast Fed Infant." *Archives of Pediatrics* 37 (1920): 278–81.

———. "An Analysis of a Series of Case Records Relative to Certain Phases of Breast Feeding." *Journal of the American Medical Association* 79 (22 July 1922): 258–72.

"Discussion." *Illinois Medical Journal* 66 (1934): 291.

"Discussion of Papers by Drs. Northrup, Graham and Chapin." *Transactions of the American Pediatric Society* 20 (1908): 145.

"Doctors to Censor Milk." *Chicago Medical Recorder* 31 (15 February 1909): 160.

Dodson, John M. "Breast Feeding—Its Vital Importance." *Bulletin Chicago School of Sanitary Instruction* 14 (13 May 1911): 6.

Doering, E. J. "Prophylaxis of Summer Complaints of Children." *Chicago Medical Recorder* 1 (July 1891): 433–38.

Douglas, Elizabeth. "Quarterly Report of the Social Service Department." *The Presbyterian Hospital Bulletin* (October 1914): 13.

Duncan, Burris, et al. "Exclusive Breast-Feeding for at Least 4 Months Protects against Otitis Media." *Pediatrics* 91 (May 1993): 867–72.

Dunn, Charles Hunter. "The Use in Practice of the Theoretical Resources Provided by Percentage Feeding." *Transactions of the American Pediatric Society* 19 (1907): 60–69.

Earle, Chas. Warrington. "Infant Feeding in Summer Complaints." *Chicago Medical Recorder* 1 (July 1891): 439–46.

———. "The Sterilization of Food for Infants." *Chicago Medical Recorder* 3 (August 1892): 472–80.

Eaton, P. J. "A Few of the Things a Pediatrician Should Teach." *Transactions of the American Pediatric Society* 21 (1909): 40–47.

"Edict Against Slop." *Chicago Tribune,* 23 September 1892, 1–2.

"Editorial." *Chicago Medical Recorder* 31 (15 January 1909): 62–63.

"Editorial. Certified Milk." *Archives of Pediatrics* 14 (1897): 54–55.

"Editorial. The Chicago Medical Society Milk Commission and Its Contract with Dairies." *Chicago Medical Recorder* 31 (15 December 1909): 837–38.

"Editorial. Preventive Medicine." *Chicago Medical Recorder* 2 (September 1891): 67.

Edsall, David L., and Charles A. Fife. "Concerning the Accuracy of Percentage Modification of Milk for Infants." *Transactions of the American Pediatric Society* 15 (1903): 59–75.

Edson, Cyrus. "Preserved Milk." *Babyhood* 11 (December 1885): 9.

———. "The Feeding of Cows and Its Effect on Milk." *Babyhood* 3 (August 1887): 293–94.

Eigher, Marvin S., and Sally Wendkos Olds. *The Complete Book of Breastfeeding.* New York: Workman Publishing, 1987.

Erdman, Henry E. *The Marketing of Whole Milk.* New York: Macmillan, 1921.

Eskay's Food Advertisement. *American Motherhood* 22 (December 1905).

"An Experiment in Infant Feeding." *American Motherhood* 38 (June 1914): 378–79.

"Feeding of Babies Registered at Infant Welfare Stations Classified by Numbers of Babies and Methods of Feeding 1926–1930." *Report of the Department of Health of the City of Chicago for the Years 1926 to 1930 Inclusive.* Chicago, 1931, 247.

"Feeding of the Baby during the First Month." *Bulletin Chicago School of Sanitary Instruction* 4 (4 June 1910): 2.

"Feeding of Infants Registered at Infant Welfare Conferences 1933." *Board of Health City of Chicago Annual Report 1933.* Chicago, 1934, 17.

Ferguson, R. R. "Certified Milk." *Illinois Medical Journal* 26 (December 1914): 579–82.

"Field Nurses—Infant Welfare Work." *Report of the Department of Health of the City of Chicago for the Year 1922.* Chicago, 1923, 147.

Fisher, Irving. "Address." *Transactions of the American Association for the Study and Prevention of Infant Mortality* (1910): 33–42.

Foley, Edna L. *Visiting Nurse Manual.* Chicago: Visiting Nurse Association of Chicago, 1914.

———. "Annual Meeting—Superintendent's Report." *Twenty-seventh Annual Report The Visiting Nurse Association of Chicago for Year Ending December 31, 1916,* 1917, 35–39.

———. "Superintendent's Report." *The Visiting Nurse Association of Chicago Twenty-ninth Annual Report for Year Ending December 31, 1918,* 1919, 15–24.

———. "Superintendent's Report." *The Visiting Nurse Association of Chicago Thirty-second Annual Report for Year Ending December 31, 1921,* 1922, 27–30.

"Fourth Annual Report of the Chicago Foundlings' Home," *The Chicago Foundlings Record* 5 (February 1875).

Freed, Gary L. "Breast-feeding: Time to Teach What We Preach." *Journal of the American Medical Association* 269 (13 January 1993): 243–45.

Freed, Gary L., et al. "National Assessment of Physicians' Breast-feeding Knowledge, Attitudes, Training and Experience." *Journal of the American Medical Association* 273 (1995): 472–76.

Freeman, Rowland G. "Remarks on the Development of Dairy Hygiene in the United States." *Proceedings of the First Annual Session of the American Association of Medical Milk Commissions, Atlantic City, June 3, 1907,* 17–18.

———. "Pasteurization of Milk." *Journal of the American Medical Association* 54 (29 January 1910): 372–73.

Fulmer, Harriet. "Report of Nurses Work for Year 1904." *Fifteenth Annual Report The Visiting Nurse Association of Chicago for Year Ending December 31, 1904,* 1905, 14–20.

———. "Visiting Nursing in a Great City," *Charities and the Commons: A Weekly Journal of Philanthropy and Social Advance* 16 (7 April 1907): 22–24.

———. "Report of Nurse's Work, 1907." *Eighteenth Annual Report The Visiting Nurse Association of Chicago for Year Ending December 31, 1907,* 1908, 28–34.

———. "Report of the Nurses' Work for the Year 1909." *Twentieth Annual Report The Visiting Nurse Association of Chicago for Year Ending December 31, 1909,* 1910, 39–44.

————. "Report of the Nurses' Work for the Year Ending December 31, 1910." *Twenty-first Annual Report The Visiting Nurse Association of Chicago for Year Ending December 31, 1910,* 1911, 37–38.

Fyffe, Edith A. H. "Modified Milk." *The Woman's Medical Journal* 6 (1897): 289–90.

Garland, Joseph, and Mabel B. Rich. "Duration of Breast Feeding: A Comparative Study." *New England Journal of Medicine* 203 (25 December 1930): 1279–82.

Garofalo, Roberto P., and Armond S. Goldman. "Expression of Functional Immunomodulatory and Anti-Inflammatory Factors in Human Milk." *Clinics in Perinatology* 26 (June 1999): 361–77.

Gaskin, Ina May. *Babies, Breastfeeding, and Bonding.* Massachusetts: Bergin & Garvey Publishers, 1987.

"General Information." *Fifteenth Annual Report The Visiting Nurse Association of Chicago For Year Ending December 31, 1904,* 1905, 48.

"God's Dealings with the Foundlings." *Faith's Record* 9 (October 1879): 82.

"God's Dealings with the Foundlings," *Faith's Record* 12 (July 1882): 51.

"God's Dealings with the Foundlings," *Faith's Record* 13 (August 1883): 58.

Gray, Paula Holmes. "Secretary's Report." *The Visiting Nurse Association of Chicago Tenth Annual Report: 1900,* 1901, 15–18.

Goldman, Armond S. "The Immune System of Human Milk: Antimicrobial, Antiinflammatory and Immunomodulating Properties." *The Pediatric Infectious Disease Journal* (August 1993): 664–72.

Greenberg, Susan H. "Nursing Trouble." *Newsweek,* Special Issue, Spring/Summer 1999.

Griffith, Albert F. "Talks with the Doctor." *American Motherhood* 24 (May 1907): 329–34.

Grulee, Clifford G. "The Use and Abuse of Carbohydrates in Infant-Feeding." *The Journal-Lancet* (15 March 1912): 141–47.

————. *Infant Feeding.* Philadelphia: W. B. Saunders Company, 1914.

————. "Infant Feeding at the Presbyterian Hospital." *The Presbyterian Hospital of the City of Chicago Bulletin* (April 1916): 9–11, Rush-Presbyterian-St. Luke's Medical Center Archives, Chicago.

————. "Colic in the Breast-Fed Infant." *Medical Clinics of North America* 3 (May 1920): 1621–28.

————. "Fundamentals of Infant Feeding." *Illinois Medical Journal* 66 (1934): 288–92.

————. "Breast Feeding." *Illinois Medical Journal* 70 (1936): 257.

Hamilton, B. Wallace. "This Is the Danger Month for Your Baby." *The Delineator* 83 (July 1913): 7.

————. "Why the Bottle Baby?" *The Delineator* 88 (April 1916): 10.

Harvey, Robert H. "Domestic Science Column Lesson No. 226—The Feeding of an Infant During Its First Year." *Chicago Tribune,* 22 May 1904, 24.

Hatfield, M. P. "The Etiology of Infantile Summer Complaints." *Chicago Medical Recorder* 1 (July 1891): 430–32.

Helliker, Kevin. "Dying for Milk: Pressure to Breast-Feed Causes Some Mothers to Inadvertently Starve Their Babies." *Wall Street Journal,* 22 July 1994, A1, A4.

Helmholz, Henry F. "Studies on Milk Sugar." *American Association for Study and*

Prevention of Infant Mortality: Transactions of the First Annual Meeting, November 9–11, 1910. New York: Arno Press, 1974, 107–14.

Helmholz, H. F., and Walter Hoffman. "An Analysis of the Mortality for 1915 in the Infant Welfare Stations of Chicago." *Journal of the American Medical Association* 67 (25 November 1916): 1567–69.

Hess, Julius H. "Uniform for the Wet Nurse." *The Modern Hospital* 7 (September 1916): 265–66.

———. "Mother's Milk—Nature's Birthday Gift to the Baby." *Hygeia* 1 (June 1923): 149–54.

———. "Give the Babies Their Rights: Healthy Babies Make Happy Homes." *Chicago's Health* (21 July 1925): 717–18.

———. *Feeding and Nutritional Disorders in Infancy and Childhood.* Philadelphia: F. A. Davis Co., 1928.

Hess, Julius H., and Evelyn Lundeen. *The Premature Infant: Medical and Nursing Care.* Philadelphia: J. B. Lippincott Company, 1941.

Hill, Lewis Webb. *Practical Infant Feeding.* Philadelphia: W. B. Saunders Company, 1923.

Hirshberg, Leonard Keene. "What You Ought to Know about Your Baby." *The Delineator* 73 (January 1909a): 106.

———. "What You Ought to Know about Your Baby." *The Delineator* 73 (February 1909b): 262.

Hogan, Louise E. "What Should be Done for Baby." *Arthur's Home Magazine* 62 (March 1892): 287.

Holmes, Bayard. "Medical History of Chicago. The Condition of Medical Thought, Medical Practice, and Hospital Service after the Great Fire and before the World's Fair: 1871–1893." *Medical Life* 34 (June 1927): 335.

Holt, L. Emmett. "A Ready Method of Calculating Milk Formulas of Various Percentages and the Caloric Value of the Same." *Transactions of the American Pediatric Society* 23 (1911): 278–84.

———. *The Care and Feeding of Children: A Catechism for the Use of Mothers and Children's Nurses.* New York: D. Appleton & Co., 1914.

Holt, L. Emmett, Angelia M. Courtney, and Helen L. Fales. "A Chemical Study of Woman's Milk, Especially Its Inorganic Constituents." *American Journal of Diseases of Children* 10 (October 1915): 229–48.

Hoobler, B. Raymond. "Problems Connected with the Collection and Production of Human Milk." *Journal of the American Medical Association* 69 (11 August 1917): 421–25.

———. "Human Milk: Its Commercial Production and Distribution." *Journal of the American Medical Association* 84 (17 January 1925): 165–66.

———. "The Production, Collection and Distribution of Human Milk." *Journal of the American Medical Association* 88 (4 June 1927): 1786–89.

Houppert, Karen. "Nursed to Death." *Salon.* Retrieved from <salon1999.com/mwt/feature/1999/05/21/nursing/index.html> on 23 May 1999.

Howe, Frederic W. "Production of Certified Milk." *Proceedings of the Thirteenth Annual Conference of the American Association of Medical Milk Commissions Held at New Orleans, Louisiana, October 27 and 28, 1919,* 202–18.

————. "Clean Natural vs. Pasteurized Milk." *Proceedings of the Fifteenth Annual Conference of The American Association of Medical Milk Commissions Held in Boston, Mass., June 6 and 7, 1921,* 398–405.

Howie, Peter W., et al. "Protective Effect of Breast Feeding against Infection." *British Medical Journal* 300 (6 January 1990): 11–16.

"Important Experiments toward Maintaining Purity of the Milk Supply." *The Mother's Nursery Guide* 9 (September 1893): 315.

"Improved in Quality Milk Is Better Since the Inspection Was Ordered." *Chicago Tribune,* 24 December 1892, 8.

"Infancy Service." *Chicago's Health* 22 (2 October 1928): 231.

"Infant Welfare." *Report of the Department of Health of the City of Chicago for the Years 1923, 1924 and 1925.* Chicago, 1926, 263–64.

"Infant Welfare Field Work." *Report and Handbook of the Department of Health of the City of Chicago for the Years 1911 to 1918 Inclusive.* Chicago, 1919, 567.

"Infant Welfare Physicians." *Report and Handbook of the Department of Health of the City of Chicago for the Years 1911 to 1918 Inclusive.* Chicago, 1919, 570–72.

"Infant Welfare Service." *Report and Handbook of the Department of Health of the City of Chicago for the Years 1911 to 1918 Inclusive.* Chicago, 1919, 561–89.

"Infant Welfare Service, 1909–1910." *Report of the Department of Health of the City of Chicago for the Years 1907, 1908, 1909, 1910.* Chicago, 1911, 170–80.

"The Infant Welfare Society." *Report of the Department of Health of the City of Chicago for the Years 1923, 1924 and 1925.* Chicago, 1926, 254.

"Infant Welfare Stations." *Bulletin Chicago School of Sanitary Instruction* 21 (28 June 1919): 101.

"Infant Welfare Stations." *Chicago's Health* 20 (29 June 1926): 173.

"Infant Welfare Stations Established." *Report of the Department of Health of the City of Chicago for the Year 1922.* Chicago, 1923, 144–45.

"Infant Welfare Station Work." *Bulletin Chicago School of Sanitary Instruction* 19 (5 February 1916): 28.

"Infant Welfare Work." *Bulletin Chicago School of Sanitary Instruction* 17 (16 May 1914): 84.

"Infant Welfare Work." *Report of the Department of Health of the City of Chicago for the Years 1919, 1920 and 1921.* Chicago, 1922, 127–32.

"Infant Welfare Work." *Report of the Department of Health of the City of Chicago for the Years 1923, 1924 and 1925.* Chicago, 1926, 228–30.

"The Influence of the Milk of Wet-Nurses." *Babyhood* 3 (October 1887): 372–73.

"Its Effects Too Slow. Operation of the Milk Ordinance. Nine Months in Force and Hardly Any Improvement Perceptible." *Chicago Herald,* 16 September 1893, 17.

Jacobi, A. *Infant Diet.* New York: G. P. Putnam's Sons, 1874.

————. "Infant Feeding and Infant Foods." *Transactions of the Medical Society of the State of New York 1807–1905* (8 February 1882): 77–99.

————. "Infant Feeding—A Review." *Pediatrics* 1 (1 January 1896): 1–10.

————. "The Gospel of Top Milk." *Journal of the American Medical Association* 51 (10 October 1908): 1216–19.

Jameson, Marnell. "A Natural Formula for Success." *Los Angeles Times,* 4 September 2000.

"January Report of Social Service." *The Presbyterian Hospital Bulletin* (January 1917): 12.

Jelliffe, Smith Ely. "Some Dangers Resulting from the Use of Cows' Milk." *Babyhood* 10 (September 1894): 294–96.

"Jewish Women." *The Daily Jewish Courier,* 8 July 1912.

Jordan, James O., and Frank E. Mott. "Condensed Milk and Its Value for General Use and for Infant Feeding." *American Journal of Public Hygiene* 6 (1910): 391–410.

Kearney, Margaret H. "Identifying Psychosocial Obstacles to Breastfeeding Success." *Journal of Obstetric, Gynecologic, and Neonatal Nursing* 17 (March–April 1988): 98–105.

Kegel, Arnold H. "Milk." *Chicago's Health* 21 (13 December 1927): 299–300.

———. "Milk and Health." *Chicago's Health.* 23 (17 September 1929): 118.

Kellogg, John H. "The Supreme Importance of Clean, Uncooked Milk for Infants and Children and the Dangers of Pasteurized Milk." *Proceedings of the Fifteenth Annual Conference of The American Association of Medical Milk Commissions Held in Boston, Mass., June 6 and 7, 1921,* 330–361.

Kennicott, Cass L. "Milk Inspection." *Report and Handbook of the Department of Health of the City of Chicago for the Years 1911 to 1918 Inclusive.* Chicago, 1919, 146–55.

Kerr, John W. "The Bearing of Communicable Diseases on the Pure Milk Movement." *Proceedings of the Third Annual Conference of the American Association of Medical Milk Commissions Held at Atlantic City, New Jersey, June 7, 1909,* 1909a, 100–06.

———. "The Relation of the Medical Milk Commission to the Establishment and Conduct of Infants' Milk Depots." *Proceedings of the Third Annual Conference of the American Association of Medical Milk Commissions Held at Atlantic City, New Jersey, June 7, 1909,* 1909b, 89–93.

"Kind of Feeding Infants Were Receiving at Time of Registration at Infant Welfare Stations." *Report of the Department of Health of the City of Chicago for the Years 1923, 1924, 1925.* Chicago, 1926, 223.

King, Ginevra F. "Report of the Nurses' Committee for 1922." *The Visiting Nurse Association of Chicago Thirty-third Annual Report for Year Ending December 31, 1922,* 1923, 14–18.

Kober, George M. *Report of the Committee on Social Betterment.* Washington, D.C.: The President's Homes Commission, 1908.

Koplik, Henry. "The Increase of Weight in Infants Fed Artificially." *Transactions of the American Pediatric Society* 11 (1899): 110–20.

Lactated Brand Infant Food Advertisement. *Ladies' Home Journal* 24 (August 1907): 37.

Ladd, Maynard. "The Need of Greater Accuracy in Prescribing Starch in Infant Feeding." *Transactions of the American Pediatric Society* 19 (1907): 101–6.

La Leche League International. *The Womanly Art of Breastfeeding.* 6th rev. ed. New York: Plume, 1997.

Leary, Warren E. "Why Fewer Blacks Choose to Breast-feed Than Do Whites." *New York Times,* 7 April 1988, B7.

Lintner, J. J. "Chicago's Pure Milk Campaign." *Chicago's Health* 21 (5 April 1927): 102–5.

"Little Mothers' Clubs." *Report of the Department of Health of the City of Chicago for the Year 1922*. Chicago, 1923, 164–75.

"The Long Arm of the Health Department." *Bulletin Chicago School of Sanitary Instruction* 23 (11 June 1921): 93–94.

Long, J. H. "Report of Chemist." *Report of the Department of Health City of Chicago for the Year 1885*. Chicago, 1886, 99–100.

"Look After the Milk." *Chicago Inter Ocean,* 10 September 1892, 4.

MacDonald, Elizabeth Stone. "Our Babies." *Modern Priscilla* 35 (March 1920): 50.

Madden-Lunsford, Kerry. "Nursing a Baby Shouldn't Be This Much of a Problem." *Los Angeles Times,* 28 April 1999, Southern California Living Section.

Marchand, Lucille, and Mary Helen Morrow. "Infant Feeding Practices: Understanding the Decision-making Process." *Family Medicine* 26 (May 1994): 319–24.

Martinez, Gilbert A., and Fritz W. Krieger. "1984 Milk-Feeding Patterns in the United States." *Pediatrics* 76 (December 1985): 1004–8.

Mason, Charles F. "The Nursing Mother." *Babyhood* 11 (September 1886): 344.

Matich, J. Renee, and Laura S. Sims. "A Comparison of Social Support Variables between Women Who Intend to Breast or Bottle Feed." *Social Science and Medicine* 34 (April 1992): 919–27.

Mayer, Elizabeth J., et al. "Reduced Risk of IDDM Among Breast-Fed Children." *Diabetes* 37 (December 1988): 1625–32.

McBride, Marion A. "For the Chidren." [*sic*] *New Crusade* (June 1897): 85–86.

McClanahan, H. M. "The Relative Morbidity of Breast and Bottle Fed Infants." *Transactions of the American Pediatric Society* 30 (1918): 185–95.

McCleary, G. F. "The Infants' Milk Depot: Its History and Function." *Journal of Hygiene* 4 (1904): 329–67.

McEwen, Floy. "Doctor and His Own Commission." *Proceedings of the Eleventh Annual Conference of the American Association of Medical Milk Commissions Held at Brooklyn, New York, June 1 and 3, 1917,* 164–69.

"Medical News." *Journal of the American Medical Association* 59 (1912): 659.

"Medical Progress." *Babyhood* 12 (April 1896): xviii-xix.

Meigs, Arthur V. "Proof that Human Milk Contains Only About One Per Cent. Casein; with Remarks upon Infant Feeding." *Archives of Pediatrics* 1 (1884): 216–41.

———. *Milk Analysis and Infant Feeding: A Practical Treatise on the Examination of Human and Cows' Milk, Cream, Condensed Milk, Etc., And Directions as to the Diet of Young Infants*. Philadelphia: P. Blakiston, Son & Co., 1885.

———. "The Artificial Feeding of Infants." *Transactions of the American Pediatric Society* 1 (1889): 71–85.

"Members of the American Association of Medical Milk Commissions." *Proceedings of the First Annual Session of the American Association of Medical Milk Commissions, Atlantic City, June 3, 1907,* 114–17.

Mellin's Food Advertisement. *Ladies' Home Journal* 19 (November 1902): 47.

Mellin's Food Company. *Diet after Weaning: A Manual for the Care and Feeding of*

Children between the Ages of One and Two Years. Boston: Mellin's Food Company, 1907.

———. *The Mellin's Food Method of Percentage Feeding.* Boston: Press of Mellin's Food Company, 1908.

Merki, Louis. "Milk Inspector's Report." *Report of the Department of Health of the City of Chicago for the Year 1877.* Chicago, 1878, 47–48.

"Methods of Milk Analysis." *Annual Report of the Department of Health of the City of Chicago for the Year Ended December 31, 1894.* Chicago, 1895, 177–79.

"Milk and Food Inspection." *Report of the Department of Health of the City of Chicago for the Year 1891.* Chicago, 1892, 41.

"The Milk Commission." *Chicago Medical Recorder* 25 (15 December 1903): 415.

"Milk Inspection and Dairy Inspection." *Report of the Department of Health of the City of Chicago for the Years 1907, 1908, 1909, 1910.* Chicago, 1911, 300–303.

"Milk Laboratory Exactness and Definite Results in Infant Feeding." *Chicago Medical Recorder* 9 (1895): lxiii.

"Milk—Magic Ration." *Housewives Magazine* 11 (May 1918): 19.

"The Milk Station at Hull House." *Hull-House Bulletin* 5 (Semi-Annual, 1902): 14.

Moak, Harris. "Certified vs. Pasteurized Milk." *Proceedings of the Ninth Annual Conference of The American Association of Medical Milk Commissions Held at San Francisco, California, June 17, 18, 19, 1915,* 138–50.

Moody, Helen Watterson. "The True Meaning of Motherhood." *Ladies' Home Journal* 16 (May 1899): 12.

Morse, John Lovett. "Directory for Wet Nurses." *Boston Medical and Surgical Journal* 179 (8 August 1918): 218.

"Mortality for 1872." *Report of the Board of Health of the City of Chicago for the Years 1870, 1871, 1872 and 1873.* Chicago, 1874, 87.

"Mothers' Breast Milk Station." *Report of the Board of Health for the Year 1940.* Chicago, 1941, 15.

"Mothers' Department. How to Nurse the Baby." *Arthur's Home Magazine* 49 (November 1881): 660.

"Mothers' Department." *Arthur's Home Magazine* 51 (January 1883): 53.

"Mother's Milk." *Hygeia* 3 (November 1925): 653–54.

"The Mother's Parliament." *Babyhood* 1 (July 1885): 246.

"The Mothers' Parliament." *Babyhood* 2 (March 1886a): 142–44.

"The Mother's Parliament." *Babyhood* 2 (April 1886b): 175–76.

"The Mother's Parliament." *Babyhood* 3 (October 1887): 383–88.

"The Mothers' Parliament," *Babyhood* 5 (June 1889): 218–19.

Nestlé's Food Advertisement. *American Motherhood* 38 (April 1914): 279.

"A New Effort for Care of Sick Babies." *Visiting Nurse Quarterly Magazine* (July 1906): 84.

Newell, Franklin S. "The Effect of Overcivilization on Maternity." *The American Journal of the Medical Sciences* 136 (1908): 532–41.

Newman, Henry Parker. "The Gynecological and Obstetrical Significance of Girlhood." *Chicago Medical Recorder* 20 (May 1901): 458–62.

"New Milk Laboratory Helps Babies." *The Presbyterian Hospital of the City of Chicago Bulletin* 28 (January 1936): 1. Rush-Presbyterian-St. Luke's Medical Center Archives, Chicago.

"New Milk Law in Effect: Better Quality Expected. Cans to Be Shipped from Country Sealed and the Responsibility for Impurities Will Rest on the Sender." *Chicago Tribune,* 1 May 1904, 7.

"News Items." *Chicago Medical Recorder* 17 (October 1899): 265.

"News Items." *Chicago Medical Recorder* 27 (December 1905): 871.

"News Items." *Chicago Medical Recorder* 30 (15 April 1908): 251–52.

"News Items." *Chicago Medical Recorder* 31 (15 June 1909): 75.

Newton, Niles Rumely, and Michael Newton. "Relationship of Ability to Breast Feed and Maternal Attitudes toward Breast Feeding." *Pediatrics* 5 (April 1950): 869–75.

Niblack, Henry C. "Public Health Point of View." *Illinois Medical Journal* 70 (1936): 259–61.

"Notes from a Talk Given by Mrs. Welles, President of the Auxiliary of Infant Welfare Society." *The Presbyterian Hospital Bulletin* (July 1915): 10.

"Nursery Problems." *Babyhood* 2 (June 1886a): 245–46.

"Nursery Problems." *Babyhood* 2 (July 1886b): 291.

"Nursery Problems." *Babyhood* 2 (November 1886c): 437.

"Nursery Problems." *Babyhood* 4 (March 1888): 126.

"Nursery Problems." *Babyhood* 5 (June 1889): 211.

"Nursery Problems." *The Mother's Nursery Guide* 9 (December 1892): 17.

Odd, W. H., et al. "Association between Breast Feeding and Asthma in 6 Year Old Children: Findings of a Prospective Birth Cohort Study." *British Medical Journal* 319 (25 September 1999): 815–19.

"Organization of Field Work." *Report and Handbook of the Department of Health of the City of Chicago for the Years 1911 to 1918 Inclusive.* Chicago, 1919, 564–65.

Ostheimer, Maurice. "Help the Mother Nurse Her Child: A Plea to Physicians Not to Begin Artificial Feeding Without First Trying to Help the Mother Maintain Her Milk Supply." *Journal of the American Medical Association* 53 (14 August 1909): 520–23.

Our Babies. Chicago: Chicago Department of Health, n.d., circa 1916, 1917.

"Our Milk Is Good." *Chicago Inter Ocean,* 24 December 1892, 9.

"Parents' Problems." *American Motherhood* 23 (August 1906): 199.

"Parents' Problems." *American Motherhood* 39 (2 August 1914): 133.

Park, Wm. H., and L. Emmett Holt. "Report upon the Results with Different Kinds of Pure and Impure Milk in Infant Feeding in Tenement Houses and Institutions of New York City: A Clinical and Bacteriological Study." *Archives of Pediatrics* 20 (December 1903): 881–909.

Parvin, Theophilus. "Diarrhoea in Children." *Archives of Pediatrics* 1 (April 1884): 242–46.

Pearson, Raymond A. "Development of Dairy Hygiene." *Proceedings of the Second Annual Session of the American Association of Medical Milk Commissions, Chicago, June 1, 1908,* 70–71.

Penfield, Geraldine K. "The Care of an Infant, from a Mother's Standpoint." *Arthur's Home Magazine* 64 (December 1894): 995.

Peterson, Christine E., and Julie DaVanzo. "Why Are Teenagers in the United States Less Likely to Breast-Feed Than Older Women?" *Demography* 29 (August 1992): 431–50.

Philbin, Edith M. "Collection and Dispensing of Breast Milk." *American Journal of Nursing* 26 (February 1926): 101–4.

Phillips, Wilbur C. "Infants' Milk Depots and Infant Mortality." *American Association for the Study and Prevention of Infant Mortality: Transactions of the First Annual Meeting, Johns Hopkins University, Baltimore, November 9–11, 1910.* New York: Arno Press, 1974, 77–88.

Pisek, Godfrey Roger. "Fallacious Standards Employed in Artificial Infant Feeding." *Journal of the American Medical Association* 51 (10 October 1908): 1214–16.

Poncher, H. G. "Relation to Supplementary Feeding in the Newborn." *Illinois Medical Journal* 70 (1936): 258–61.

Pooler, H. A. "The Milk Supply of Large Cities, and the Improper Mode in Which It Is Conducted." *The Medical News* 49 (23 October 1886): 470–72.

Potter, Nathaniel. "Observations on Cholera Infantum." *Baltimore Medical and Surgical Journal and Review* (October 1833): 104–25.

"The Preservation of Milk." *Babyhood* 3 (June 1897): 226–27.

"Principal Health Ordinances Passed since 1910." *Report and Handbook of the Department of Health of the City of Chicago for the Years 1911–1918 Inclusive.* Chicago, 1919, 301.

Pryor, Karen. *Nursing Your Baby.* New York: Pocket Books, 1973.

"Quarterly Report—Social Service Work April–July." *The Presbyterian Hospital of the City of Chicago Bulletin* (July 1916): 21. Rush-Presbyterian-St. Luke's Medical Center Archives, Chicago.

"Questions and Answers." *Hygeia* 2 (March 1924): 201.

Radetsky, Peter. "Got Cancer Killers." *Discover* 20 (June 1999): 70–75.

Raisler, Jeanne, et al. "Breast-Feeding and Infant Illness: A Dose-Response Relationship?" *American Journal of Public Health* 89 (January 1999): 25–30.

Rassin, D. K., et al. "Incidence of Breastfeeding in a Low Socioeconomic Group of Mothers in the United States: Ethnic Patterns." *Pediatrics* 73 (1984): 132.

Ravenel, Mazyck P. "The Transmission of Tuberculosis through Milk." *Proceedings of the Second Annual Session of The American Association of Medical Milk Commissions, Chicago, June 1, 1908,* 56–58.

Reilly, F. W. "Hot Weather Care of Infants and Young Children." *Biennial Report of the Department of Health of the City of Chicago Being for the Years 1895 and 1896.* Chicago, 1897, 112–16.

"Report of Health Department Infant Welfare Stations, 1923–1925 Inclusive." *Report of the Department of Health of the City of Chicago for the Years 1923, 1924, 1925.* Chicago, 1926, 230–31.

"Report of the Health Department Laboratories for 1905." *Biennial Report of the Department of Health of the City of Chicago for the Years 1904–1905.* Chicago, 1906, 6.

"Report of the Municipal Laboratory: 1894." *Annual Report of the Department of*

Health of the City of Chicago for the Year Ended December 31, 1894. Chicago, 1895, 145–46.

"Report of the Progress in the Prevention of Needless Neonatal Deaths." *Report of the Chicago Health Department for the Year 1951*. Chicago, 1952, 152.

"Report of the Sanitary Milk Commission of Chicago." *Bulletin Chicago School of Sanitary Instruction* 10 (28 September 1907): 5–7.

"Requirement in Regard to Refrigeration of Milk in Transit Passed Upon." *Report and Handbook of the Department of Health of the City of Chicago for the Years 1911 to 1918 Inclusive*. Chicago, 1919, 308–12.

Reynolds, Arthur R. "Speech by Arthur R. Reynolds." *Fifth Annual Report of The Visiting Nurse Association of Chicago*, 1895, 25–26.

Riordan, Jan, and Kathleen G. Auerbach. *Breastfeeding and Human Lactation*. Sudbury, MA: Jones and Bartlett Publishers, 1999.

Robertson, John Dill. "Foreword." *Report and Handbook of the Department of Health of the City of Chicago for the Years 1911–1918 Inclusive*. Chicago, 1919, xiii–xxxviii.

Rohtge, M. "Report from the Children's Ward." *The Presbyterian Hospital of the City of Chicago Bulletin* (July 1914): 11. Rush-Presbyterian-St. Luke's Medical Center Archives.

Rorer, S. T. "Milk: Its Use and Abuse." *Ladies' Home Journal* 16 (May 1899): 34.

Ross Laboratories. *Ross Laboratories Mothers' Surveys, Recent Trends in Breast Feeding*, Columbus, OH: Ross Laboratories, 1991.

Rotch, Thomas Morgan. "The Management of Human Breast-Milk in Cases of Difficult Infantile Digestion." *Transactions of the American Pediatric Society* 2 (1890): 88–100.

———. "The Value of Milk Laboratories for the Advancement of Our Knowledge of Artificial Feeding." *Archives of Pediatrics* 10 (February 1893): 97–111.

———. *Pediatrics: The Hygienic and Medical Treatment of Children*. Philadelphia: J. B. Lippincott Company, 1896.

———. "Some Considerations Regarding Substitute Feeding during the First Year." *Transactions of the American Pediatric Society* 16 (1904): 41–55.

———. "An Historical Sketch of the Development of Percentage Feeding." *New York Medical Journal* 85 (23 March 1907): 532–37.

———. "Modern Laboratory Feeding and the Wide Range of Resources Which It Provides." *Transactions of the American Pediatric Society* 20 (1908): 105–18.

———. "The Cardinal Principles for the Successful Feeding of Infants." *Interstate Medical Journal* 17 (1910): 305–15.

"Rules for the Nurses of the Visiting Nurse Association." *The Visiting Nurse Association of Chicago Eleventh Annual Report*, 1901, 10–12.

Ryan, Alan S. "The Resurgence of Breastfeeding in the United States." *Pediatrics* 99 (4 April 1997). Available at: <http://www.pediatrics.org/cgi/content/full/99/4/e12>.

Ryan, Alan S., et al. "The Recent Decline in Breastfeeding." *Pediatrics* (1991): 873–74.

"Scarcely Any Pure Milk." *Chicago Daily News*, 1 September 1892, 2.

"Scoring of Sanitary Conditions." *Report and Handbook of the Department of Health of the City of Chicago for the Years 1911 to 1918 Inclusive.* Chicago, 1919, 580–83.

Scovil, Elisabeth Robinson. "The Truth about Baby Foods." *Ladies' Home Journal* 19 (August 1902): 26.

Sears, Roebuck and Co. *1902 Edition of the Sears, Roebuck Catalogue.* New York: Bounty Books, 1969.

"Second Session." *Proceedings of the Second Annual Session of the American Association of Medical Milk Commissions, Chicago, June 1, 1908,* 38.

Sedgwick, Julius Parker "The Care of Certified Milk Immediately after Delivery." *Proceedings of the Ninth Annual Conference of the American Association of Medical Milk Commissions Held at San Francisco, California, June 17, 18, 19, 1915,* 161–75.

———. "Establishment, Maintenance, and Reinstitution of Breast Feeding." *Journal of the American Medical Association* 69 (11 August 1917): 417–18.

———. "A Preliminary Report of the Study of Breast Feeding in Minneapolis." *Transactions of the American Pediatric Society* 32 (1920): 279–91.

Shaw, Henry L.K., and Frank J. Williams. "Acid Milk in Infant Feeding." *Transactions of the American Pediatric Society* 34 (1922): 46–56.

Sheard, Nancy F. "Breastfeeding Protects against Otitis Media." *Nutrition Reviews* 51 (September 1993): 275–77.

Short, R. V. "What the Breast Does for the Baby, and What the Baby Does for the Breast." *The Australian and New Zealand Journal of Obstetrics and Gynaecology* 34 (June 1994): 262–64.

Shortridge, K. F., et al. "Protective Potential of Colostrum and Early Milk against Prospective Influenza Viruses." *Journal of Tropical Pediatrics* 36 (April 1990): 94–95.

Shu, Xiao Ou, et al. "Breastfeeding and Risk of Childhood Acute Leukemia." *Journal of the National Cancer Institute* 91 (20 October 1999): 1765–72.

"'Six Months Law' Has Good Results." *Hygeia* 3 (July 1925): 413.

"Slaughter of the Innocents." *Chicago Tribune,* 23 August 1892, 6.

Smith, J. Lewis. "Recent Improvements in Infant Feeding." *Transactions of the American Pediatric Society* 1 (1889): 86–94.

Snedeker, Lendon. "Some Thoughts on Breast Feeding." *Public Health Nursing* 27 (December 1935): 648–51.

Snyder, J. Ross. "The Breast Milk Problem." *Journal of the American Medical Association* 51 (10 October 1908): 1212–14.

"Social Service." *The Presbyterian Hospital Bulletin* (April 1914): 7–9.

"Social Service Report." *Presbyterian Hospital Bulletin* (July 1915a): 6.

"Social Service Report." *The Presbyterian Hospital Bulletin* (October 1915b): 12.

"Social Service Report." *The Presbyterian Hospital Bulletin* (January 1916): 9.

"Social Service Report April–June." *The Presbyterian Hospital Bulletin* (July 1917): 15.

"Social Service Report July–September." *The Presbyterian Hospital Bulletin* (October 1918): 17–19.

"Social Service Report—October 1916." *The Presbyterian Hospital Bulletin* (October 1916): 22.

"Society Proceedings." *Chicago Medical Recorder* 1 (July 1891): 473–74.

"Some General Rules in the Maternity Work Carried On by the Chicago Nurse Association." *Visiting Nurse Quarterly Magazine* (October 1905): 20.

Southworth, Thomas S. "The Improvement of Breast-Milk and the Prolongation of Lactation." *Journal of the American Medical Association* 39 (2 August 1902): 249–52.

———. "High Fat Percentages in Infant Feeding." *Journal of the American Medical Association* 51 (10 October 1908): 1219–24.

Southworth, Thomas S., and Oscar M. Schloss. "The Hard Curds of Infant Stools; Their Origin, Nature and Transformation." *Transactions of the American Pediatric Society* 20 (1908): 119–27.

"State of Chicago's Health." *Bulletin Chicago School of Sanitary Instruction* 12 (10 July 1909): 2.

"State of Chicago's Health." *Bulletin Chicago School of Sanitary Instruction* 13 (26 March 1910a): 2–5.

"State of Chicago's Health." *Bulletin Chicago School of Sanitary Instruction* 13 (14 May 1910b): 5.

"State of Chicago's Health." *Bulletin Chicago School of Sanitary Instruction* 13 (21 May 1910c): 2.

"State of Chicago's Health, Week Ended September 12, 1908." *Bulletin Chicago School of Sanitary Instruction* 11 (12 September 1908): 2–4.

"State of Chicago's Health, Week Ended July 17, 1909." *Bulletin Chicago School of Sanitary Instruction* 12 (17 July 1909): 2.

"State of Chicago's Health, Week Ended July 9, 1910." *Bulletin Chicago School of Sanitary Instruction* 13 (9 July 1910a): 2.

"State of Chicago's Health, Week Ended August 13, 1910." *Bulletin Chicago School of Sanitary Instruction* 13 (13 August 1910b): 3–4.

Stephens, Elizabeth L. "Sacredness and Responsibility of Motherhood." *New Crusade* (February 1897): 272.

"Sterilized Milk Station." *Hull-House Bulletin* 6 (Mid-Winter, 1903–4): 15.

Stickel, W. J. "A Day Back of the Yards." *Visiting Nurse Quarterly Magazine* (July 1906): 80–81.

Stitt, Pauline George. "Breast Feeding." *Pediatric Clinics of North America* 8 (May 1961): 627–37.

"Stop the Bogus Milk Traffic." *Chicago Tribune,* 23 September 1892, 4.

"Summer Infant Welfare Field Work—1919." *Report of the Department of Health of the City of Chicago for the Years 1919, 1920 and 1921.* Chicago, 1922, 128.

"Summer Milk Stations in New York." *Archives of Pediatrics* 28 (July 1911): 561–62.

"Syllabus of Courses Given to Little Mothers' Clubs." *Report and Handbook of the Department of Health of the City of Chicago for the Years 1911–1918 Inclusive.* Chicago, 1919, 593–95.

"Table LXXI. Infant Welfare Field Work." *Report and Handbook of the Department of*

Health of the City of Chicago for the Years 1911 to 1918 Inclusive. Chicago, 1919, 567.

Talbot, Fritz B. "A Directory for Wet-Nurses: Its Experiences for Twelve Months." *Journal of the American Medical Association* 56 (10 June 1911): 1715–17.

———. "The Wet-Nurse Problem." *National Conference on Infant Mortality, Report of the Proceedings,* 1913, 324–31.

———. "Directory for Wetnurses." *Boston Medical and Surgical Journal* 196 (21 April 1927): 653–54.

———. "An Organization for Supplying Human Milk." *New England Journal of Medicine* 199 (27 September 1928): 610–11.

"Talks with the Doctor." *American Motherhood* 24 (May 1907): 332.

Taylor, J. Madison. "The Curative Powers in Human Milk." In American Academy of Medicine, *Prevention of Infant Mortality: Being the Papers and Discussions of a Conference Held at New Haven, Conn., November 11, 12, 1909,* 66–73.

Tenney, Eleanor F. "Secretary's Report to the Visiting Nurse Association of Chicago and the Staff of Nurses." *Nineteenth Annual Report The Visiting Nurse Association of Chicago For Year Ending December 31, 1908,* 1909, 16.

"Test the Milk." *Bulletin Chicago School of Sanitary Instruction* 10 (12 October 1907): 5.

"The Theory and Practice of Visiting Nursing, and the Attitude of the Profession towards It." *The American Journal of Nursing* 6 (July 1906): 821–23.

"They Water and Color the Milk." *Chicago Tribune,* 9 August 1894, 7.

Tobey, James A. "Know Your Foods: The Part Milks Plays in Your Diet as Considered by the Nutritionist." *Modern Priscilla,* 42 (October 1928): 25.

———. "A New Foster-Mother." *Hygeia* (1929): 1110–12.

Tonks, Eliza, and Elisabeth Shirley Enochs. "Development of Breastfeeding Education in the United States." *The Trained Nurse and Hospital Review* 87 (1931): 36–41.

"To Secure Pure Milk What Is Done in Chicago to Prevent Adulteration." *Chicago Tribune,* 21 July 1894, 14.

Tow, Abraham. "The Rationale of Breast Feeding: A Modern Concept." *Hygeia* 12 (1934): 406–8.

Tuley, Henry Enos. "Legislation as a Factor in the Production of Clean Milk." *Proceedings of the Second Annual Session of the American Association of Medical Milk Commissions, Chicago, June 1, 1908,* 65–69.

"Twenty Dairy Suggestions." *Bulletin Chicago School of Sanitary Instruction* 14 (19 August 1911): 234–35.

"United Report of the Woman's Auxiliary Board of the Presbyterian Hospital of Chicago for 1917." *The Presbyterian Hospital of the City of Chicago Bulletin* (January 1918): 27. Rush-Presbyterian-St. Luke's Medical Center Archives, Chicago.

U.S. Department of Labor Children's Bureau. *Infant Care.* Washington, D.C.: GPO, 1927.

Van Derslice, James Warren. "Infant Feedings with Especial Reference to the Use of Citrate of Soda." *Chicago Medical Recorder* 29 (August 1907): 471–79.

———. "Gastro-Intestinal Disorders of Infancy and Early Childhood." *Illinois Medical Journal* 19 (January 1911): 23–34.

———. "The Making of a Milk Commission." *Proceedings of the Ninth Annual Con-*

ference of the American Association of Medical Milk Commissions Held at San Francisco, California, June 17, 18, 19, 1915, 167–75.

Van Doozer, B. "Letter to Dr. Ben C. Miller, Sanitary Superintendent Chicago Health Department, 1 January 1876." *Report of the Board of Health of the City of Chicago, for the Years 1874 and 1875.* Chicago, 1876, 69–70.

Vaughan, Victor C. "Summer Diarrhea of Infants." *Hygeia* 1 (June 1923): 145–48.

Veeder, Borden S. "Periods in the Life of the American Pediatric Society: Infancy." *Transactions of the American Pediatric Society* 50 (1938): 49–55.

Verdon, Lexie. "When Breast-Feeding Fails." *The Washington Post,* 12 June 2000.

Vinton, Maria M. "Baby's First Month." *Mother's Nursery Guide* 9 (February 1893): 69.

"Visiting Nurse." *Hull House Bulletin* 1 (January 1896).

"Visiting Nurses' Association of Chicago." *American Journal of Nursing* 1 (1901): 882–84.

"Visiting of New-Born Babies." *Report of the Department of Health of the City of Chicago for the Years 1923, 1924 and 1925.* Chicago, 1926, 260–61.

"Vital Statistics." *Biennial Report of the Department of Health of the City of Chicago for the Years 1904–1905.* Chicago, 1906, 259–345.

"Vital Statistics of Chicago." *Biennial Report of the Department of Health of the City of Chicago for the Years 1897 and 1898.* Chicago, 1899, 251–67.

"Vital Statistics of Chicago: 1893." *Annual Report of the Department of Health of the City of Chicago for the Year Ended December 31, 1893.* Chicago, 1894, 41–73.

von Meysenbug, Ludo. "Breast Feeding with Especial Reference to Some of Its Problems." *New Orleans Medical and Surgical Journal* 87 (1934–35): 738–43.

Wallace, Emma Gary. "The Care and Feeding of Children." *American Motherhood* 38 (3 March 1914): 181.

Walls, Frank X. "Food Disorders in Infancy." *The Quarterly Bulletin of the Northwestern Medical School* 11 (June 1909): 69–81.

Walker, Jerome. "Is Nursing by the Mother to Be Encouraged?" *The Archives of Pediatrics* 2 (January 1885): 1–10.

Watson, William T. "A Plea for a Square Deal for the Wet Nurse." *Journal of the American Medical Association* 47 (8 December 1906): 1909–11.

Waugh, William F. "Treatment of Summer Complaint." *Chicago Medical Recorder* 7 (August 1894): 102–6.

Wells, Helen Raymond. "Suggestions for the Young Mother." *American Motherhood* 24 (May 1907): 295.

Wentworth, A. H. "The Importance of Milk Analysis in Infant Feeding." *Boston Medical and Surgical Journal* 146 (26 June 1902a): 683–86.

———. "The Importance of Milk Analysis in Infant Feeding." *Boston Medical and Surgical Journal* 147 (3 July 1902b): 5–10.

Westphal, Mary E. "Superintendent's Report." *Fifty-third Annual Report of The Visiting Nurse Association of Chicago,* 1942, 6–11.

———. "Superintendent's Report." *Sixty-first Annual Report of The Visiting Nurse Association of Chicago,* 1950, 18–24.

Westcott, Thompson S. "Modified Wet Nursing." *Transactions of the American Pediatric Society* 18 (1906): 15–22.

————. "Modified Wet Nursing." *Archives of Pediatrics* 24 (March 1907): 192–98.

"What Other Women Have Found Out." *Ladies' Home Journal* 24 (June 1907): 28.

Whitman, Ross C. "Office Examination of Human and Cow's Milk." *Chicago Medical Recorder* 27 (July 1905): 487–90.

Wieman, Constance M., et al. "Racial/ethnic Differences in the Decisions to Breast-feed among Adolescent Mothers." *Pediatrics* 101 (June 1998). Available at: <http://www.pediatrics.org/cgi/content/full/101/6/e11>

Wile, Ira S. "Educational Responsibilities of a Milk Depot." *Prevention of Infant Mortality, Being the Papers and Discussions of a Conference Held at New Haven, Connecticut, November 11, 12, 1909,* 139–53.

"Will Have Pure Milk." *The Chicago Evening Post,* 28 September 1892, 1.

"Will Sue Milkman Ryan." *The Chicago Evening Post,* 26 September 1892, 1.

Winters, Joseph Edcil. "The Relative Influences of Maternal and Wet-Nursing on Mother and Child." *The Medical Record: A Weekly Journal of Medicine and Surgery* 30 (6 November 1886): 505–14.

Wolcott, Elsie P. *Use and Cost of Ice in Families with Children.* Chicago, 1925.

Wold, Agnes E., and Lars Å. Hanson. "Defense Factors in Human Milk." *Current Opinion in Gastroenterology* 10 (November 1994): 652–58.

Wood, Mrs. Ira Couch. "Address of Mrs. Ira Couch Wood, President of the Board of the Illinois Training School for Nurses." *The Presbyterian Hospital of the City of Chicago Bulletin* (April 1915): 21, Rush-Presbyterian-St. Luke's Hospital Medical Center Archives, Chicago.

Wood-Allen, Mary. "Baby's Firsts." *Mother's Friend* (September 1895): 13–16.

————. "Physical Nurture." *New Crusade* (October 1896): 180–81.

————. "Parents' Problems." *American Motherhood* 24 (February 1907): 129.

Yale, Leroy M. "Summer Complaint." *Babyhood* 1 (June 1885): 203.

————. "Private Interests and Public Duty in Guarding the Milk Supply." *The Mother's Nursery Guide* 9 (February 1893): 74.

————. "The Meaning of Clean Milk." *Babyhood* 14 (July 1898): 183–85.

"The Youngest Member of the Family." *Arthur's Home Magazine* 59 (February 1889): 107.

Secondary Sources

Apple, Rima D. "'To Be Used Only under the Direction of a Physician': Commercial Infant Feeding and Medical Practice, 1870–1940." *Bulletin of the History of Medicine* 54 (Fall 1980): 402–17.

————. *Mothers and Medicine: A Social History of Infant Feeding, 1890–1950.* Madison: University of Wisconsin Press, 1987.

————. "The Medicalization of Infant Feeding in the United States and New Zealand: Two Countries, One Experience." *Journal of Human Lactation* 10 (1994): 31–37.

————. "Constructing Mothers: Scientific Motherhood in the Nineteenth and Twentieth Centuries." *Social History of Medicine* (1995): 161–78.

————. *Vitamania: Vitamins in American Culture.* New Brunswick: Rutgers University Press, 1996.

Baker, Jeffrey P. *The Machine in the Nursery: Incubator Technology and the Origins of Newborn Intensive Care.* Baltimore: Johns Hopkins University Press, 1996.

Beaver, M. W. "Population, Infant Mortality and Milk." *Population Studies* 27 (July 1973): 243–54.

Bell, Martin L. *A Portrait of Progress: A Business History of the Pet Milk Company from 1885–1960.* St. Louis: Pet Milk Company, 1962.

Berkow, Ira. *Maxwell Street: Survival in a Bazaar.* New York: Doubleday & Company, 1977.

Blum, Linda M. *At the Breast: Ideologies of Breastfeeding and Motherhood in the Contemporary United States.* Boston: Beacon Press, 1999.

Bonner, Thomas Neville. *Medicine in Chicago, 1850–1950: A Chapter in the Social and Scientific Development of a City.* Urbana: University of Illinois Press, 1991.

Brodie, Janet Farrell. *Contraception and Abortion in Nineteenth-Century America.* Ithaca: Cornell University Press, 1994.

Brosco, Jeffrey P. "The Early History of the Infant Mortality Rate in America: 'A Reflection upon the Past and a Prophecy of the Future.'" *Pediatrics* 103 (February 1999): 478–85.

Brumberg, Joan Jacobs. "From Psychiatric Syndrome to 'Communicable' Disease: The Case of Anorexia Nervosa." In *Framing Disease: Studies in Cultural History,* ed. Charles E. Rosenberg and Janet Golden, 134–54. New Brunswick: Rutgers University Press, 1992.

————. *The Body Project: An Intimate History of American Girls.* New York: Random House, 1997.

Buder, Stanley. *Pullman: An Experiment in Industrial Order and Community Planning, 1880–1930.* New York: Oxford University Press, 1967.

Caulfield, Ernest. "Infant Feeding in Colonial America." *The Journal of Pediatrics* 41 (December 1952): 673–87.

Cheney, Rose A. "Seasonal Aspects of Infant and Childhood Mortality: Philadelphia, 1865–1920." *Journal of Interdisciplinary History* 14 (Winter 1984): 561–85.

Cone, Thomas. *200 Years of Feeding Infants in America.* Columbus, OH: Ross Laboratories, 1976.

Crosby, Alfred W. *Ecological Imperialism: The Biological Expansion of Europe, 900–1900.* Cambridge: Cambridge University Press, 1986.

Curry, Lynne. *Modern Mothers in the Heartland: Gender, Health, and Progress in Illinois, 1900–1930.* Columbus: Ohio State University Press, 1999.

Damon-Moore, Helen. *Magazines for the Millions: Gender and Commerce in the "Ladies' Home Journal" and the "Saturday Evening Post," 1880–1910.* Albany: State University of New York Press, 1994.

D'Emilio, John, and Estelle B. Freedman. *Intimate Matters: A History of Sexuality in America.* Chicago: University of Chicago Press, 1997.

Devitt, Neal. "The Transition from Home to Hospital Birth in the United States, 1930–1960." *Birth and the Family Journal* (1977): 47–58.

Duffy, John. "Social Impact of Disease in the Late Nineteenth Century." *Bulletin of the New York Academy of Medicine* 47 (1971): 797–811.

———. *The Sanitarians: A History of American Public Health.* Urbana: University of Illinois Press, 1990.

Duis, Perry R. *Challenging Chicago: Coping with Everyday Life, 1837–1920.* Urbana: University of Illinois Press, 1998.

Fildes, Valerie. *Wet Nursing: A History from Antiquity to the Present.* New York: Basil Blackwell, 1988.

Golden, Janet. "Trouble in the Nursery: Physicians, Families, and Wet Nurses at the End of the Nineteenth Century." In *"To Toil the Livelong Day": America's Women at Work, 1780–1980,* ed. Carol Groneman and Mary Beth Norton, 125–137. Ithaca: Cornell University Press, 1987.

———. "From Wet Nurse Directory to Milk Bank: The Delivery of Human Milk in Boston, 1909–1927." *Bulletin of the History of Medicine* 62 (Winter 1988), 589–605.

———. *A Social History of Wet Nursing in America: From Breast to Bottle.* Cambridge: Cambridge University Press, 1996; Columbus: Ohio State University Press, 2001.

Gordon, Linda. *Woman's Body, Woman's Right: Birth Control in America.* New York: Penguin Books, 1990.

Gordon, Sarah, ed. *All Our Lives: A Centennial History of Michael Reese Hospital and Medical Center 1881–1891.* Chicago: Michael Reese Hospital and Medical Center, 1981.

Grant, Julia. *Raising Baby by the Book: The Education of American Mothers.* New Haven: Yale University Press, 1998.

Halpern, Sydney A. *American Pediatrics: The Social Dynamics of Professionalism, 1880–1908.* Berkeley: University of California Press, 1988.

Hammonds, Evelynn Maxine. *Childhood's Deadly Scourge: The Campaign to Control Diphtheria in New York City, 1880–1930.* Baltimore: Johns Hopkins University Press, 1999.

Heer, Jean. *World Events, 1866–1966: The First Hundred Years of Nestlé.* Switzerland: Chateau de Glerolles-Rivaz, 1966.

Holli, Melvin G. "The Great War Sinks Chicago's German *Kultur.*" In *Ethnic Chicago,* Melvin G. Holli and Peter d'A. Jones, ed. Grand Rapids: William B. Eerdman's, 1984.

Hoy, Suellen M. *Chasing Dirt: The American Pursuit of Cleanliness.* New York: Oxford University Press, 1995.

Jones, Kathleen W. "Sentiment and Science: The Late Nineteenth Century Pediatrician as Mother's Adviser." *Journal of Social History* 17 (Fall 1983): 79–96.

Klaus, Alisa. *Every Child a Lion: The Origins of Maternal and Infant Health Policy in the United States and France, 1890–1920.* Ithaca: Cornell University Press, 1993.

Knodel, John. *Demographic Behavior in the Past.* Cambridge: Cambridge University Press, 1988.

Koven, Seth, and Sonya Michel. "Womanly Duties, Maternalist Politics and the Origins of Welfare States in France, Germany, Great Britain, and the United States, 1880–1920." *American Historical Review* 95 (October 1990): 1076–1108.

Ladd-Taylor, Molly. *Raising a Baby the Government Way: Mothers' Letters to the Children's Bureau, 1915–1932*. New Brunswick: Rutgers University Press, 1986.

———. "'Grannies' and 'Spinsters': Midwife Education under the Sheppard-Towner Act." *Journal of Social History* 22 (Winter 1988): 255–75.

———. "'My Work Came Out of Agony and Grief': Mothers and the Making of the Sheppard-Towner Act." In *Mothers of a New World: Maternalist Politics and the Origins of Welfare States*, ed. Seth Koven and Sonya Michel, 321–42. New York: Routledge, 1993.

———. *Mother-Work: Women, Child Welfare, and the State, 1890–1930*. Urbana: University of Illinois Press, 1994.

Leavitt, Judith Walzer. *Brought to Bed: Childbearing in America, 1750–1950*. New York: Oxford University Press, 1986.

———. "Joseph B. DeLee and the Practice of Preventive Obstetrics." *American Journal of Public Health* 78 (October 1988): 1353–61.

———. *The Healthiest City: Milwaukee and the Politics of Health Reform*. Madison: University of Wisconsin Press, 1996a.

———. *Typhoid Mary: Captive to the Public's Health*. Boston: Beacon Press, 1996b.

Levenstein, Harvey. "'Best for Babies' or 'Preventable Infanticide'? The Controversy over Artificial Feeding of Infants in America, 1880–1920." *The Journal of American History* 70 (June 1983): 75–94.

Lindenmeyer, Kriste. "Saving Mothers and Babies: The Sheppard-Towner Act in Ohio, 1921–1929." *Ohio History* 99 (Summer/Autumn 1990): 105–34.

———. *"A Right to Childhood": The U.S. Children's Bureau and Child Welfare, 1912–46*. Urbana: University of Illinois Press, 1997.

Marion, John Francis. *The Fine Old House*. Philadelphia: SmithKline Corporation, 1980.

Mayer, Harold M., and Richard C. Wade. *Chicago: Growth of a Metropolis*. Chicago: University of Chicago Press, 1969.

McCarthy, Kathleen D. *Noblesse Oblige: Charity and Cultural Philanthropy in Chicago, 1849–1929*. Chicago: University of Chicago Press, 1982.

McClary, Andrew. "Germs Are Everywhere: The Germ Threat as Seen in Magazine Articles, 1890–1920." *Journal of American Culture* 3 (Spring 1980): 33–46.

Meckel, Richard A. *Save the Babies: American Public Health Reform and the Prevention of Infant Mortality, 1850–1929*. Baltimore: Johns Hopkins University Press, 1990.

Melvin, Patricia Mooney. "Milk to Motherhood: The New York Milk Committee and the Beginning of Well-Child Programs." *Mid-America* 65 (October 1983): 111–34.

Millard, Ann V. "The Place of the Clock in Pediatric Advice: Rationales, Cultural Themes, and Impediments to Breastfeeding." *Social Science and Medicine* 31 (1990): 211–21.

Miller, Donald L. *City of the Century: The Epic of Chicago and the Making of America*. New York: Simon & Schuster, 1996.

Miller, Julie. "To Stop the Slaughter of the Babies: Nathan Straus and the Drive for Pasteurized Milk, 1893–1920." *New York History* 74 (1993): 159–84.

Pernick, Martin. *The Black Stork: Eugenics and the Death of "Defective" Babies in American Medicine and Motion Pictures since 1915.* New York: Oxford University Press, 1996.

———. "Eugenics and Public Health in American History." *American Journal of Public Health* 87 (November 1997): 1767–72.

Preston, Samuel H., and Michael R. Haines. *Fatal Years: Child Mortality in Late Nineteenth-Century America.* Princeton: Princeton University Press, 1991.

Rodkin, Dennis. "Mothers Know Best Forty Years Ago, the Founders of La Leche League Proved It." *Chicago Tribune Magazine,* 20 October 1996, 20–22.

Rosen, George. *A History of Public Health.* Baltimore: Johns Hopkins University Press, 1993.

Rosenberg, Charles E. *The Cholera Years: The United States in 1832, 1849, and 1866.* Chicago: University of Chicago Press, 1962.

———. "Social Class and Medical Care in 19th-Century America: The Rise and Fall of the Dispensary." *Journal of the History of Medicine and Allied Sciences* 29 (1974): 32–54.

———. "Pathologies of Progress: The Idea of Civilization as Risk." *Bulletin of the History of Medicine* 72 (Winter 1998): 714–30.

Rothman, Sheila M. *Living in the Shadow of Death: Tuberculosis and the Social Experience of Illness in American History.* New York: Basic Books, 1994.

Salmon, Marylynn. "The Cultural Significance of Breastfeeding and Infant Care in Early Modern England and America." *Journal of Social History* 28 (Winter 1994): 247–69.

Scanlon, Jennifer. *Inarticulate Longings: "The Ladies' Home Journal," Gender, and the Promises of Consumer Culture.* New York: Routledge, 1995.

Schnucker, R. V. "The English Puritans and Pregnancy, Delivery and Breast Feeding." *History of Childhood Quarterly* 1 (Spring 1974): 637–58.

Sherwood, Joan. "Treating Syphilis: The Wetnurse as Technology in an Eighteenth-Century Parisian Hospital." *Journal of the History of Medicine and Allied Sciences* 50 (July 1995): 315–39.

Smith-Rosenberg, Carroll. *Disorderly Conduct: Visions of Gender in Victorian America.* New York: Oxford University Press, 1985.

Sullivan-Fowler, Micaela. "Doubtful Theories, Drastic Therapies: Autointoxication and Faddism in the Late Nineteenth and Early Twentieth Centuries." *Journal of the History of Medicine and Allied Sciences* 50 (July 1995): 364–90.

Sussman, George D. *Selling Mother's Milk: The Wet-Nursing Business in France, 1715–1914.* Urbana: University of Illinois Press, 1982.

Theriot, Nancy M. *Mothers and Daughters in Nineteenth-Century America: The Biosocial Construction of Femininity.* Lexington: The University Press of Kentucky, 1996.

Tomes, Nancy. "The Private Side of Public Health: Sanitary Science, Domestic Hygiene, and the Germ Theory, 1870–1900." *Bulletin of the History of Medicine* 64 (1990): 509–39.

————. *The Gospel of Germs: Men, Women, and the Microbe in American Life*. Cambridge, MA: Harvard University Press, 1998.

Treckel, Paula A. "Breastfeeding and Maternal Sexuality in Colonial America." *Journal of Interdisciplinary History* 20 (Summer 1989): 25–51.

Tully, Julia, and Kathryn G. Dewey. "Private Fears, Global Loss: A Cross-Cultural Study of the Insufficient Milk Syndrome." *Medical Anthropology* 9 (Summer 1985): 225–43.

Ulrich, Laurel Thatcher. *A Midwife's Tale: The Life of Martha Ballard, Based on Her Diary, 1785–1812*. New York: Vintage Books, 1990.

Viner, Russell. "Politics, Power, and Pediatrics." *The Lancet* 353 (16 January 1999): 232–34.

Waserman, Manfred J. "Henry L. Coit and the Certified Milk Movement in the Development of Modern Pediatrics." *Bulletin of the History of Medicine* (July–August 1972): 359–90.

Watkins, Susan Cotts. "Markets, States, Nations, and Bedrooms in Western Europe, 1870–1960." In *Macro-Micro Linkages in Sociology,* ed. Joan Huber, 263–79. Newbury Park, CA: Sage Publications, 1991.

Weaver, John D. *Carnation: The First 75 Years, 1899–1974*. Los Angeles: Anderson, Ritchie & Simon, 1974.

Weiner, Lynn Y. "Reconstructing Motherhood: The La Leche League in Postwar America." *The Journal of American History* (March 1994): 1357–81.

Weiss, Nancy Pottishman. "The Mother-Child Dyad Revisited: Perceptions of Mothers and Children in Twentieth Century Child-Rearing Manuals." *Journal of Social Issues* 34 (1978): 29–45.

White, Cynthia L. *Women's Magazines, 1693–1968*. London: Michael Joseph, 1970.

Wolf, Jacqueline H. "'Let Us Have More Mother-Fed Babies': Early Twentieth-Century Breastfeeding Campaigns in Chicago and Minneapolis." *Journal of Human Lactation* 15 (June 1999): 1–5.

————. "The Social and Medical Construction of Lactation Pathology." *Women and Health* 30 (2000): 93–109.

Zelizer, Viviana A. *Pricing the Priceless Child: The Changing Social Value of Children*. New York: Basic Books, 1985.

Zuckerman, Mary Ellen. *A History of Popular Women's Magazines in the United States, 1792–1995*. Westport, CT: Greenwood Press, 1998.

Index

Chicago and North Western Railroad: and cows' milk, refrigeration of, 66

Chicago Board of Health. *See* Chicago Department of Health

Chicago Board of Health Mothers' Breast Milk Station, xvii, 133, 153–55, 156. *See also* human milk, stations

Chicago Department of Health, 121–30; and artificial food, 17, 40, 129–30, 166, 190, 194; and bovine tuberculosis, 61–62, 63; and breastfeeding, xv, xvi, 1, 16, 17–18, 20, 46, 104, 105, 122, 126–30, 190–91, 195; and breastfeeding rates, xv, 17; and Herman Bundesen, xvi, 128, 129, 130, 166; and Chicago Milk Commission, 179; and cows' milk, 46, 50–51, 52, 53–54, 55–59, 60–64, 67–70, 71, 126, 127 fig. 16, 158; and the feeding question, 6; on feeding schedules, 32, 35; and field surveys, xv, 17, 18 fig. 1, 122–26; and human milk, xvi, 190; on infant care, 193; and infant diarrhea, xiv, 43 fig. 4, 48–49, 122–23; and infant mortality, xiv, 1, 20, 43 fig. 4; and infant welfare campaigns, xv, 17, 25, 26, 27, 43 fig. 4, 122–31; and Infant Welfare Society, 113, 115; and infant welfare stations, xv, xvi, 103, 126, 128, 129–30, 194; on lactation failure, 38; and Little Mothers' Clubs, 120–21; and mothers, 122, 124, 158, 193; and Mothers' Breast Milk Station, xvii, 133, 153–55, 156; on overfeeding, 36; on pasteurization, 52, 64–65, 67–68, 123; and proprietary food salesmen, 166; Revised Code of 1931, xvi, 153, 193, 195; and swill milk, 51–53; and visiting nurses, xvi, 122–24, 125–26, 129; on wet nursing, 137

Chicago Ethical Society, 105. *See also* Visiting Nurse Association

Chicago Foundlings Home, wet nurses in, 136, 138, 156

Chicago Herald: on milk inspection, 56–57, 58

Chicago Hope, 7, 201

Chicago Inter Ocean: on milk inspection, 56

Chicago Lying-In Dispensary. *See* Chicago Maternity Center

Chicago Maternity Center, 248 n. 37; and breastfeeding, 194

Chicago Medical Recorder: ads for wet nurses in, 138; on Chicago Milk Commission, 177; on philanthropy, 102–3

Chicago Milk Commission, xv, 175–81; and baby tents, 110; and breastfeeding, 112, 180; on certified milk, 72; compared with Infant Welfare Society, 114; and Hull House, 171; and physicians, 176, 179; on working-class mothers, 19–20. *See also* Infant Welfare Society

Chicago Pediatric Society, xiv, 11, 59, 84, 89, 176; and wet nurses, 147

Chicago Relief and Aid Society: and baby tents, xiv, 109–10

Chicago School Board: and Chicago Milk Commission, 176

Chicago's Health: on breastfeeding, 130

Chicago Tribune: ads for wet nurses in, 135, 143; and Chicago Milk Commission, 177; on cows' milk, 44, 50; on lactation failure, 31, 38

Chicago Woman's Club: and Chicago Milk Commission, 175; and Infant Welfare Society, 120

child-rearing: theories of, 220 n. 91

Children's Hospital Society of Chicago, xiv, 19; and Chicago Milk Commission, 112, 175–76; and wet nurses, 147

Children's Memorial Hospital: and acid milk, 192; and evaporated milk, 192; wet nurses in, xv, 150

cholera infantum. *See* infant diarrhea

Christopher, W. S.: on cows' milk, 51; on wet nurses, 140

Churchill, Frank Spooner: on artificial food, 77, 91, 98; and Chicago Medical Society Milk Commission, 181; and Chicago Milk Commission, 176; on feeding schedules, 97; on human milk analysis, 93–94; and Infant Welfare Society, 116; on lactation failure, 97; on milk laboratories, 168, 170; on mothers, 14, 97; on percentage feeding, 83; on proprietary infant foods, 163; on weaning, 14; on wet nurses, 138, 149, 150

Civic Federation of Chicago: and infant feeding, 104, 125

CMC. *See* Chicago Milk Commission

Coit, Henry: and certified milk, xiv, 172–73, 174; on feeding milk of one species to another, 76; on pasteurization, 64–65. *See also* certified milk

Coit, John Summerfield, 172

colostrum, 91–92, 191, 229 n. 91, 229 n. 92

commercial infant foods. *See* proprietary infant foods

complementing. *See* artificial food, complementing with

condensed milk, 159–62, 240 n. 5; advertising of, 161–62; cost of, 162; dilution of, 79, 162; and infant mortality, 221 n. 11; use of by mothers, 14. *See also* cows' milk; evaporated milk

Women and Health Series: Cultural and Social Perspectives
Rima D. Apple and Janet Golden, Editors

The series examines the social and cultural construction of health practices and policies, focusing on women as subjects and objects of medical theory, health services, and policy formulation.

Mothers and Motherhood: Readings in American History
  Edited by Rima D. Apple and Janet Golden

Modern Mothers in the Heartland: Gender, Health, and Progress in Illinois, 1900–1930
  Lynne Curry

Making Midwives Legal: Childbirth, Medicine, and the Law, second edition
  Raymond G. DeVries

A Social History of Wet Nursing in America: From Breast to Bottle
  Janet Golden

Travels with the Wolf: A Story of Chronic Illness
  Melissa Anne Goldstein

The Selling of Contraception: The Dalkon Shield Case, Sexuality, and Women's Autonomy
  Nicole J. Grant

Women in Labor: Mothers, Medicine, and Occupational Health in the United States, 1890–1980
  Allison L. Hepler

Crack Mothers: Pregnancy, Drugs, and the Media
  Drew Humphries

And Sin No More: Social Policy and Unwed Mothers in Cleveland, 1855–1990
Marian J. Morton

Women and Prenatal Testing: Facing the Challenges of Genetic Technology
Edited by Karen H. Rothenberg and Elizabeth J. Thomson

Women's Health: Complexities and Differences
Edited by Sheryl Burt Ruzek, Virginia L. Olesen, and Adele E. Clarke

Bodies of Technology: Women's Involvement with Reproductive Medicine
Edited by Ann R. Saetnan, Nelly Oudshoorn, and Marty Kirejczyk

Motherhood in Bondage
Margaret Sanger. Foreword by Margaret Marsh

Listen to Me Good: The Life Story of an Alabama Midwife
Margaret Charles Smith and Linda Janet Holmes

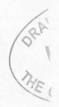